Undiagnosed and Rare Diseases

Editors

BRETT J. BORDINI
ROBERT M. KLIEGMAN

CLINICS IN PERINATOLOGY

www.perinatology.theclinics.com

Consulting Editor
LUCKY JAIN

March 2020 • Volume 47 • Number 1

ELSEVIER

1600 John F. Kennedy Boulevard • Suite 1800 • Philadelphia, Pennsylvania, 19103-2899

http://www.theclinics.com

CLINICS IN PERINATOLOGY Volume 47, Number 1
March 2020 ISSN 0095-5108, ISBN-13: 978-0-323-71143-2

Editor: Kerry Holland
Developmental Editor: Casey Potter

Clinics in Perinatology (ISSN 0095-5108) is published quarterly by Elsevier Inc., 360 Park Avenue South, New York, NY 10010-1710. Months of issue are March, June, September, and December. Business and Editorial Offices: 1600 John F. Kennedy Blvd., Ste. 1800, Philadelphia, PA 19103-2899. Customer Service Office: 3251 Riverport Lane, Maryland Heights, MO 63043. Periodicals postage paid at New York, NY and additional mailing offices. Subscription prices are $312.00 per year (US individuals), $610.00 per year (US institutions), $365.00 per year (Canadian individuals), $747.00 per year (Canadian institutions), $435.00 per year (international individuals), $747.00 per year (international institutions), $100.00 per year (US and Canadian students), and $195.00 per year (International students). International air speed delivery is included in all Clinics subscription prices. All prices are subject to change without notice. **POSTMASTER:** Send address changes to *Clinics in Perinatology*, Elsevier Health Sciences Division, Subscription Customer Service, 3251 Riverport Lane, Maryland Heights, MO 63043. **Customer Service: Telephone: 1-800-654-2452** (U.S. and Canada); **1-314-447-8871** (outside U.S. and Canada). **Fax: 1-314-447-8029. E-mail: journalscustomerservice-usa@elsevier.com** (for print support); **journalsonlinesupport-usa@elsevier.com** (for online support).

Reprints. For copies of 100 or more, of articles in this publication, please contact the Commercial Reprints Department, Elsevier Inc., 360 Park Avenue South, New York, NY 10010-1710. Tel. 212-633-3874; Fax: 212-633-3820; E-mail: reprints@elsevier.com.

Clinics in Perinatology is also published in Spanish by McGraw-Hill Interamericana Editores S.A., P.O. Box 5-237, 06500 Mexico D.F., Mexico.

Clinics in Perinatology is covered in *MEDLINE/PubMed (Index Medicus) Current Contents, Excepta Medica, BIOSIS and ISI/BIOMED.*

Contributors

CONSULTING EDITOR

LUCKY JAIN, MD, MBA
George W. Brumley Jr Professor and Chair, Emory University School of Medicine, Department of Pediatrics, Chief Academic Officer, Children's Healthcare of Atlanta, Executive Director, Emory and Children's Pediatric Institute, Atlanta, Georgia

EDITORS

BRETT J. BORDINI, MD
Associate Professor, Department of Pediatrics, Section of Hospital Medicine, Nelson Service for Undiagnosed and Rare Diseases, Children's Hospital of Wisconsin, Medical College of Wisconsin, Children's Corporate Center, Milwaukee, Wisconsin

ROBERT M. KLIEGMAN, MD
Professor and Chair Emeritus, Department of Pediatrics, Nelson Service for Undiagnosed and Rare Diseases, Children's Hospital of Wisconsin, Medical College of Wisconsin, Children's Corporate Center, Milwaukee, Wisconsin

AUTHORS

DONALD BASEL, MBBCh, FACMG
Associate Professor and Chief of Genetics, Department of Pediatrics, Division of Genetics, Nelson Service for Undiagnosed and Rare Diseases, Children's Hospital of Wisconsin, Medical College of Wisconsin, Milwaukee, Wisconsin

CHRISTINA M. BENCE, MD
Pediatric Surgery Research Fellow, Division of Pediatric Surgery, Medical College of Wisconsin, Children's Hospital of Wisconsin, Milwaukee, Wisconsin

BRETT J. BORDINI, MD
Associate Professor, Department of Pediatrics, Section of Hospital Medicine, Nelson Service for Undiagnosed and Rare Diseases, Children's Hospital of Wisconsin, Medical College of Wisconsin, Children's Corporate Center, Milwaukee, Wisconsin

YVONNE E. CHIU, MD
Associate Professor, Departments of Dermatology (Pediatric Dermatology) and Pediatrics, Medical College of Wisconsin, Milwaukee, Wisconsin

ZACHARY A. COLVIN, DO
Maternal Fetal Medicine Fellow, Department of Obstetrics and Gynecology, Medical College of Wisconsin, Milwaukee, Wisconsin

JOHN C. DENSMORE, MD
Associate Professor, Division of Pediatric Surgery, Medical College of Wisconsin, Children's Hospital of Wisconsin, Milwaukee, Wisconsin

MICHAEL G. EARING, MD
Department of Pediatrics, Medical College of Wisconsin, Herma Heart Institute, Children's Hospital of Wisconsin, Section of Adult Cardiovascular Medicine, Department of Internal Medicine, Milwaukee, Wisconsin

ABDUL AZIZ ELKADRI, MD
Assistant Professor of Pediatrics, Medical College of Wisconsin, Milwaukee, Wisconsin

GABRIELLE C. GEDDES, MD
Department of Pediatrics, Medical College of Wisconsin, Herma Heart Institute, Children's Hospital of Wisconsin, Milwaukee, Wisconsin

MATTHEW HARMELINK, MD
Assistant Professor, Department of Neurology, Medical College of Wisconsin, Milwaukee, Wisconsin

PATRICE K. HELD, PhD
Assistant Professor, Department of Pediatrics, Wisconsin State Laboratory of Hygiene, University of Wisconsin-Madison School of Medicine and Public Health, Madison, Wisconsin

ROBERT M. KLIEGMAN, MD
Professor and Chair Emeritus, Department of Pediatrics, Nelson Service for Undiagnosed and Rare Diseases, Children's Hospital of Wisconsin, Medical College of Wisconsin, Children's Corporate Center, Milwaukee, Wisconsin

LEAH E. LALOR, MD
Assistant Professor, Departments of Dermatology (Pediatric Dermatology) and Pediatrics, Medical College of Wisconsin, Milwaukee, Wisconsin

CATHERINE LARSON-NATH, MD
Assistant Professor of Pediatrics, Pediatric Gastroenterology, Hepatology and Nutrition, University of Minnesota, Minneapolis, Minnesota

STEVEN R. LEUTHNER, MD, MA
Professor of Pediatrics, Neonatology, Professor of Bioethics, Wauwatosa, Wisconsin

LYNN MALEC, MD, MSc
Associate Investigator, Versiti Blood Research Institute, Assistant Professor, Medical College of Wisconsin, Milwaukee, Wisconsin

JAMES J. NOCTON, MD
Professor, Department of Pediatrics, Section of Rheumatology, Nelson Service for Undiagnosed and Rare Diseases, Children's Hospital of Wisconsin, Medical College of Wisconsin, Milwaukee, Wisconsin

JOHN ROUTES, MD
Professor, Pediatrics, Medical College of Wisconsin, Milwaukee, Wisconsin

SAI-SUMA SAMUDRALA, BS
Department of Cell Biology, Neurobiology and Anatomy, Medical College of Wisconsin, Milwaukee, Wisconsin

JESSICA SCOTT SCHWOERER, MD
Associate Professor, Department of Pediatrics, Division of Genetics and Metabolism, University of Wisconsin Hospital and Clinics, Madison, Wisconsin

NISSIM G. STOLBERG, DO
Division of Rheumatology, Department of Pediatrics, Medical College of Wisconsin, Milwaukee, Wisconsin

CORINNE SWEARINGEN, MD
Neonatology Fellow, Department of Pediatrics, Medical College of Wisconsin, Wauwatosa, Wisconsin

MATTHEW TALLAR, MD
Assistant Professor, Pediatrics, Medical College of Wisconsin, Milwaukee, Wisconsin

JAMES W. VERBSKY, MD, PhD
Division of Rheumatology, Department of Pediatrics, Medical College of Wisconsin, Milwaukee, Wisconsin

BERNADETTE E. VITOLA, MD, MPH
Associate Professor of Pediatrics, Pediatric Gastroenterology, Hepatology and Nutrition, Medical College of Wisconsin, Milwaukee, Wisconsin

KATIE B. WILLIAMS, MD, PhD
Medical Genetics Fellow, Department of Pediatrics, University of Wisconsin Hospital and Clinics, Madison, Wisconsin

Contents

> Critically ill neonates experience high rates of morbidity and mortality. Major diagnostic errors are identified in up to 20% of autopsied neonatal intensive care unit deaths. Neonates with undiagnosed or rare congenital disorders may mimic critically ill neonates with more common acquired conditions. The context of the diagnostic evaluation can introduce unique biases that increase the likelihood of diagnostic error. Herein is presented a framework for understanding diagnostic errors in perinatal medicine, and individual, team, and systems-based solutions for improving diagnosis learned through the implementation and administration of an undiagnosed and rare disease program.

> Dysmorphology is the practice of defining the morphologic phenotype of syndromic disorders. Genomic sequencing has advanced our understanding of human variation and molecular dysmorphology has evolved in response to the science of relating embryologic developmental implications of abnormal gene signaling pathways to the resultant phenotypic presentation. Machine learning has enabled the application of deep convoluted neural networks to recognize the comparative likeness of these phenotypes relative to the causal genotype or disrupted gene pathway.

> Neonatal acute liver failure (NALF) is a rare disease with a few known primary causes: gestational alloimmune liver disease (GALD), viral infections, metabolic diseases, and ischemic injury. Many cases still do not have a known cause. Laboratory evaluation may suggest a diagnosis. Most of the known causes have disease-specific treatments that improve outcomes. Survival is improving with better knowledge about and treatment options for GALD; however, overall mortality for NALF is still 24%. Liver

transplant remains an important option for neonates with an indeterminate cause of NALF and those who do not respond to established treatments.

Autoinflammatory disorders are rare genetic defects that result in inflammation in the absence of an infectious or autoimmune disease. Although very rare, these disorders can occur in the perinatal period, and recognizing their presentation is important because there are often long-term complications and effective targeted therapies for these disorders. Most of these disorders present with rash, fevers, and laboratory evidence of inflammation. Importantly, these disorders can now be separated into their pathophysiologic mechanisms of action, which can also guide therapies. The article reviews the different mechanisms of autoinflammatory disorders and highlights those disorders that can present in the newborn period.

Numerous disorders present with vesiculopustular eruptions in the neonatal period, ranging from benign to life-threatening. Accurate and prompt diagnosis is imperative to avoid unnecessary testing and treatment for benign eruptions, while allowing for adequate treatment of potentially fatal disorders. In this review, we highlight several rare blistering diseases of the newborn. A diagnostic approach is outlined to provide clinicians with a framework for approaching a neonate with vesicles, pustules, or ulcers.

Severe combined immunodeficiency (SCID) encompasses a group of genetic defects. T cell development is universally affected and has alteration of B and/or NK cells. We present the case of a 5-day-old boy with combined heterozygous frame shift (c.256_257del, p.(Lys86Valfs*33)) and missense (c.1186C>T, p.(Arg396Cys)) variations in the RAG1 gene. He was admitted to our institution because of 0 TREC on Newborn Screen and worsening rash. Initially thought to have Omenn syndrome versus maternal engraftment with graft versus host disease, DNA analysis identified the noted mutations and he subsequently received a bone marrow transplant from a matched sibling.

Congenital diarrheal disorders are heterogeneous conditions characterized by diarrhea with onset in the first years of life. They range from simple temporary conditions, such as cow's milk protein intolerance to irreversible complications, such as microvillous inclusion disease with significant morbidity and mortality. Advances in genomic medicine have improved our understanding of these disorders, leading to an ever-increasing list of identified causative genes. The diagnostic approach to these conditions consists of establishing the presence of diarrhea by detailed review of the history, followed by characterizing the composition of the diarrhea, the response to fasting, and with further specialized testing.

administered a high glucose infusion rate with isotonic fluids to reverse catabolism. Combined advanced biochemical and molecular testing is often needed to identify specific metabolic disorders and guide ongoing treatment.

Heterotaxy is a generalized term for patients who have an abnormality of laterality that cannot be described as situs inversus. Infants with heterotaxy can have significant anatomic and medical complexity and require personalized, specialized care, including comprehensive anatomic assessment. Common and rare anatomic findings are reviewed by system to help guide a thorough phenotypic evaluation. General care guidelines and considerations unique to this patient population are included. Future directions for this unique patient population, particularly in light of improved neonatal survival, are discussed.

Neonatal appendicitis is a rare disease with a high mortality rate. Appendicitis is difficult to diagnose in neonatal and infant populations because it mimics other more common conditions in these age groups. Furthermore, signs and symptoms of appendicitis are often nonspecific in nonverbal patients and a high index of suspicion is necessary to initiate the appropriate diagnostic work-up. The keys to successful management of appendicitis in infants include keeping the diagnosis on the differential in the setting of unexplained intra-abdominal sepsis, following a diagnostic algorithm in the work-up of infant abdominal pathology, and performing appendectomy once the diagnosis is confirmed.

The congenital muscular dystrophies and congenital myopathies are a heterogenous group of diseases with a wide variety of presentations and outcomes. With the growing understanding of genetic involvement, and developing therapies, having a genetically confirmed diagnosis with phenotype correlation is essential. To achieve this, a structured approach is warranted to each child to ensure that mimickers are excluded. By structuring the evaluation appropriately, the clinician can help expedite the evaluation of these infants in a cost-effective manner. Understanding the pitfalls of each step of testing will allow the clinician to better understand variants in presentation and avoid cognitive errors in the process.

PROGRAM OBJECTIVE

The goal of *Clinics in Perinatology* is to keep practicing perinatologists, neonatologists, obstetricians, practicing physicians and residents up to date with current clinical practice in perinatology by providing timely articles reviewing the state of the art in patient care.

TARGET AUDIENCE

Perinatologists, neonatologists, obstetricians, practicing physicians, residents and healthcare professionals who provide patient care utilizing findings from *Clinics in Perinatology*.

LEARNING OBJECTIVES

Upon completion of this activity, participants will be able to:
1. Review diagnosis strategies to minimize diagnostic errors
2. Discuss approaches intended to expedite diagnosis
3. Recognize characteristic signs and symptoms of rare disorders that mimic more common congenital and acquired conditions

ACCREDITATION

The Elsevier Office of Continuing Medical Education (EOCME) is accredited by the Accreditation Council for Continuing Medical Education (ACCME) to provide continuing medical education for physicians.

The EOCME designates this journal-based CME activity for a maximum of 14 *AMA PRA Category 1 Credit*(s)™. Physicians should claim only the credit commensurate with the extent of their participation in the activity.

All other health care professionals requesting continuing education credit for this enduring material will be issued a certificate of participation.

DISCLOSURE OF CONFLICTS OF INTEREST

The EOCME assesses conflict of interest with its instructors, faculty, planners, and other individuals who are in a position to control the content of CME activities. All relevant conflicts of interest that are identified are thoroughly vetted by EOCME for fair balance, scientific objectivity, and patient care recommendations. EOCME is committed to providing its learners with CME activities that promote improvements or quality in healthcare and not a specific proprietary business or a commercial interest.

The planning committee, staff, authors and editors listed below have identified no financial relationships or relationships to products or devices they or their spouse/life partner have with commercial interest related to the content of this CME activity:
Christina M. Bence, MD; Brett J. Bordini, MD; Yvonne E. Chiu, MD; Zachary A. Colvin, DO; John C. Densmore, MD; Michael G. Earing, MD; Abdul Aziz Elkadri, MD; Gabrielle C. Geddes, MD; Patrice K. Held, PhD; Kerry Holland; Alison Kemp; Robert M. Kliegman, MD; Leah E. Lalor, MD; Catherine Larson-Nath, MD; Steven R. Leuthner, MD, MA; Swaminathan Nagarajan; James J. Nocton, MD; Sai-Suma Samudrala, BS; Jessica Scott-Schwoerer, MD; Nissim G. Stolberg, DO; Corinne Swearingen, MD; Matthew Tallar, MD; Bernadette E. Vitola, MD, MPH; Katie B. Williams, MD, PhD.

The planning committee, staff, authors and editors listed below have identified financial relationships or relationships to products or devices they or their spouse/life partner have with commercial interest related to the content of this CME activity:
Donald Basel, MBBCh, FACMG: is a consultant/advisor for FDNA, Inc.

Matthew Harmelink, MD: is a consultant/advisor for AveXis, Inc., Biogen, Blueprint Partnership, Connected Research, Emerging Therapy Solutions, ETS Consulting, Magnolia Innovation, MarketPlus, PTC Therapeutics, Sanderson Market Plus; is a consultant/advisor and receives research support from Sarepta Therapeutics.

Lynn Malec, MD, MSc: is a consultant/advisor for Bayer AG, CSL, Spark Therapeutics, Inc., and Takeda Pharmaceutical Company Limited; is a consultant/advisor, participates in speakers bureau, and receives research support from Genzyme Corporation.

John Routes, MD: is a paid speaker for Takeda Pharmaceutical Company Limited and a clinical investigator for CSL.

James Verbsky, MD, PhD: receives royalties and/or holds patents from UpToDate, Inc.

UNAPPROVED/OFF-LABEL USE DISCLOSURE

The EOCME requires CME faculty to disclose to the participants:

1. When products or procedures being discussed are off-label, unlabelled, experimental, and/or investigational (not US Food and Drug Administration [FDA] approved); and
2. Any limitations on the information presented, such as data that are preliminary or that represent ongoing research, interim analyses, and/or unsupported opinions. Faculty may discuss information about pharmaceutical agents that is outside of FDA-approved labelling. This information is intended solely for CME and is not intended to promote off-label use of these medications. If you have any questions, contact the medical affairs department of the manufacturer for the most recent prescribing information.

TO ENROLL

To enroll in the *Clinics in Perinatology* Continuing Medical Education program, call customer service at 1-800-654-2452 or sign up online at http://www.theclinics.com/home/cme. The CME program is available to subscribers for an additional annual fee of 245 USD.

METHOD OF PARTICIPATION

In order to claim credit, participants must complete the following:

1. Complete enrolment as indicated above.
2. Read the activity.
3. Complete the CME Test and Evaluation. Participants must achieve a score of 70% on the test. All CME Tests and Evaluations must be completed online.

CME INQUIRIES/SPECIAL NEEDS

For all CME inquiries or special needs, please contact elsevierCME@elsevier.com.

CLINICS IN PERINATOLOGY

SERIES OF RELATED INTEREST

Pediatric Clinics
https://www.pediatric.theclinics.com/

THE CLINICS ARE AVAILABLE ONLINE!
Access your subscription at:
www.theclinics.com

Erratum

An error was made in the December 2019 issue (Volume 46, Issue 4, December 2019, Pages 709-30) *Clinics in Perinatology* issue. In the article "Nonpharmacological Management of Pain During Common Needle Puncture Procedures in Infants: Current Research Evidence and Practical Considerations: An Update," the author listing Marsha Campbell Yeo RN, PhD, NNP-BC should be listed as Marsha Campbell-Yeo RN, PhD, NNP-BC.

Clin Perinatol 47 (2020) xv
https://doi.org/10.1016/j.clp.2019.12.002
perinatology.theclinics.com

Foreword

Finding a Needle in a Haystack Can be Challenging

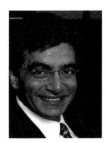

Lucky Jain, MD, MBA
Consulting Editor

The idiom *"looking for a needle in a haystack"* is often used to denote something exceptionally challenging to find. It is based on the idea that a sewing needle in a pile of dry grass would be hard to find. Indeed, such is the case with many rare diseases which display considerable phenotypic and geographical heterogeneity even when traced back to their genetic origin. Collectively, diseases affecting fewer than 1 in 2000 individuals are referred to as rare diseases. It is estimated that up to 300 million people worldwide are afflicted with a rare disease and 80% of these have a genetic origin.[1]

There is a second reason why the idiom *"looking for a needle in a haystack"* is appropriate to this conversation. Way back then, farmers probably worried about the consequences of a needle or some other tiny sharp object that escaped attention and was swallowed by a horse or a cow. Undetected, rare diseases can similarly exert considerable toll. Children are affected in 50-75% of rare diseases, often with multisystem involvement (**Fig. 1**).[2] Collectively, these diseases account for significant morbidity and mortality in early childhood and impose a sizeable burden on strained healthcare systems. As a result of these challenges, many hospital systems have initiated specialized programs for rare diseases. The expertise and resources required for such programs lend themselves to centralized programs that can serve as referral centers. Data from these regional centers can be collated by global organizations which can then serve as a resource for centers seeking validation of challenging diagnoses. Orphanet is one such organization (www.orpha.net) that has evolved into a 37-country network co-founded by the European Commission, as is the International Rare Disease Research Consortium (IRDiRC).[3]

These and many other important issues related to rare diseases have been covered in great depth in this issue of the Clinics edited by Drs. Kliegman and Bordini. As

Clin Perinatol 47 (2020) xvii–xix
https://doi.org/10.1016/j.clp.2019.12.003
0095-5108/20/© 2019 Elsevier Inc. All rights reserved.

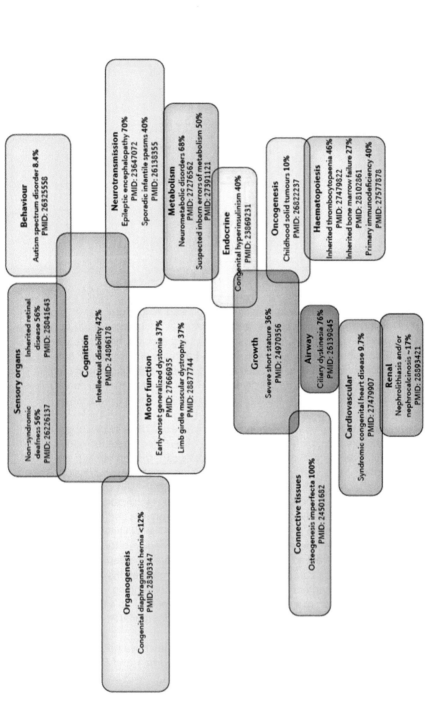

Fig. 1. Available diagnostic rates based on whole-exome sequencing in classes of pediatric genomic diseases. The diagnostic rate of whole-exome sequencing is given for each phenotype class, with the associated PubMed identification (PMID) number; only case series ≥10 were used, and only pathogenic or likely pathogenic variants in probable or known disease genes are included. There were remarkably few studies available in the published literature for many of the broad classes of disease with the exception of neurodevelopmental disorders. Box sizes are approximately proportionate to the prevalence of the phenotypes in pediatric practice. (*From Wright CF, FitzPatrick DR, Firth HV. Pediatric genomics: diagnosing rare disease in children.* Nature Reviews Genetics. 2018;19:253-268. p. 254.)

always, I am grateful to the publishing staff at Elsevier including Kerry Holland and Casey Potter for their support in making this important resource available for you.

Lucky Jain, MD, MBA
Emory University School of Medicine, and Children's Healthcare of Atlanta
2015 Uppergate Drive NE
Atlanta, GA 30322, USA

E-mail address:
ljain@emory.edu

REFERENCES

1. Wakap SN, Lambert DM, Olry A, et al. Estimating cumulative point prevalence of rare diseases: analysis of the Orphanet database. Eur J Hum Genet 2019. https://doi.org/10.1038/s41431-019-0508-0.
2. Wright CF, Ftizpatrick DR, Firth HV. Paediatric genomics: diagnosing rare disease in children. Nat Rev Genet 2018;19:253–68.
3. Austin CP, Cutillo CM, Lau LPL, et al, International Rare Diseases Research Consortium (IRDiRC). Future of rare diseases research 2017-2027: an IRDiRC perspective. Clin Transl Sci 2018;11:21–7.

Preface

Undiagnosed and Rare Diseases in Perinatal Medicine: Uncommon Manifestations or Mimics of Neonatal Disorders

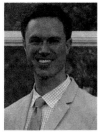 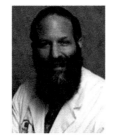

Brett J. Bordini, MD   Robert M. Kliegman, MD
Editors

The first two decades of the twenty-first century have witnessed remarkable advances in perinatal outcomes, with increasingly sophisticated diagnostic modalities allowing for improved detection of congenital disorders, and breakthroughs in medical and surgical therapies allowing for impressive reductions in mortality and morbidity for both congenital and acquired conditions.[1] Despite these advances, congenital disorders continue to be the leading cause of infant mortality in the United States, and diagnosis remains challenging: the spectrum of congenital disorders is broader in perinatal medicine, and yet, phenotypic variability is often narrower, with many conditions presenting subtly or with features that mimic disorders more routinely encountered in ill neonates. Compounding these challenges are the rapidly progressive nature of many congenital disorders and the multitude of systems-based and individual cognitive biases that can pervade the neonatal intensive care unit and contribute to diagnostic error.[2]

In this issue of *Clinics in Perinatology*, we present a predominantly single center's experience in approaching undiagnosed and rare diseases in perinatal medicine. Of particular interest are those rare disorders that mimic more common congenital and acquired conditions, as well as those common disorders that may present in an uncommon manner or with atypical symptoms. Herein, we emphasize approaches intended to expedite diagnosis so as to decrease morbidity in survivable conditions and allow for reproductive counseling and comfort care as indicated in those disorders not compatible with life. The challenge for clinicians under these circumstances is deciding when a patient's course warrants further diagnostic evaluation or reconsideration of a

Clin Perinatol 47 (2020) xxi–xxii
https://doi.org/10.1016/j.clp.2019.12.001
0095-5108/20/© 2020 Elsevier Inc. All rights reserved.

working diagnosis, and which of the increasingly numerous and robust diagnostic modalities to implement.

Continual refinements in understanding the cognitive science of diagnosis and the cause of diagnostic error, combined with ongoing advances in diagnostic modalities, particularly more comprehensive and rapidly available molecular genetics techniques, hold considerable promise in further improving outcomes in perinatal medicine. We hope this issue will bring clinicians and the patients and families for which they care greater mindfulness of the spectrum of undiagnosed and rare diseases in perinatal medicine, as well as strategies to minimize diagnostic delays and errors.

Brett J. Bordini, MD
Department of Pediatrics
Medical College of Wisconsin
Children's Hospital of Wisconsin
Children's Corporate Center
999 North 92nd Street–Suite C560
Milwaukee, WI 53226, USA

Robert M. Kliegman, MD
Department of Pediatrics
Medical College of Wisconsin
Children's Hospital of Wisconsin
Children's Corporate Center
999 North 92nd Street–Suite C450
Milwaukee, WI 53226, USA

E-mail addresses:
bbordini@mcw.edu (B.J. Bordini)
rkliegma@mcw.edu (R.M. Kliegman)

REFERENCES

1. Ely DM. Infant mortality by age at death in the United States, 2016. NCHS Data Brief 2018;(326):8.
2. Custer JW, Winters BD, Goode V, et al. Diagnostic errors in the pediatric and neonatal ICU: a systematic review. Pediatr Crit Care Med 2015;16(1):29–36.

Undiagnosed and Rare Diseases in Perinatal Medicine

Lessons in Context and Cognitive Diagnostic Error

Brett J. Bordini, MD[a],*, Robert M. Kliegman, MD[b],
Donald Basel, MBBCh[b], James J. Nocton, MD[c]

KEYWORDS

- Diagnostic error • Cognitive bias • Context errors • Diagnostic calibration
- Cognitive forcing functions • Perinatal medicine • Neonatal intensive care unit

KEY POINTS

- Neonates with undiagnosed or rare congenital disorders may mimic critically ill neonates with more common acquired conditions.
- Patients in neonatal intensive care settings are at risk of diagnostic error, and the context of the diagnostic evaluation may introduce unique biases that can increase the likelihood of diagnostic error.
- Improving diagnosis requires comprehensive individual, team, and systems-based solutions that identify and minimize cognitive biases and foster more analytical approaches to diagnosis.
- Clinical contexts at increased risk of introducing cognitive biases benefit from the use of cognitive forcing functions and additional systematic approaches to reduce diagnostic error.

Since the publication of *To Err is Human: Building a Safer Health System* by the Institute of Medicine in 2000 and the seminal *Improving Diagnosis in Health Care* by the National Academies of Science-Engineering-Medicine in 2015, diagnostic error has

[a] Department of Pediatrics, Section of Hospital Medicine, Nelson Service for Undiagnosed and Rare Diseases, Children's Hospital of Wisconsin, Medical College of Wisconsin, 999 North 92nd Street, Suite C560, Milwaukee, WI 53226, USA; [b] Department of Pediatrics, Nelson Service for Undiagnosed and Rare Diseases, Children's Hospital of Wisconsin, Medical College of Wisconsin, 999 North 92nd Street, Suite C560, Milwaukee, WI 53226, USA; [c] Department of Pediatrics, Section of Rheumatology, Nelson Service for Undiagnosed and Rare Diseases, Children's Hospital of Wisconsin, Medical College of Wisconsin, 999 North 92nd Street, Suite C465, Milwaukee, WI 53226, USA
* Corresponding author.
E-mail address: bbordini@mcw.edu

Clin Perinatol 47 (2020) 1–14
https://doi.org/10.1016/j.clp.2019.10.002
0095-5108/20/© 2019 Elsevier Inc. All rights reserved.
perinatology.theclinics.com

become an intense focus in improving patient safety. The degree to which diagnostic error is implicated in adverse patient outcomes is less well defined than more readily quantified sources, such as medication errors,[1] although in perinatal medicine, major diagnostic errors are identified in up to 20% of autopsied neonatal intensive care unit deaths.[2] Although outcomes have improved significantly over the past generation, patients cared for in neonatal intensive care settings continue to be at high risk for both mortality and morbidity,[3–5] and not solely as a function of prematurity or low birth weight.[6–8] In the United States, the most common cause of death for infants up to 1 year of age is congenital anomalies (**Fig. 1**),[9] despite only 3% of neonates having a major congenital anomaly.[10] Currently, only 15% of neonates with major congenital anomalies will have an identifiable genetic cause on routine genetic testing[11]; improved diagnosis holds considerable promise for optimal outcomes in those conditions that are compatible with life.

Some congenital disorders are overt in their presentation, with features that allow for prenatal or rapid postnatal diagnosis, whereas others are subtler and may mimic the perturbations in homeostasis common to many infants born prematurely, with low birth weight, or otherwise critically ill. In critically ill neonates, supporting appropriate physiology and extrauterine development is a challenge fraught with subtle clinical changes that can portend major complications. Appreciating when these perturbations in homeostasis are driven not solely by prematurity or exogenous factors, such as infection or meconium aspiration, but rather by a rare and potentially heritable disorder, is a significant diagnostic challenge that requires timeliness and carries major therapeutic implications. These infants are at high risk of *diagnostic error*, particularly when presenting features are subtle, are slowly progressive, or mimic findings commonly encountered in perinatal medicine. Maintaining too high an index of

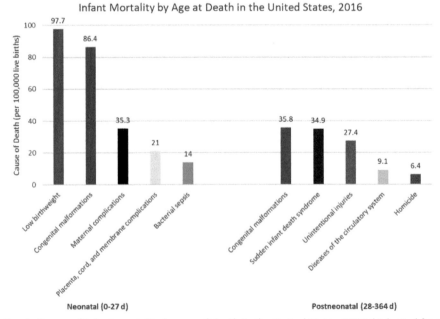

Fig. 1. Causes of infant mortality by age of death in the United States, 2016. (*Adapted from* Ely DM, Driscoll AK, Matthews TJ. Infant Mortality by Age at Death in the United States, 2016. *NCHS Data Brief*. (326):8; 2018.)

suspicion for a rare disorder risks excessive testing, diagnosing, and intervening, as well as creating undue parental worry; conversely, maintaining an insufficient index of suspicion risks diagnostic error and improper treatment, with their attendant morbidity and mortality. Appropriate diagnosis offers an opportunity for prompt and specific intervention, decreased parental anxiety, decreased resource utilization, and timely transition to comfort care and reproductive counseling when indicated.[12]

Improving diagnosis requires understanding not only the root causes of diagnostic error, but also the manners in which these causes may be mitigated. Cognitive psychology has provided a broad conceptual framework for comprehending those factors that alone or in aggregate result in diagnostic error; evidence-based solutions to improving diagnosis remain nascent.[13] In our Undiagnosed and Rare Disease (URD) program, we have developed a process and an environment designed to identify the risk or actuality of diagnostic error and provide a method for improved diagnostic accuracy. In the process of evaluating critically ill neonates with diagnostic dilemmas, we have recognized that delays or errors in diagnosis are oftentimes the result of context-related biases[14] in which the setting of the diagnostic evaluation itself, the neonatal intensive care unit, can produce or contribute to cognitive errors in which rare, often heritable disorders may not be given appropriate or timely consideration in the differential diagnosis, particularly when presenting features mimic findings commonly encountered in perinatal medicine, such as sustained hypoxia, hypoglycemia, acidosis, or temperature instability (**Table 1**). Once diagnostic error occurs, context also can perpetuate a diagnostic momentum that precludes consideration of alternate diagnoses,[15] despite patients failing to respond to treatment or otherwise progress as expected, such as an infant we evaluated with a presumed diagnosis of culture-negative bacterial meningitis whose fevers and cerebrospinal fluid pleocytosis persisted in spite of broad-spectrum anti-infective therapies and multiple negative microbiologic assays, whom we ultimately diagnosed with interleukin-1 receptor antagonist deficiency, an autoinflammatory condition that improved with administration of anakinra. Recognizing that the context of a diagnostic evaluation can unduly influence its outcome allows clinicians to engage more analytical approaches in their diagnostic formulations and can improve the timeliness or accuracy of diagnosis. The lessons learned in the administration of our URD program offer further insights into developing an evidentiary basis for improving diagnosis and can be leveraged to improve outcomes in perinatal medicine.

COGNITIVE BIASES AND DIAGNOSTIC ERROR

Diagnostic error may be considered from a variety of perspectives. The *type* of error may consist of a missed, delayed, or wrong diagnosis, whereas the *root cause* may be a *systems-based error*, a *no-fault error*, in which disease features are sufficiently subtle or mimic another disorder so as to preclude proper diagnosis, or a *cognitive diagnostic error*, in which faulty knowledge, data gathering, or synthesis results in erroneous diagnosis. Diagnostic errors are often multifactorial with respect to root cause, although cognitive errors, alone or in combination with systems-based errors, comprise up to 75% of all diagnostic errors.[16,17] Although faulty knowledge and data gathering may contribute to cognitive diagnostic errors, most of these errors are related to the cognitive processes clinicians use in medical reasoning and synthesis, and the ways in which these processes can become susceptible to *bias*.[16,18]

Dual process theory holds that clinicians engaging in medical reasoning typically use either a predominantly intuitive approach, termed a *system 1 process*, or a more analytical approach, termed a *system 2 process*. System 1 processes are

Table 1
Examples of neonatal diagnostic errors from our program and selected examples from the literature

Initial Diagnosis	Final Diagnosis
Cardiopulmonary	
Heart failure without heart murmur	Supraventricular tachycardia
	Heart block
	Cardiomyopathy
	Severe aortic stenosis
	Anomalous coronary artery
	Vein of Galen malformation
	Pulmonary embolus
	Intracardiac thrombus
	Myocardial infarction
	Severe anemia
Persistent transient tachypnea of the newborn	Primary ciliary dyskinesia
	Neuroendocrine cell hyperplasia
	Pulmonary hemosiderosis
	Interstitial lung disorders
Respiratory distress syndrome	Blastomycosis[46]
	Anomalous pulmonary venous return
	Alveolar-capillary dysplasia
	Pulmonary hypoplasia
	Lymphangiectasia
	Surfactant protein deficiency
Congenital pulmonary airway malformation	Pleuropulmonary blastoma[47]
Laryngomalacia	Subglottic stenosis
	Hemangioma
	Papillomatosis
	Vocal cord paralysis
	Vascular ring or sling
Gastrointestinal/Hepatic	
Abdominal distension	Inguinal hernia
	Rectovaginal fistula
	Malrotation
	Hirschsprung disease
	Hydronephrosis
	Polycystic kidney disease
	Ascites
Esophageal reflux	Volvulus
	Pyloric stenosis
	Inguinal hernia
	Congenital adrenal hyperplasia
	Increased intracranial pressure
	Inborn error of metabolism
Physiologic jaundice	Biliary atresia
	TORCH infection
	Alagille syndrome
	Byler syndrome
	Red cell membrane or enzyme defect
	Hemophagocytic lymphohistiocytosis
	Neonatal hemochromatosis
	Thrombotic thrombocytopenic purpura

(continued on next page)

Table 1
(continued)

Initial Diagnosis	Final Diagnosis
Omphalocele	Fetus-in-fetu[48]
Draining umbilicus/ umbilical granuloma	Urachal cyst Omphalomesenteric cyst
Pyloric stenosis	Alpha-1-antitrypsin deficiency
Dermatologic	
Blueberry muffin rash	Congenital leukemia Langerhans cell histiocytosis Blue rubber bleb nevus syndrome Neuroblastoma Red cell aplasia Spherocytosis Twin-twin transfusion (donor twin) Erythroblastosis fetalis
Congenital dermal melanocytosis	Child maltreatment GM$_1$ gangliosidosis Hurler syndrome Hunter syndrome Mucolipidosis Niemann-Pick disease Segmental café-au-lait macules
Neurologic	
Neonatal abstinence syndrome	Gaucher disease
Spasticity/hypoxic ischemic encephalopathy	Gaucher disease
Erb palsy/ pseudoparalysis	Septic arthritis Osteomyelitis Fracture
Infectious	
Bacterial sepsis	Congenital enterovirus Herpes simplex virus Infant botulism Volvulus Ductal-dependent congenital heart disease Inborn error of metabolism
Herpes simplex	Incontinentia pigmenti Cutis aplasia
TORCH infection	Hemophagocytic lymphohistiocytosis Langerhans cell histiocytosis Aicardi-Goutières syndrome
Conjunctivitis	Herpes simplex Ophthalmia neonatorum secondary to *Neisseria gonorrhoeae* Congenital glaucoma

Abbreviation: TORCH, toxoplasmosis, other, rubella, cytomegalovirus, herpes simplex.

based in *heuristics*, which rely on pattern recognition and rules of thumb to rapidly sort large amounts of clinical information into an *illness script* that allows for the quick elaboration of a diagnosis. System 2 processes, on the other hand, rely on deliberate counter-factual reasoning and hypothesis generation tailored to individual patient circumstances to arrive at a more robust differential diagnosis. Although clinicians predominantly engage system 1 processes and achieve relatively accurate diagnoses for most patients under most circumstances,[18] heuristics can fail when patient presentations are multisystem, complex, or evolving, instead becoming a form of bias that can result in diagnostic error (**Table 2**). Biases may also be the result of *errors of attribution*, in which perceived characteristics or motivations of patients, family members, or members of the medical evaluation team are given undue weight in the diagnostic formulation. These factors can influence the affective state of the clinician and the integrity of cognition, increasing the likelihood of error.[19] Examples of attribution-related errors are listed in **Table 3**.

Finally, cognitive bias may be a product of the context in which a diagnostic evaluation takes place. With *context-related biases*, the setting of the diagnostic evaluation influences how clinicians perceive and process the information used in medical decision-making. External factors, such as an increased patient volumes, higher patient acuity, or staffing shortages, as well as internal factors, such as sleep deprivation, stress, and physician burnout, can amplify individual cognitive burden and increase the likelihood of diagnostic error.[20–22] Independent of cognitive burden, context can introduce bias by causing physicians to consciously or subconsciously deemphasize relevant information and amplify impertinent information while formulating a diagnosis. Most common among context-related biases is the *framing effect*,[23] in which the manner or setting of a patient's presentation implicitly restricts the breadth of differential diagnoses considered. This framing effect is often more prominent in contexts in

Table 2
Cognitive biases related to heuristic failure

Bias	Definition
Anchoring	Locking into a diagnosis based on initial presenting features, failing to adjust diagnostic impressions when new information becomes available.
Confirmation bias	Looking for and accepting only evidence that confirms a diagnostic impression, rejecting or not seeking contradictory evidence.
Diagnostic momentum	Perpetuating a diagnostic label over time, usually by multiple providers both within and across health care systems, despite the label being incomplete or inaccurate.
Expertise bias/yin-yang out	Believing that a patient who has already undergone an extensive evaluation will have nothing more to gain from further investigations, despite the possibility that the disease process or diagnostic techniques may have evolved so as to allow for appropriate diagnosis.
Overconfidence bias	Believing one knows more than one does, acting on incomplete information or hunches, and prioritizing opinion or authority, as opposed to evidence.
Premature closure	Accepting the first plausible diagnosis before obtaining confirmatory evidence or considering all available evidence. "*When the diagnosis is made, thinking stops.*"
Unpacking principle	Failing to explore primary evidence or data in its entirety and subsequently failing to uncover important facts or findings, such as accepting a biopsy report or imaging study report without reviewing the actual specimen or image.

From Bordini BJ, Stephany A, Kliegman R. Overcoming Diagnostic Errors in Medical Practice. J Pediatr. 2017;185:19-25.e1. https://doi.org/10.1016/j.jpeds.2017.02.065; with permission.

Table 3 Cognitive biases related to errors of attribution	
Bias	**Definition**
Affective bias	Allowing emotions to interfere with a diagnosis, either positively or negatively; dislikes of patient types (eg, "frequent flyers").
Appeal to authority	Deferring to authoritative recommendations from senior, supervising, or "expert" clinicians, independent of the evidentiary support for such recommendations.
Ascertainment bias	Maintaining preconceived expectations based on patient or disease stereotypes.
Countertransference	Being influenced by positive or negative subjective feelings toward a specific patient.
Outcome bias	Minimizing or overemphasizing the significance of a finding or result, often based on subjective feelings about a patient, a desired outcome, or personal confidence in one's own clinical skills; the use of "slightly" to describe abnormal results.
Psych-out bias	Maintaining biases about people with presumed mental illness.

From Bordini BJ, Stephany A, Kliegman R. Overcoming Diagnostic Errors in Medical Practice. J Pediatr. 2017;185:19-25.e1. https://doi.org/10.1016/j.jpeds.2017.02.065; with permission.

which patient handoffs occur frequently and diagnostic labels can take on an independent momentum, leaving little opportunity for physicians to challenge their appropriateness,[15] or in specialty care settings, in which patient symptoms are more likely to be considered primarily within the scope of that specialty's pathophysiologic mechanisms.[24] Specialty-specific settings also may increase the risk of *availability bias*, in which familiar and more frequently encountered diagnoses are more readily recalled and are given greater weight in the differential diagnosis. When framing effects and availability heuristics are invoked early, they may perpetuate anchoring biases and result in a diagnostic momentum that precludes consideration of alternate diagnoses,[25] producing both erroneous diagnoses and significant delays in proper diagnosis. Further examples of context-related biases are listed in **Table 4**.

CONTEXT-RELATED BIASES AND DIAGNOSTIC ERROR IN PERINATAL MEDICINE

Advances in prenatal molecular genetic testing, including the use of cell-free fetal DNA screening for aneuploidy and single-gene disorders, chromosomal microarray analysis, and fetal exome sequencing, have resulted in improved prenatal identification of inherited major congenital anomalies, including in up to 2% of advanced-maternal-age pregnancies without abnormalities on ultrasound and with a normal karyotype.[26–28] Nonetheless, depending on the underlying disorder, up to 30% of inherited congenital anomalies may remain undiagnosed prenatally,[11,29] and this rate increases substantially in instances of functional disorders, such as inborn errors of metabolism,[30] or in circumstances in which prenatal screening programs and diagnostic procedures are not universally applied or available.[26] In disorders with phenotypic features that are subtle or nonspecific, postnatal diagnosis may be delayed or may not be established antemortem.

Both the rate of and mortality related to congenital anomalies are higher in preterm neonates compared with term neonates[31,32]; prompt and proper postnatal diagnosis allows for personalized approaches to patient care that can include initiation of evidence-based therapies in disorders with established treatments, consideration of

Table 4
Cognitive biases related to errors of context

Bias	Definition
Availability bias	Basing decisions on the most recent patient with similar symptoms, preferentially recalling recent and more common diseases.
Base-rate neglect	Over- or underestimating the prevalence of a disease, typically overestimating the prevalence of common diseases and underestimating the prevalence of rare diseases.
Framing effect	Being influenced by how or by whom a problem is described, or by the setting in which the evaluation takes place.
Frequency bias	Believing that common things happen commonly and are usually benign in general practice.
Hindsight bias	Reinforcing diagnostic errors once a diagnosis is discovered in spite of these errors. May lead to a clinician overestimating the efficacy of his or her clinical reasoning and may reinforce ineffective techniques.
Posterior probability error	Considering the likelihood of a particular diagnosis in light of a patient's prior or chronic illnesses. New headaches in a patient with a history of migraines may in fact be a tumor.
Representative bias	Basing decisions on an expected typical presentation. Not effective for atypical presentations. Overemphasis on disease diagnostic criteria or "classic" presentations. "Looks like a duck, quacks like a duck."
Sutton slip	Ignoring alternate explanations for "obvious" diagnoses (Sutton law is that one should first consider the obvious).
Thinking in silo	Restricting diagnostic considerations to a particular specialty or organ system. Each discipline has a set of diseases within its comfort zone, which reduces diagnostic flexibility or team-based communication.
Zebra retreat	Lacking conviction to pursue rare disorders even when suggested by evidence.

From Bordini BJ, Stephany A, Kliegman R. Overcoming Diagnostic Errors in Medical Practice. J Pediatr. 2017;185:19-25.e1. https://doi.org/10.1016/j.jpeds.2017.02.065; with permission.

investigational therapies in rarer disorders or in instances in which effective therapies are actively under investigation, individualized genetic counseling, and compassionate withdrawal of support in disorders in which survival is not feasible.[12]

Recent advances in next-generation sequencing technologies notably include the introduction of a 26-hour genome sequencing protocol that has produced clinically actionable results in little more than a day and that is anticipated to significantly improve morbidity and mortality[12,33]; refinements in metabolomics have allowed for earlier and more precise identification of metabolic disorders and more rapid introduction of specialized diets or enzyme replacement therapy.[34] The challenge under these circumstances is determining when patients warrant such evaluation, and when clinicians need to engage more analytical diagnostic approaches while simultaneously focusing on and reacting to tenuous physiology as critically ill neonates transition to extrauterine life. Given the magnitude of this challenge, it may be exceedingly difficult to recognize when bias may be impeding appropriate diagnosis, or when confidence in a proposed or working diagnosis may be misplaced. The degree of concordance between diagnostic confidence and diagnostic accuracy is termed *diagnostic calibration*. In the context of a busy neonatal intensive care unit with high patient acuity, a variety of cognitive biases may result in poor diagnostic calibration, either as a result of bias-induced overconfidence or cognitive burden–related complacency, in which a clinician may be aware of the possibility of diagnostic error, but underestimates or otherwise trivializes its frequency or impact.[35] These biases may interfere with the ability to recognize when a patient's physiology or response to treatment fails to support the proposed diagnosis, such as when difficulty ventilating indicates interstitial lung disease or surfactant protein deficiency as opposed to bronchopulmonary dysplasia, or when red flags such as persistent acidosis indicate a more intensely time-sensitive diagnosis, such as an inborn error of metabolism or a ductal-dependent cardiac lesion.

IMPROVING DIAGNOSIS: INDIVIDUAL AND SYSTEMS-BASED APPROACHES

Diagnosis is a dynamic, iterative process that is intrinsically enmeshed in the context within which it occurs. That context is unique to each patient encounter and includes not only the cognitive and affective circumstances of the clinician in that moment, but also the circumstances of the patient, the patient's family, and other members of the evaluation team, as well as those of the clinic or hospital unit in which the evaluation is being conducted. This unique combination of factors invariably carries the risk of producing bias that may result in diagnostic error, and yet, most physicians maintain a *bias blind spot*, in which they perceive themselves as being less susceptible to bias, despite bias being a universal "operating characteristic of the diagnosing brain."[13,18,36–38] Furthermore, patients may improve sufficiently in spite of diagnostic error, oftentimes resulting in clinician overconfidence,[35] in which failures in reasoning are reinforced because the clinician is unaware of the diagnostic errors that occurred and uses the fact that the patient improved as confirmation that medical reasoning was sound.

Operationalizing an awareness of bias into improved patient outcomes remains challenging.[18,38] In our URD program, we have consciously confronted a tendency to minimize or misperceive bias by implementing a process and an environment designed to enhance diagnostic calibration. Primary among these strategies is the use of *cognitive forcing functions*,[39] which allows us to regularly question the appropriateness of any diagnostic labels that have accumulated in the course of a patient evaluation. To do so, we implement diagnostic checklists at regular intervals, following any diagnostic test or therapeutic intervention, with any change in patient status, and, perhaps most importantly, with any patient handoff or change in attending provider or team members. These structured opportunities allow for the interruption of diagnostic momentum and form part of a feedback system that over time improves individual and collective diagnostic calibration.[35,39,40] Over the course of each patient evaluation, we regularly use the following checklist[41]:

1. Have we gathered sufficient information on which to base our analysis?
2. Have we unpacked that information and processed it in an objective and bias-free manner?
3. What is the ultimate phenotype suggested by the patient's complaints and findings?
4. Does that phenotype suggest one underlying disease process or multiple disease processes occurring simultaneously?
5. Have we generated plausible hypotheses regarding the pathophysiology of these complaints and findings?
6. Have we implemented a directed diagnostic testing strategy using sufficiently sensitive and specific diagnostic assays that will allow us to discern among these diagnostic hypotheses in a Bayesian probabilistic fashion, as opposed to a dichotomous, "rule in, rule out" fashion?

7. Have we checked for additional sources of bias?
8. Have we considered alternate diagnoses sufficiently, and in particular, "do-not-miss" diagnoses?

In addition to the use of cognitive forcing functions, such as diagnostic checklists, proposals designed to improve diagnostic reasoning at the level of the individual clinician are multifaceted and diverse. Rajkomar and Dhaliwal[42] proffered a 3-tiered approach: (1) Recurring, individualized feedback on diagnostic accuracy; too often once a physician attains sufficient training to allow for independent practice, whether that be by the completion of a residency training program or additional fellowship-based specialty training, recurring opportunities for formalized feedback diminish. (2) Deliberate practice, in which simulated cases are discussed slowly and intentionally, with the physician actively engaging the cognitive processes that would allow for the development of working, differential, and refined diagnoses. At our institution, we engage in this practice weekly via our recurring "Professor's Rounds" forum, in which a third-year pediatrics resident presents a difficult or challenging case from his or her training and has multiple attending physicians reason through the case in real time, providing a nice complement to the more standard morning report format commonly encountered in medical student and residency training and offering a more direct opportunity for modeling clinical reasoning. (3) Metacognition is proposed as the third rail in the individual approach to improving diagnosis, in which students are instructed in the cognitive science of diagnosis so as to improve insight into the role bias can play in producing diagnostic error. Oftentimes, medical education fails to provide this framework for improving diagnosis. This lack of feedback and deliberate practice risks the development of the "experienced nonexpert," who by virtue of failing to engage in self-reflection, fails to develop a context-sensitive fund of knowledge that would allow for more timely and appropriate engagement of analytical diagnostic approaches.[42,43]

Beyond improving diagnostic calibration at the level of the individual, efforts to promote a *team-based approach* to diagnosis can enhance diagnostic accuracy beyond that achieved even by individual senior expert clinicians.[40] The primary aphorism that has driven the evaluation of each patient in our program is that "none of us is as smart as all of us"; indeed, collective intelligence-based medical decision-making has consistently and significantly outperformed even the most accurate diagnosticians in certain clinical contexts.[40] In our URD group, each patient evaluation team is composed not only of generalists and those specialists whose area of expertise is directly related to the patient's primary concerns, but also of additional specialists from a wide breadth of disciplines. In doing so, we foster a collective knowledge base that can mitigate context-related biases by soliciting perspectives on pathophysiology and differential diagnoses that may not have otherwise been considered were the patient evaluated within the silos of individual specialty settings. This collaborative and more deliberate approach to diagnosis additionally encourages the use of system 2 processes by actively promoting the generation of multiple diagnostic hypotheses and testing strategies. The end goal and product of this process is the *group phenotype*, in which the evaluation team has collectively, as a *group*, analyzed the patient's primary concerns, physical findings, and objective data into discrete phenotypic phenomena. These phenomena can then be explored further in attempts to uncover underlying and unifying pathophysiologic mechanisms and can additionally serve as high-quality phenotypic data that can better inform the interpretation of molecular genetic studies.[44]

Beyond the level of individual and team-based approaches, health care systems can prioritize improved diagnosis through the use of data-driven tools and enhanced focus on cognitive psychology as a foundational concept in medical education. In much the same way that health care institutions, and particularly intensive care settings, have implemented procedural time-outs, central line safety checklists, and other data-driven tools, such as sepsis trigger warnings, as an extension of the patient safety movement, individual clinicians, teams, and health care systems can leverage the collective experiences of the patient safety movement and cognitive psychology to create an environment and a process that foster optimal diagnosis and hone well-calibrated diagnosticians.[13,42] Improving pipelines for molecular diagnostics, including more rapid next-generation sequencing technologies, can additionally improve outcomes when time-to-diagnosis is of paramount importance; however, in our experience, when biochemical or otherwise functional assays may provide more rapid diagnosis, those approaches should be favored.[45] Over time, this approach will result in the entirety of the medical team having such engagement in the diagnostic process that improved calibration will become second nature: "Expertise is characterized by the ability to recognize when one's initial impression is wrong and to having back-up strategies readily available when the initial strategy does not work."[35]

Perinatal medicine comprises an exceedingly high-risk population that by virtue of the context of their diagnostic evaluation, are at an increased risk of diagnostic error. Emerging technologies, especially more widely and rapidly available genetic testing, as well as systems-based patient safety interventions, hold great potential to improve diagnosis. In addition, interventions designed to better attune the individual clinician and patient care team to the need for diagnostic pauses and more deliberate analytical approaches may result in further improvements in perinatal medicine. The lessons learned here are not specific to neonates and can improve outcomes in all of pediatrics.

DISCLOSURE STATEMENT

The authors have nothing to disclose.

REFERENCES

1. Diagnostic errors | AHRQ Patient Safety Network. Available at: https://psnet.ahrq.gov/primers/primer/12/diagnostic-errors. Accessed April 4, 2019.
2. Custer JW, Winters BD, Goode V, et al. Diagnostic errors in the pediatric and neonatal ICU: a systematic review. Pediatr Crit Care Med 2015;16(1):29–36.
3. Products - Data Briefs - Number 320 - September 2018. 2019. Available at: https://www.cdc.gov/nchs/products/databriefs/db326.htm. Accessed April 4, 2019.
4. Ely D. Fetal, perinatal, and infant mortality. Presented at the: Secretary's Advisory Committee on Infant Mortality. Division of Vital Statistics; National Center for Health Statistics, December 4, 2018. Available at: https://www.hrsa.gov/sites/default/files/hrsa/advisory-committees/infant-mortality/meetings/12042018/Fetal-Perinatal-IM-Ely.pdf. Accessed April 4, 2019.
5. Mathews TJ, MacDorman MF, Menacker F. Infant mortality statistics from the 1999 period: linked birth/infant death data set. Natl Vital Stat Rep 2002;50(4):1–28.
6. Tracy SK, Tracy MB, Sullivan E. Admission of term infants to neonatal intensive care: a population-based study. Birth 2007;34(4):301–7.
7. Harrison W, Goodman D. Epidemiologic trends in neonatal intensive care, 2007-2012. JAMA Pediatr 2015;169(9):855–62.
8. Schulman J, Braun D, Lee HC, et al. Association between neonatal intensive care unit admission rates and illness acuity. JAMA Pediatr 2018;172(1):17–23.

9. Ely DM, Driscoll AK, Matthews TJ. Infant mortality by age at death in the United States, 2016. NCHS Data Brief 2018;(326):8.

10. Nelson K, Holmes LB. Malformations due to presumed spontaneous mutations in newborn infants. N Engl J Med 1989;320(1):19–23.

11. Moorthie S, Blencowe H, Darlison MW, et al. Estimating the birth prevalence and pregnancy outcomes of congenital malformations worldwide. J Community Genet 2018;9(4):387–96.

12. Petrikin JE, Willig LK, Smith LD, et al. Rapid whole genome sequencing and precision neonatology. Semin Perinatol 2015;39(8):623–31.

13. Improving Diagnosis in Health Care. Committee on Diagnostic Error in Health Care; Board on Health Care Services; Institute of Medicine; The National Academies of Sciences, Engineering, and Medicine. Balogh EP, Miller BT, Ball JR, editors. Washington, DC: National Academies Press (US); 2015.

14. Shafer GJ, Suresh G. Diagnostic errors in the neonatal intensive care unit: a case series. AJP Rep 2018;08(4):e379–83.

15. Berkwitt A, Grossman M. Cognitive bias in inpatient pediatrics. Hosp Pediatr 2014;4(3):190–3.

16. Graber ML, Franklin N, Gordon R. Diagnostic error in internal medicine. Arch Intern Med 2005;165(13):1493–9.

17. Zwaan L, de Bruijne M, Wagner C, et al. Patient record review of the incidence, consequences, and causes of diagnostic adverse events. Arch Intern Med 2010; 170(12):1015–21.

18. Croskerry P. Bias: a normal operating characteristic of the diagnosing brain. Diagnosis (Berl) 2014;1(1):23–7.

19. Croskerry P. Diagnostic failure: a cognitive and affective approach. In: Henriksen K, Battles JB, Marks ES, et al., editors. Advances in Patient Safety: From research to implementation (Volume 2: Concepts and Methodology). Rockville (MD): Agency for Healthcare Research and Quality (US); 2005.

20. Cognitive overload in the ICU | AHRQ Patient Safety Network. Available at: https://psnet.ahrq.gov/webmm/case/380/Cognitive-Overload-in-the-ICU. Accessed May 31, 2019.

21. Patel VL, Zhang J, Yoskowitz NA, et al. Translational cognition for decision support in critical care environments: a review. J Biomed Inform 2008;41(3): 413–31.

22. Sweller J. Cognitive load theory, learning difficulty, and instructional design. Learn Instr 1994;4(4):295–312.

23. Saposnik G, Redelmeier D, Ruff CC, et al. Cognitive biases associated with medical decisions: a systematic review. BMC Med Inform Decis Mak 2016;16. https://doi.org/10.1186/s12911-016-0377-1.

24. Ogdie AR, Reilly JB, Pang WG, et al. Seen through their eyes: residents' reflections on the cognitive and contextual components of diagnostic errors in medicine. Acad Med 2012;87(10):1361–7.

25. Anchoring bias with critical implications | AHRQ Patient Safety Network. Available at: https://psnet.ahrq.gov/webmm/case/350/anchoring-bias-with-critical-implications. Accessed May 7, 2019.

26. Van den Veyver IB. Recent advances in prenatal genetic screening and testing. F1000Res 2016;5. https://doi.org/10.12688/f1000research.9215.1.

27. Talkowski ME, Ordulu Z, Pillalamarri V, et al. Clinical diagnosis by whole-genome sequencing of a prenatal sample. N Engl J Med 2012;367(23): 2226–32.

28. Wapner RJ, Martin CL, Levy B, et al. Chromosomal microarray versus karyotyping for prenatal diagnosis. N Engl J Med 2012;367(23):2175–84.

29. EUROCAT. EUROCAT Prenatal Detection Rates: prenatal diagnosis of 18 selected congenital anomaly subgroups for registries with complete data from 2013 to 2017. 2019. Available at: http://www.eurocat-network.eu/newprevdata/showPDF.aspx?winx=1896&winy=957&file=pd1.aspx. Accessed June 7, 2019.

30. Diukman R, Goldberg JD. Prenatal diagnosis of inherited metabolic diseases. West J Med 1993;159(3):374–81.

31. Field D, Boyle E, Draper E, et al. Towards reducing variations in infant mortality and morbidity: a population-based approach. Southampton (UK): NIHR Journals Library; 2016. (Programme Grants for Applied Research, No. 4.1.) Chapter 3, The Late And Moderately preterm Birth Study. Available at: https://www.ncbi.nlm.nih.gov/books/NBK349423/. Accessed June 7, 2019.

32. Tomashek KM, Shapiro-Mendoza CK, Davidoff MJ, et al. Differences in mortality between late-preterm and term singleton infants in the United States, 1995–2002. J Pediatr 2007;151(5):450–6.e1.

33. Saunders CJ, Miller NA, Soden SE, et al. Rapid whole-genome sequencing for genetic disease diagnosis in neonatal intensive care units. Sci Transl Med 2012;4(154):154ra135.

34. Jackson F, Georgakopoulou N, Kaluarachchi M, et al. Development of a pipeline for exploratory metabolic profiling of infant urine. J Proteome Res 2016;15(9): 3432–40.

35. Berner ES, Graber ML. Overconfidence as a cause of diagnostic error in medicine. Am J Med 2008;121(5, Supplement):S2–23.

36. Schiff GD, Kim S, Abrams R, et al. Diagnosing Diagnosis Errors: Lessons from a Multi-institutional Collaborative Project. In: Henriksen K, Battles JB, Marks ES, et al., editors. Advances in Patient Safety: From Research to Implementation (Volume 2: Concepts and Methodology). Rockville (MD): Agency for Healthcare Research and Quality (US); 2005. Available at: https://www.ncbi.nlm.nih.gov/books/NBK20492/. Accessed September 19, 2016.

37. Holmboe ES, Durning SJ. Assessing clinical reasoning: moving from in vitro to in vivo. Diagnosis (Berl) 2014;1(1):111–7.

38. West RF, Meserve RJ, Stanovich KE. Cognitive sophistication does not attenuate the bias blind spot. J Pers Soc Psychol 2012;103(3):506–19.

39. Ely JW, Graber ML, Croskerry P. Checklists to reduce diagnostic errors. Acad Med 2011;86(3):307.

40. Wolf M, Krause J, Carney PA, et al. Collective intelligence meets medical decision-making: the collective outperforms the best radiologist. PLoS One 2015;10(8):e0134269.

41. Bordini BJ, Stephany A, Kliegman R. Overcoming diagnostic errors in medical practice. J Pediatr 2017;185:19–25.e1.

42. Rajkomar A, Dhaliwal G. Improving diagnostic reasoning to improve patient safety. Perm J 2011;15(3):68–73.

43. Bereiter C, Scardamalia M. Surpassing ourselves: an inquiry into the nature and implications of expertise. Chicago: Open Court Publishing Company; 1993.

44. Lu JT, Campeau PM, Lee BH. Genotype–phenotype correlation — promiscuity in the era of next-generation sequencing. N Engl J Med 2014;371(7):593–6.

45. Konersman CG, Bordini BJ, Scharer G, et al. BAG3 myofibrillar myopathy presenting with cardiomyopathy. Neuromuscul Disord 2015;25(5):418–22.

46. Bradsher RW. The endemic mimic: blastomycosis an illness often misdiagnosed. Trans Am Clin Climatol Assoc 2014;125:188–203.
47. Zucker EJ, Epelman M, Newman B. Perinatal thoracic mass lesions: pre- and postnatal imaging. Semin Ultrasound CT MR 2015;36(6):501–21.
48. Erdogdu E, Arısoy R, Kumru P, et al. Unusual presentation of fetus in fetu in triplet pregnancy mimicking abdominal wall defect. Case Rep Perinat Med 2015;4(2): 135–6.

Dysmorphology in a Genomic Era

Donald Basel, MBBCh

KEYWORDS

- Dysmorphology • Phenotype • HPO

KEY POINTS

- Clinical dysmorphology evolved out of the need to standardize descriptive terminology used to define human variation, primarily in the context of malformations and syndromic disorders.
- DNA analysis may provide the genotype and confirm a diagnosis, but it cannot define the phenotype.
- The advances made in molecular technology have led to the identification and ongoing discovery of the underlying genetic pathoetiology of many syndromes.

INTRODUCTION

Clinical dysmorphology evolved out of the need to standardize descriptive terminology used to define human variation, primarily in the context of malformations and syndromic disorders. The classic dysmorphology approach of establishing a clear history and, through detailed examination, listing abnormal findings ordered in a sequence ranked by perceived importance and then using these data to aid in establishing a working clinical diagnosis, is tried and tested but effective in only a small subset of recognized syndromes. This science and art of syndrome recognition is gradually being lost as newer technologies both blur the margins between various syndromes and enable syndrome recognition through the application of various computational tools. In this article, we review the utility of deep phenotyping and the application of dysmorphology in a genomic era.

DNA analysis may provide the genotype and confirm a diagnosis, but it cannot define the phenotype the advances made in molecular technology have led to the identification and ongoing discovery of the underlying genetic pathoetiology of many syndromes. The field of molecular dysmorphology grew out of the fusion of knowledge of normal human embryologic development and aberrations in gene signaling pathways giving rise to syndromic disorders.[1] Many of these pathways interact, either directly or indirectly, and thus syndromes previously considered

Department of Pediatrics, Division of Genetics, Medical College of Wisconsin, 9000 West Wisconsin Avenue, MS #716, Milwaukee, WI 53226, USA
E-mail address: dbasel@mcw.edu

Clin Perinatol 47 (2020) 15–23
https://doi.org/10.1016/j.clp.2019.10.009
0095-5108/20/© 2019 Elsevier Inc. All rights reserved.

distinct entities now share common or overlapping genetic etiologies, which has further compounded the challenge of clearly defining syndromes. As a result, the era of the gene-x-opathy descriptor is our current reality. A commonly used example of this involves the RAS pathway. RASopathies represent disorders impacting the RAS-MEK-ERK pathway, which includes a diverse group of disorders, including neurofibromatosis type I, Legius, Noonan with and without multiple lentigines, Costello, and cardiofaciocutaneous syndromes, as represented in **Fig. 1**. Noonan syndrome has the greatest overlap, and certain genes within the pathway may present as either Noonan syndrome or cardiofaciocutaneous syndrome. Neurofibromatosis is associated only with neurofibromin, and Costello syndrome is similarly seen only with pathogenic variants in HRAS. In addition to the genetic heterogeneity of common pathways, disorders that use metabolites in signal transduction can share common pathoetiology through these common factors. Disorders of cholesterol metabolism are a good representation of such syndromic overlap. Aside from cholesterol being a key precursor in the general steroid biosynthesis pathway, it is additionally a key signaling molecule in the Sonic Hedgehog pathway, and as such is implicated in related syndromic disorders that include Smith Lemli Opitz, Gorlin syndrome, Rubinstein Taybi, holoprosencephaly, and Pallister Hall and Greig syndromes.

VARIATION AND ONTOLOGY

Human variation is estimated at approximately 0.1%, which equates to roughly 6 coding variants per gene. Sequencing of the human genome clarified that humans have

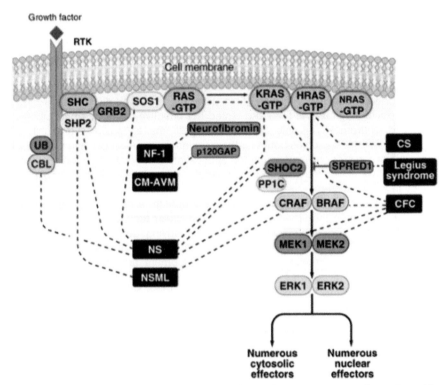

Fig. 1. The RASK/MAPK signal transduction pathway. (*From* Rauen KA. The RASopathies, Annu Rev Genom Hum Genet 14:355–369, 2013; with permission.)

close to 23,000 genes, of which only 5500 have corresponding phenotype data. Given that approximately two-thirds of our genes do not have a clear disease association, it is apparent that we need tools to facilitate and assist in the identification of disorders in undiagnosed and rare diseases. There is still much to learn about our genetic code, let alone how tertiary chromatin structure impacts disease and gene regulation. Even if we could perform genomic sequencing on every patient, in most patients the molecular diagnosis would remain elusive. The current diagnostic rate for exome sequencing is approximately 25%, this increases to approximately 30% with exome trio analysis in which selected relatives are sequenced and the additional data are used to assess allele segregation with the phenotype. It should not be inferred from this that genomic sequencing has limited clinical utility, as clinically actionable decisions are made in most cases undergoing sequencing, either through direct pathophysiological mechanisms in a positive result or through exclusion in negative test outcomes.

Sequencing in isolation of supportive phenotypic data significantly limits the analyst's ability to undertake a comprehensive evaluation of variants identified through sequencing. Several publications have highlighted the value of supportive phenotype data in focusing the analysis to identify causal variants in genomic sequencing.[2–4] Gripp and colleagues[5] published a unique twist on this concept by using artificial intelligence (AI) to aid variant identification. This automated phenotyping through facial recognition software will be discussed in greater detail.

To standardize phenotype terminology and create a structured hierarchical basis for computational analysis, the Human Phenotype Ontology (HPO) was developed in 2008 and through ongoing international collaboration with the Monarch Initiative and other organizations, several tools have been developed to aid diagnostics in undiagnosed diseases.[6] Using HPO terminology, developmental malformations can be cross referenced across a number of different species, which can in turn help define function in human genes. Conversely, genes identified in undiagnosed human malformations can be evaluated for plausible disease association by comparing phenotypic presentations across various species[7] (**Fig. 2**).

There are too many analytical tools available to allow for a detailed discussion of them all. It would, however, be useful to outline a few of the more common tools used in clinical practice. In general, these tools help define a differential diagnosis based on HPO terminology derived from a thorough dysmorphic evaluation. The details of how to approach a dysmorphic examination have been previously covered[8,9] and are not detailed here, but it is helpful to conceptualize the etiologic basis of the deformity, as outlined in **Fig. 3**.

To adequately phenotype a patient, it is expected that a detailed head-to-toe evaluation is undertaken, capturing all major (**Table 1**) and minor anomalies (**Table 2**). In addition, a complete review of the medical record is required to understand the historical progression and extract the phenotypic elements provided through medical investigation.

An international initiative to standardize the nosology used in clinical dysmorphology has been adapted to the Internet as an online resource supported by the National Human Genome Research Institute: https://elementsofmorphology.nih.gov/. These terms provide the basis for the HPO definitions, which can then be applied to computational tools such as Phenomizer (http://compbio.charite.de/phenomizer/), a tool that creates ranked lists of diseases from OMIM (Online Mendelian Inheritance in Man; www.omim.org) based on the probability of the HPO terms listed presenting concurrently (**Fig. 4**). It is important to realize that none of the computational tools provide diagnoses, rather they present ranked lists of possible disorders to consider in the

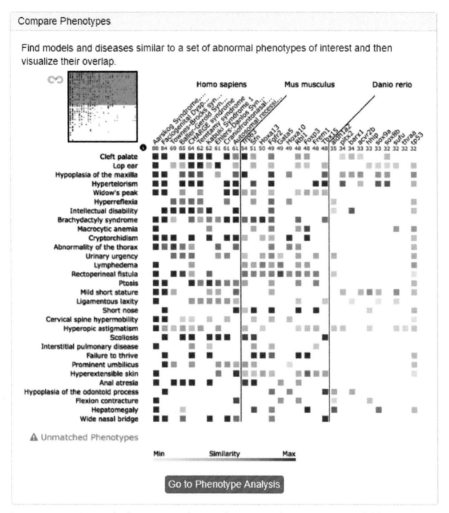

Fig. 2. Comparison of phenotypes. (*From* the Monarch Intiative. Available at: https://monarchinitiative.org/.)

differential diagnosis. The onus for making a diagnosis relies on the critical thinking of the physician.

OMIM can be searched directly using any phenotypic descriptor. This character string is processed through a Boolean search engine of its internal database to define the rank list of probable disorders based on the characters used in the search. The lists generated are highly dependent on the search terms used and are, in general, less accurate than implementing specific HPO terms.

ARTIFICIAL INTELLIGENCE IN DYSMORPHOLOGY

Evolving beyond the reliance of the evaluating physician to accurately define dysmorphic ontological terminology, several groups are working on facial recognition software for syndromic identification. These tools too are not diagnostic, but offer

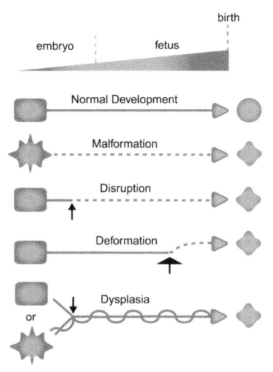

Fig. 3. Etiologic mechanisms for congenital anomalies. (*Adapted from* Spranger J, Benirschke K, Hall JG, Errors of morphogenesis: concepts and terms. Recommendations of an international working group. J Pediatr. 1982 Jan;100(1):160-5; with permission.)

Table 1
Major malformations[a]

Neurologic	Abdominal wall
• Severe hydrocephalus	• Gastroschisis
• Lissencephaly	• Omphalocele
• Schizencephaly	Craniofacial
• Megalencephaly	• Craniosynostosis
• Neural tube defect	• Facial cleft
• Spina bifida	• Cleft lip and palate
• Meningomyelocele	• Structural eye defect
• Encephalocele	• Coloboma
Cardiovascular	• Aniridia
• Various congenital heart malformations	• Structural ear defects
• Cardiomyopathy	• Microtia
• Severe arrhythmia	• Aplasia of the auditory canal
Genitourinary	Limb
• Ambiguous genitalia	• Amelia
• Kidney malformations	• Split/hand foot malformation
• Urachal defects	
Respiratory	
• Congenital pulmonary airway malformation	
• Tracheoesophageal fistula	

[a] Not an inclusive list.

Table 2
Minor malformations[a]

Craniofacial
- Large fontanel
- Flat or low nasal bridge
- Saddle nose, upturned nose
- Micrognathia
- Cutis aplasia of the scalp

Eye
- Palpebral fissures
  - Telecanthus or epicanthus
  - Up or down slanting
- Hypertelorism
- Brushfield spots

Ear
- Posteriorly rotated pinna
- Lack of helical fold
- Preauricular with or without auricular skin tags
- Small pinna
- Auricular (preauricular) pit or sinus
- Folding of helix
- DARWINIAN tubercle
- Crushed (crinkled) ear
- Asymmetric ear sizes
- Low-set ears

Skin
- Dimpling over the bones
- Capillary hemangioma (face/posterior neck)
- Dermal melanosis (African, Asian)
- Sacral dimple
- Pigmented nevi
- Redundant skin folds
- Cutis marmorata
- Café au lait macules

Hand
- Simian crease
- Bridged upper palmar creases
- Fifth finger clinodactyly
- Joint hypermobility (hyperextension of thumb)
- Cutaneous syndactyly
- Polydactyly
- Short, broad thumb
- Narrow or hyperconvex nails
- Hypoplastic nails
- Camptodactyly
- Short fourth metacarpal

Foot
- Syndactyly of second/third toe
- Asymmetric toe length
- Clinodactyly of second toe
- Overlapping toes
- Nail hypoplasia
- Wide gap between hallux and second toe
- Deep plantar crease between hallux and second toe

Other
- Mild calcaneovalgus
- Hydrocele
- Shawl scrotum
- Hypospadias
- Hypoplasia of labia majora
- Supernumerary nipples
- Undescended testes
- Tongue tie

[a] Not an inclusive list.

rank-listed possibilities for diagnostic consideration. There are various machine learning tools used (eg, Support Vector Machines, KNearest Neighbors, Deformable Models, Hidden Markov Models) that yield variable results. The class of machine learning architectures called Deep Learning, such as convolutional neural networks, have seen substantial gains in recent years. These methods extract features from training images and perform classification of images, often identifying features, such as image texture, that would not have been chosen by diagnosticians. A classic critique of machine learning methods is that they are black-box; meaning that it can be difficult to understand why it arrived at a particular outcome once it has been trained. New algorithms, such as attention-based networks, allow the possibility of opening the box to understand why the classifier made its decision. These new features provide a robust data set for comparative analysis. One of the more widely implemented tools is the free resource: Face2Gene, which in addition to the facial computational analysis, enables adjunct HPO terminology to be entered to further refine the phenotype. The depiction in **Fig. 5** outlines the process implemented by FDNA Inc. to establish a bioinformatic reference for comparative image analysis.[10]

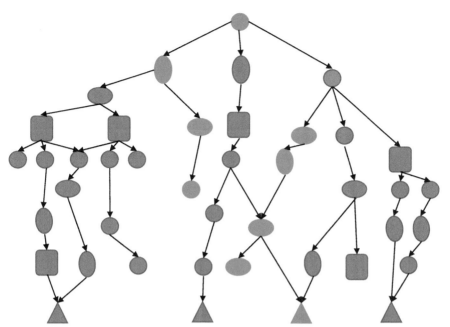

Fig. 4. HPO features linking searched terms with disease-associated findings. (*Data from* Köhler S, Schulz MH, Krawitz P, et al. Clinical diagnostics in human genetics with semantic similarity searches in ontologies. Am J Hum Genet 2009;85(4):457-64; Köhler S, Vasilevsky NA, Engelstad M, et al. The Human Phenotype Ontology in 2017. Nucleic Acids Res 2017;45(D1):D865-76.

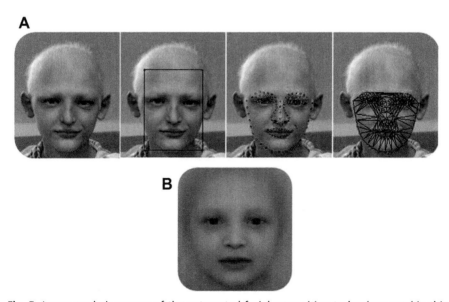

Fig. 5. Image analysis process of the automated facial recognition technology used in this study. (*A*) A face is detected in the frontal image and anatomic points are automatically identified. The face is divided into multiple regions, whose appearance is analyzed. (*B*) Last, a mask depicting the characteristic appearance of each syndrome is created. (*From* Hadj-Rabia S, Schneider H, Navarro E, et al. Automatic recognition of the XLHED phenotype from facial images. Am J Med Genet A. 2017 Sep;173(9):2408-2414. https://doi.org/10.1002/ajmg.a.38343. Epub 2017 Jul 10; with permission.)

The machine learning aspect of these tools ensures that, over time, their accuracy will improve. The knowledge base is continually expanded through "crowdsourcing" the expertise of recognized experts who continue to train the system by entering molecularly confirmed diagnoses. The AI utility of Face2Gene has been termed DeepGestalt, and in a recent publication Gurovich and colleagues[11] have shown that this tool is able to list the correct diagnosis within the top 10 differential 91% of the time. The model also has been shown to be able to differentiate the numerous genotypes causing Noonan syndrome with high accuracy in addition to being able to differentiate disorders within a common pathway (eg, RASopathies). Pascolini and colleagues[12] describe similarities in phenotype in various disorders associated with chromatin remodeling that were identified through DeepGestalt. There is some overlap in the context of the epigenetic modification that occurs at a molecular level, but phenotypic overlap had not been previously appreciated. The next evolution of this technology is to incorporate the data derived from phenotyping and apply that directly to machine learning tools used for variant identification and classification. In a recent publication, Hsieh and colleagues described such an approach to variant prioritization termed PEDIA (prioritization of exome data by image analysis) in which data from DeepGestalt is used within the variant analysis pipeline to improve the likelihood of identifying causal variants in genomic analysis.[13]

CLOSING CONSIDERATIONS

The development of these various tools and their application to molecular dysmorphology will change the way that we approach phenotyping as a whole. Computer-assisted image processing can be applied to histology, radiology, and any other data sets that allow for a digital reference to be established. This "next-generation phenotyping" will become the basis for comparative analysis to aid further understanding of genomic data. Where is the limit? Vocal analysis, gait analysis, handwriting, visual tracking; there are many avenues for phenotype expansion and with the power of cloud computing and integration of machine learning, we are limited only by our imagination.

DISCLOSURE

D. Basel is an unpaid member of the FDNA Scientific Advisory Board.

REFERENCES

1. Biesecker LG. Molecular dysmorphology. In: Jorde L, Little P, Dunn M, et al, editors. Encyclopedia of genetics, genomics, proteomics, and bioinformatics. Hoboken (NJ): Wiley-Blackwell; 2005.
2. Seaby EG, Pengelly RJ, Ennis S. Exome sequencing explained: a practical guide to its clinical application. Brief Funct Genomics 2016;15(5):374–84.
3. Maver A, Lovrecic L, Volk M, et al. Phenotype-driven gene target definition in clinical genome-wide sequencing data interpretation. Genet Med 2016;18(11):1102–10.
4. Tomar S, Sethi R, Lai PS. Specific phenotype semantics facilitate gene prioritization in clinical exome sequencing. Eur J Hum Genet 2019;27(9):1389–97.
5. Gripp KW, Baker L, Telegrafi A, et al. The role of objective facial analysis using FDNA in making diagnoses following whole exome analysis. Report of two patients with mutations in the BAF complex genes. Am J Med Genet A 2016;170(7):1754–62.

6. Robinson PN1, Köhler S, Bauer S, et al. The Human Phenotype Ontology: a tool for annotating and analyzing human hereditary disease. Am J Hum Genet 2008; 83(5):610–5.
7. Robinson PN, Köhler S, Oellrich A, et al, Sanger Mouse Genetics Project. Improved exome prioritization of disease genes through cross-species phenotype comparison. Genome Res 2014;24(2):340–8.
8. Basel D. Dysmorphology. In: Kliegman R, Lye PS, Bordini B, et al, editors. Nelson Pediatric Symptom-Based Diagnosis. Elsevier; 2018. p.393-410.e1.
9. Davies DP, Evans DJR. Clinical dysmorphology: understanding congenital abnormalities. Curr Paediatrics 2003;13:288–97.
10. Hadj-Rabia S, Schneider H, Navarro E, et al. Automatic recognition of the XLHED phenotype from facial images. Am J Med Genet A 2017;173(9):2408–14.
11. Gurovich Y, Hanani Y, Bar O, et al. Identifying facial phenotypes of genetic disorders using deep learning. Nat Med 2019;25:60–4.
12. Pascolini G, Fleischer N, Ferraris A, et al. The facial dysmorphology analysis technology in intellectual disability syndromes related to defects in the histones modifiers. J Hum Genet 2019;64(8):721–8.
13. Hsieh TC, Mensah MA, Pantel JT, et al. PEDIA: prioritization of exome data by image analysis. Genet Med 2019. https://doi.org/10.1038/s41436-019-0566-2.

Neonatal Acute Liver Failure

Catherine Larson-Nath, MD[a], Bernadette E. Vitola, MD, MPH[b],*

KEYWORDS

- Neonatal • Liver failure • Gestational alloimmune liver disease • Liver transplant

KEY POINTS

- Neonatal acute liver failure is a life-threatening condition that may present with subtle signs such as poor feeding, lethargy, and fever.
- Timely identification of the cause is critical because treatment is often disease specific and lifesaving.
- The primary known causes include gestational alloimmune liver disease, viral infections, metabolic diseases, and shock.
- Outcomes have improved with better understanding of the mechanism of injury and treatment of gestational alloimmune liver disease.
- Mortality for neonates with acute liver failure is twice that of older children.

INTRODUCTION

Neonatal acute liver failure (NALF) is a rare and not well-understood disease. The diagnosis, prognosis, and management have changed over the last 10 to 15 years based on the growing knowledge of the cause and treatment of one of the most common known causes of NALF, gestational alloimmune liver disease (GALD). This article is based on the limited data that exist on this entity as well as other known causes of NALF and is derived mostly from national studies on pediatric acute liver failure, which includes neonates.

DEFINITION

The definition of acute liver failure (ALF) in adults is an international normalized ratio (INR) of greater than or equal to 1.5 without correction with vitamin K level in the presence of hepatic encephalopathy occurring within 8 weeks of the onset of jaundice in a person without preexisting liver disease. Because encephalopathy is difficult to determine in infants and is often a late finding in children, the Pediatric Acute Liver Failure Study Group, a multicenter, prospective study initiated in 1999 that collects data on children less than 18 years old with ALF from 24 participating centers in the United

[a] Pediatric Gastroenterology, Hepatology & Nutrition, University of Minnesota, 2450 Riverside Avenue, Minneapolis, MN 55454, USA; [b] Pediatric Gastroenterology, Hepatology & Nutrition, Medical College of Wisconsin, 8701 Watertown Plank Road, Milwaukee, WI 53226, USA
* Corresponding author.
E-mail address: bvitola@mcw.edu

Clin Perinatol 47 (2020) 25–39
https://doi.org/10.1016/j.clp.2019.10.006
0095-5108/20/© 2019 Elsevier Inc. All rights reserved.

States, Canada, and the United Kingdom, created a second definition for inclusion into their study: an INR greater than or equal to 2 without correction with vitamin K with or without encephalopathy.[1]

Because neonates are considered to be any children from birth to 4 weeks, liver failure in a neonate is automatically considered ALF simply based on age and duration of disease. Although neonates may have had injury in utero leading to cirrhosis before birth, which would, by definition, exclude ALF, time in utero is not considered in the 8-week time frame.

PRESENTATION

Presenting signs of NALF may vary depending on the cause. However, a study by Sundaram and collegues[2] of 148 infants less than or equal to 90 days of life with ALF showed that the most common presenting signs and symptoms were:

- Lethargy (49%)
- Fever (20%)
- Nausea/vomiting (20%)
- Hepatomegaly (71%)
- Splenomegaly (41%)
- Ascites (39%)
- Peripheral edema (38%)

This same study revealed that, overall, young infants had lower median transaminase levels in general compared with older children (alanine transaminase [ALT], 156 IU/L; aspartate transaminase [AST], 215 IU/L vs ALT, 1616 IU/L, AST, 1778 IU/L; $P<.0001$), especially the subgroup diagnosed with GALD (ALT, 35 IU/L; AST, 85 IU/L) versus other causes of NALF (ALT, 211 IU/L; AST, 289 IU/L; $P<.0001$).[2]

OUTCOMES

Survival in NALF varies based on cause and availability of treatment. However, overall survival in this population correlates strongly with the absence of encephalopathy. Based on the studies by Sundaram and collegues[2] and Ng and colleagues,[3] spontaneous survival in infants with no encephalopathy at presentation was approximately 66%, whereas spontaneous survival of infants with moderate (grade 3 or 4) encephalopathy was half that regardless of cause.[2,3] Fewer young infants were listed for transplant compared with the older cohort (41% vs 58%; $P = .008$).[2] The mortality of infants less than or equal to 90 days old was twice that of older children (24% vs 10.5%; $P = .001$), and was most often caused by multiorgan failure (64%).[2]

MECHANISMS

The mechanisms of NALF vary by cause, but many different causes lead to acute hepatic necrosis, including viral infections, ischemic injury from circulatory failure or congenital cardiac defects, toxic injury, and immune dysregulation caused by hemophagocytic lymphoproliferative histiocytosis.[4] Exceptions to this include hepatocyte replacement by an infiltrative process caused by congenital leukemia or myelodysplasia; organelle dysfunction secondary to mitochondrial cytopathy; steatosis and cholestasis caused by toxic injury, galactosemia, and tyrosinemia; and impaired development of hepatocytes and/or destruction caused by membrane attack complex formation caused by alloimmune injury in utero as a result of GALD.[4,5]

| Table 1 | | |
| Differential diagnosis for neonatal liver failure | | |
Infectious	**Metabolic**	**Other**
HSV	Galactosemia	GALD
Enterovirus	Tyrosinemia	Ischemic
CMV	Hereditary fructose intolerance	Toxic
Other viruses	Mitochondrial	Leukemia
Sepsis	Disorders of fatty oxidation	
	DNA duplication syndromes	
	Respiratory chain defects	
	Niemann-Pick	
	Urea cycle defect	

Abbreviations: CMV, cytomegalovirus; HSV, herpes simplex virus.
Data from Sundaram SS, Alonso EM, Narkewicz MR, et al. Characterization and outcomes of young infants with acute liver failure. *J Pediatr* 2011;159:813-818e1; with permission.

CAUSES

There are several causes of NALF that have been found in multiple studies (**Table 1**). However, the most common cause is still indeterminate (37.8%). The other common causes are metabolic disorders (18.9%, all combined), viral infections (16.2%), GALD (13.5%), and shock (4.1%).[2]

Neonatal Hemochromatosis

Neonatal hemochromatosis (NH) accounts for 13.5% to 16.2% of cases of neonatal liver failure.[2,6] NH is the term given to extrahepatic siderosis associated with liver disease in the neonatal period. The most common cause of NH is GALD. Other causes of NH account for less than 2% of cases.[7] Causes of NH include:

- GALD
- Infection
- Trisomy 21
- Deoxyguanosine kinase (DGUOK) gene mutations
- Bile acid synthetic defect delta 4-3-oxosterid 5 beta-reductase deficiency (SRD5B1)
- GRACILE (growth retardation, aminoaciduria, cholestasis, iron overload, lactic acidosis, and early death) syndrome (BCS1L mutation)
- Myofibromatosis
- Trichohepatoenteric syndrome
- Martinez-Frias syndrome

Gestational alloimmune liver disease

GALD is the most common known cause of NH and NALF.[2,6] GALD results from maternal production of immunoglobulin (Ig) G against fetal antigen. Maternal IgG crosses the placenta, binds to hepatocyte antigen, and leads to activation of the compliment cascade, which results in liver injury and dysfunction.[5] This injury leads to decreased production of hepcidin, which results in increased transport of placental iron into the liver, decreased transferrin production, and increased iron uptake into extrahepatic tissues.[8] Tissues commonly affected by siderosis include:

- Pancreas
- Salivary glands
- Thyroid
- Myocardium

Diagnosis is made with documentation of extrahepatic siderosis (MRI or buccal biopsy) in the setting of severe liver disease. Most often children present within hours of birth, but presentation can occur up to 3 months of age. Other laboratory (**Table 2**) and imaging findings can help differentiate the causes. Laboratory findings in GALD include[9]:

- Normal to mildly increased transaminase levels
- Significantly increased INR
- Hyperbilirubinemia
- Increased alpha fetoprotein level for gestational age
- Increased transferrin saturation with low transferrin level
- Increased ferritin level

There is often a maternal history of unexplained fetal death, miscarriage, or unexplained illness or liver disease in an infant sibling. Findings on history and examination include:

- Edema or hydrops
- Prematurity
- Ascites
- Intrauterine growth restriction
- Oligohydramnios
- Jaundice

Because of the severity and rapid progression of disease, providers should have a low threshold for initiating treatment with IV immunoglobulin (IVIG) (1 g/kg) as the diagnosis is being determined. Once diagnosis is confirmed, infants should undergo double volume exchange transfusion and a second dose of IVIG (1 g/kg).[7,10,11] With this approach, centers report survival without transplant of 75% to 80% compared with 10% to 20% based on historical controls.[7,10] Normalization of INR in GALD can take up to 6 weeks.[10]

Transplant may be considered if medical treatment fails. Transplant is difficult in these patients because of their small size and overall illness severity. Because recovery may take several weeks, if there is evidence of improvement with treatment, patience is warranted before proceeding with transplant.

Because GALD is related to maternal-fetal alloimmunity, disease may be prevented or decreased in severity in future pregnancies with administration of IVIG 1 g/kg weekly to the mother starting at 18 weeks of gestation. In 1 study, this approach led to positive outcomes in 99% of cases.[12] Without treatment, recurrence of GALD in subsequent pregnancies is 92% based on historical controls.[12]

Infectious

Viral

Viral infections are a common cause of NALF (16.2%), with herpes simplex virus (HSV) (12.8%) the most commonly identified viral cause.[2]

Herpes simplex Neonatal HSV infection is typically acquired during passage via the birth canal, although postnatal infection can occur from any active lesions on the skin or lips. Early presenting signs can be subtle, including poor feeding and lethargy,

Table 2
Typical laboratory findings in neonatal liver failure

	GALD	HLH	Mitochondrial	Viral	Ischemic
Transaminase Levels (IU/L)	Normal/mild increase<100	Moderate/significant increase (>1000)	Moderate increase (100–500)	Significant increase (>1000)	Significant increase (>1000–6000)
INR	Significant increase	Moderate/significant increase	Moderate/significant increase	Moderate/significant increase	Moderate/significant increase
Ferritin Level (ng/mL)	800–7000	Significant increase (>20,000)	Variable	Significant increase (>20,000)	Variable depending on underlying cause of ischemia
Triglyceride Levels	Normal	Increased	Normal	Normal	Normal
Hypoglycemia	Yes	Often	Yes	Often	Variable
Lactic Acidosis	Normal	Normal	Increased	Normal	Often
Alpha Fetoprotein Level (for Age)	Increased	Normal	Normal/increased	Normal	Normal
Cholestasis	Progressive after birth	Moderate/significant	Moderate	None/mild at presentation	Mild/moderate

Abbreviation: HLH, hemophagocytic lymphohistiocytosis.

Data from Sundaram, et al. *J Pediatr* 2011;159:813-818; Taylor, et al. *Liver Transpl.* 2016;22(5):677-685; Bitar, et al. *J Pediatr Gastroenterol Nutr.* 2017;64(1):70-75; Fellman, et al. *Semin Fetal Neonatal Med.* 2011;16(4):222-228.

with fever in some patients within the first 2 weeks of birth.[13] There is not always a history of herpes in one of the parents.

Diagnosis can be made with polymerase chain reaction (PCR) from blood, skin, eye, cerebrospinal fluid (CSF), and mucous membranes. Immediate initiation of therapy with acyclovir is imperative because of the high (80%) mortality of this infection.[13] Human herpes virus 6 has also been associated with NALF but is usually less severe.

Enterovirus Enteroviruses are another viral cause of NALF (2.7%).[2] Neonates with enterovirus may have more generalized symptoms, including respiratory distress, diarrhea, poor feeding, rash, and fever.[14] Because enteroviruses have also been reported in neonates with necrotizing enterocolitis (NEC), any newborn with both NALF and NEC raises suspicion for infection with enterovirus.[15] Diagnosis can be made with PCR from blood, CSF, and stool. Treatment includes supportive care.

Metabolic

NALF caused by metabolic disorders is common and often treatable with dietary adjustments. These conditions should, therefore, be screened for. Some conditions are tested for on the newborn screen, but many are not, or they can present before the newborn screen being reported.

Galactosemia

Galactosemia is an autosomal recessive inborn error of carbohydrate metabolism caused by a deficiency of galactose 1-phosphate uridyltransferase.[16] Infants with galactosemia can be identified based on newborn screening in which the transferase enzyme is assayed, or from presentation within the first days to weeks of life with the following clinical symptoms[17,18]:

- Vomiting
- Failure to thrive
- Anorexia
- Jaundice
- Hepatomegaly
- Ascites
- Coagulopathy
- *Escherichia coli* sepsis
- Cataracts

Galactosemia is one of the most common metabolic diseases to cause NALF (8.1%).[2] Treatment of galactosemia is immediate elimination of lactose and galactose from the diet because ongoing milk exposure can quickly lead to death. Even with a diet free of lactose and galactose, complications have still been reported, including cognitive impairment, ovarian failure, neurologic impairments, and decreased bone density; routine screening for complications is recommended.[19–21]

Diagnosis of galactosemia can be made with newborn screening. Enzyme activity can also be detected in a variety of tissues, including erythrocytes, liver, cultured fibroblasts, and leukocytes.[22] Genetic testing can be pursued as well, which is helpful for prenatal testing for subsequent children born to parents with a child diagnosed with galactosemia. Interestingly, a recent Cochrane Review could not identify any studies to evaluate the efficacy of newborn screening for galactosemia to reduce morbidity or mortality in infants or to decrease complications in older children.[23] Obtaining urine for reducing substances may be helpful because it will be positive, but the urinalysis will not show glycosuria. This test is only reliable if the infant has been fed milk for at least

24 to 48 hours. Milk can be removed from the diet while confirmatory testing is pending. Without exposure to milk, galactosemia cannot be the cause of NALF.

Tyrosinemia type 1

Tyrosinemia type 1 (hepatorenal) is an autosomal recessive disorder resulting from a defect in fumarylacetoacetate hydrolase and is the cause of NALF in approximately 2% of patients.[2,18] Incidence is highest in French-Canadians and Scandinavians. Clinical presentation can be acute or chronic. Most patients present early in infancy with ALF. Presenting signs and symptoms may include:

- Jaundice
- Ascites
- Abdominal distention
- Hepatomegaly
- Acute gastrointestinal bleeding
- Hypoglycemia
- Failure to thrive
- Coagulopathy
- Increased alpha fetoprotein level for age
- Renal Fanconi syndrome
- Nephromegaly
- Hypophosphatemic, vitamin D–resistant rickets
- Peripheral neuropathy
- Neurologic crises (autonomic dysfunction, pain, weakness, seizures)
- Boiled-cabbage odor

Those infants who present with chronic liver disease have typical findings including:

- Cirrhosis
- Splenomegaly
- Esophageal varices
- Increased risk and early development of hepatocellular carcinoma (as early as 2 years of age)

Diagnosis of tyrosinemia type 1 is typically made based on increased levels of succinylacetone in the urine. Enzymatic activity can also be tested in lymphocytes, cultured fibroblasts, and cultured amniocytes or chorionic villus material.[24] Molecular testing is available to confirm a diagnosis.

Treatment of tyrosinemia type 1 includes dietary restriction of tyrosine and phenylalanine as well as use of 2(2-nitro-4-trifluoromethylbenzoyl)-1,3-cyclohexanedione (NTBC), which is an inhibitor of p-hydroxyphenylpyruvate dioxygenase.[18,25] Before the availability of NTBC, prognosis was poor, with 75% of children surviving past 2 years of age and few children surviving past age 12 years.[26] Hepatic and renal function have been shown to improve significantly and neurologic crises are decreased with use of NTBC.[27,28] Despite treatment, progressive liver disease and hepatocellular carcinoma (HCC) may still develop. With ALF and HCC, liver transplant may be the only option.

Hereditary fructose intolerance

Hereditary fructose intolerance (HFI) is an autosomal recessive disorder caused by a deficiency in aldolase B (fructose-1,6-bisphosphate aldolase), which leads to a toxic accumulation of fructose-1 phosphate. This accumulation traps phosphate, leading to decreased production of ATP, and blocks both glycolysis and gluconeogenesis, thereby limiting glucose production.[18,29] HFI may present as NALF but is more likely to present in older infants after fruit and juice are introduced to the diet. However, neonates may present from exposure to fructose or sucrose in formula or use of other sucrose-containing products such as sorbitol. Signs and symptoms of HFI include[18,29,30]:

- Postprandial hypoglycemia
- Vomiting
- Diarrhea
- Lactic acidosis
- Jaundice
- Hepatomegaly
- Coagulopathy
- Renal failure
- Seizures
- Coma

Diagnosis of HFI can be made through molecular testing of the *ALDOB* gene. Aldolase B enzymatic activity can also be measured in the liver.

Treatment of HFI is strict avoidance of fructose-containing and sucrose-containing food and products such as sorbitol.

Mitochondrial disorders

Mitochondrial liver disease accounts for 2% to 12% of NALF.[2,31] Mitochondrial diseases that may present as ALF include[32]:

- Disorders of fatty oxidation; for example, carnitine palmitoyltransferase II (CPTII) deficiency
- DNA depletion syndromes; for example, deoxyguanosine kinase (DGUOK) deficiency, *MPV17* mutations
- Other respiratory chain defects; for example, *BCS1L* mutation (GRACILE syndrome)

Laboratory and examination findings that suggest mitochondrial disease include:

- Lactic acidosis, which may worsen with glucose provision
- Hypoketotic hypoglycemia
- Multiorgan involvement
- Hypotonia
- Seizures
- Failure to thrive
- Poor suck

Carnitine palmitoyl transferase II deficiency Because the enzyme carnitine palmitoyl transferase II (CPTII) is required for transportation of long-chain acylcarnitine across the mitochondrial membrane, deficiency leads to accumulation of acylcarnitine inside the mitochondria and blood.[33] There are 3 forms of CPTII deficiency, with the lethal neonatal and severe infantile hepatocardiomuscular forms possible causes of NALF.

Associated symptoms and findings in the lethal neonatal form include cardiomyopathy, arrhythmias, seizures, cystic kidneys, and facial abnormalities.[33] Diagnosis is made by assessment of CPTII enzyme activity in cultured skin fibroblasts or muscle biopsy or with genetic testing. Reduced serum total and free carnitine and increased long-chain acylcarnitine and lipid levels are also findings that suggest CPTII deficiency but are not specific for the disease.[33] The lethal neonatal form is uniformly fatal and can be distinguished from the infantile hepatocardiomuscular form by the associated dysmorphisms and brain and kidney abnormalities.[34]

Disease-specific treatment of metabolic decompensation in the severe infantile form includes provision of glucose at a glucose infusion rate (GIR) of 5 to 10 mg/kg/min and avoidance of catabolism.[34]

Deoxyguanosine kinase deficiency DGUOK deficiency, a form of mitochondrial DNA depletion, results in impaired energy production and organ dysfunction.[35] It presents in the neonatal period as a multisystem (hepatocerebral) disorder or later in infancy with isolated liver disease.[35]

Symptoms of the hepatocerebral form include liver failure, nystagmus, and hypotonia.[35,36] There is variable phenotypic presentation even within siblings who have the same mutation.[36]

Patients can present with increased tyrosine and phenylalanine levels on the newborn screen.[36] Diagnosis of mitochondrial depletion syndrome is made through identification of reduced copy number of mitochondrial DNA in liver or muscle. Confirmation of DGUOK deficiency is through identification of the genetic mutation.[35]

Treatment of children with DGUOK deficiency is focused on supporting the hepatic and neurologic manifestations.[35]

MPV17 mutations

The *MPV17* gene codes for a mitochondrial inner membrane protein responsible for mitochondrial DNA maintenance; thus, mutations in this gene lead to mitochondrial DNA depletion.[32,37] Signs and symptoms include liver failure, hypoglycemia, lactic acidosis, poor growth, and neurologic symptoms. Phenotypic presentation depends on the exact MPV17 mutation and liver failure precede neurologic symptoms in some cases.[37]

BCS1L mutation (GRACILE syndrome)

The *BCS1L* gene is needed for proper formation of complex III of the respiratory transport chain.[32] GRACILE syndrome results from a homozygous point mutation in the BCS1L gene and results in intrauterine growth restriction, renal Fanconi syndrome, lactic acidosis, cholestasis, hepatic siderosis, cirrhosis, and death in the first few months of life.[32] This mutation is associated with coagulopathy, but it is postulated that death is secondary to energy depletion and not liver failure.[32,38]

Other

Hemophagocytic lymphohistiocytosis

Approximately 3% of NALF results from hemophagocytic lymphohistiocytosis (HLH).[2,6] HLH can be primary or secondary and results in altered natural killer cell and cytotoxic T-cell function and decreased immune-mediated apoptosis.[39,40] Familial HLH presents in the first few weeks to years of life and, without treatment, is universally fatal.[40] Secondary HLH results from overstimulation of the immune system, typically from an infection.[40]

Examination and laboratory findings suggestive of HLH include fever, splenomegaly, increased ferritin level (>20,000 ng/mL), increased triglyceride levels, decreased fibrinogen level, and cytopenias.

Diagnosis is made by fulfilling criteria from HLH-2004[40] (**Box 1**), although, if a patient does not meet full criteria but there is high suspicion, a consult to bone marrow transplant is warranted.

Box 1
Diagnostic criteria for hemophagocytic lymphohistiocytosis

1. Molecular diagnosis consistent with HLH

Or

2. 5 of the following:
   - Fever
   - Splenomegaly
   - Cytopenia (affecting ≥2 of 3 lineages in the peripheral blood)
     ○ Hemoglobin level less than 90 g/L in infants less than 4 weeks old
     ○ Platelet level less than 100×10^9/L
     ○ Neutrophil level less than 1×10^9/L
   - Hypertriglyceridemia and/or hypofibrinogenemia (fasting triglyceride levels ≥3 mmol/L, fibrinogen level ≤1.5 g/L)
   - Hemophagocytosis in bone marrow, ascitic fluid, liver, spleen, or lymph nodes; no evidence of malignancy
   - Low or absent natural killer cell activity (according to local laboratory reference)
   - Ferritin level greater than or equal to 500 μg/L
   - Soluble CD25 (cluster of differentiation 25; ie, soluble interleukin-2 receptor) level greater than or equal to 2400 U/mL

From Henter, JI, Horne A, Aricó M, et al. HLH-2004: Diagnostic and therapeutic guidelines for hemophagocytic lymphohistiocytosis. *Pediatr Blood Cancer.* 2007;48(2):124-131; with permission.

Treatment of HLH includes use of dexamethasone and etoposide per established chemotherapy protocols. Children with familial HLH or those who do not respond to chemotherapy are candidates for hematopoietic stem cell transplant.[40] In general, liver transplant is not undertaken in HLH because of the stimulated immune system and frequent multisystemic organ failure. In addition, the liver failure typically improves with treatment of HLH.

Ischemic liver injury

Decreased blood flow to the liver can result in increased transaminase levels and coagulopathy and accounts for 4% of NALF.[2] Risk factors for hypoxic liver injury include perinatal asphyxia, hypovolemic or cardiogenic shock, and right-sided heart failure. Transaminase levels in the setting of an acute ischemic injury can increase to more than 6000 IU/L with a mild increase in bilirubin level. In 1 study, peak transaminase levels were seen 48 hours after the ischemic event and resolution occurred 5 to 9 days from the event.[41] Survival for NALF secondary to ischemic injury was 61.5% in 1 study.[42] Treatment of ischemia-associated NALF centers on supportive care. In severe, nonresponsive cases, investigation for other causes of NALF should be initiated and liver transplant should be considered.

Toxic injury

Toxins and medications need to be considered as possible causes of NALF, including[43]:

- Antiinfectives
  ○ Isoniazid
  ○ Antifungal agents
  ○ Amoxicillin/clavulanic acid
  ○ Ampicillin
  ○ Sulfonamides (trimethoprim/sulfamethoxazole)
- Antiseizure medications
  ○ Phenobarbital

- ○ Phenytoin
- ○ Valproic acid
- ○ Carbamazepine
- Other
  - ○ Acetaminophen (in excessive doses or chronic use)
  - ○ Propylthiouracil

Mechanism of liver injury depends on the agent causing the injury. In addition to supportive care, treatment includes removal of the offending agent and, with acetaminophen-induced injury, administration of *N*-acetylcysteine. Transplant may be considered in cases that do not respond to removal of the causative agent and supportive care.

MANAGEMENT
Supportive Care

Any child with an identified cause of liver failure should receive disease-specific treatment if available. In addition, there are general supportive measures for NALF.[44]

Fluids/electrolytes

- Carefully monitor fluid status; patients are at risk for cerebral edema, so aim for total fluids of 80% to 90% maintenance
- Avoid hyponatremia and extreme hypernatremia.

Glucose homeostasis

- Maintain glucose between 90 and 120 mg/dL; may need a GIR of 10 to 15 mg/kg/min because of impaired gluconeogenesis
- Frequent glucose monitoring

Nutrition

- Avoid catabolism by providing adequate enteral or parenteral nutrition
- Provide 2 to 3 g/kg/d of protein; may need to decrease based on ammonia level

Neurologic

- Monitor clinically for encephalopathy, which can be difficult to detect in infants (**Table 3**)
- Serial assessment of ammonia level
- Start lactulose (via nasogastric tube or enema) for any encephalopathy or increase of ammonia level
- Minimize stimulation

Coagulopathy

- Administer vitamin K
- Only give blood products for procedures or active bleeding
- Consider monitoring for intracranial hemorrhage with head ultrasonography

Gastrointestinal

- Start acid suppression

Infectious disease

- Initiate broad-spectrum antibiotics for any concerns for bacterial infection
- Initiate acyclovir until HSV is ruled out

Table 3
Hepatic encephalopathy grading scale (for patients <3 years of age)

Stage	Clinical	Asterixis/Reflexes	Neurologic Signs
Early (I and II)	Inconsolable crying, sleep reversal, inattention to task	Unreliable/normal or hyper-reflexic	Untestable
Mid (III)	Somnolence, stupor, combativeness	Unreliable/ hyper-reflexic	Most likely untestable
Late (IV)	Comatose, arouses with painful stimuli (IVa), or no response (IVb)	Absent	Decerebrate or decorticate

From Squires RH and Alonso EM. Acute Liver Failure. In: Suchy FJ, Sokol RJ and Balistreri WF, eds. *Liver Disease in Children.* 4th ed. New York: Cambridge University Press; 2014:32-50; with permission.

Liver Transplant

Transplant is a consideration for neonates with ALF who are not showing signs of recovery or who have a low chance for recovery without liver transplant. Approximately 15% to 16% of neonates with ALF require transplant.[2,6] Contraindications to transplant include sepsis or irreversible multisystemic disease, such as some forms of mitochondrial disease. Liver transplant should only be considered in diseases for which there is treatment, such as GALD, if the neonate is not responding to therapy.

Because of their small size, neonates often receive a left lateral segment. ABO-incompatible liver transplants are also a possibility for neonates because of their lack of blood group sensitization. Given the difficulty of obtaining grafts small enough for a neonate, using ABO-incompatible grafts increases the donor pool. Neonates who undergo transplant require more frequent reoperations, have more infections, and have longer hospital stays and duration of mechanical ventilation compared with older children.[45] One-year posttransplant graft survival in neonates who underwent liver transplant is reported at 76% and patient survival is reported at 88%.[45] Liver transplant is an important option for a select group of neonates with irreversible liver failure.

SUMMARY

NALF is a rare, life-threatening disease primarily caused by GALD, viral infections, metabolic diseases, and ischemic injury. Many cases still do not have a known cause. Laboratory evaluation may help suggest a diagnosis. Most of the known causes have disease-specific treatments that improve outcomes with early intervention. However, supportive care during diagnostic evaluation may be critical to maintain survival to specific treatment or liver transplant. Mortality is decreasing with better knowledge about and treatment options for GALD; however, overall mortality for NALF is still 24%. Liver transplant remains an important option for neonates with an indeterminate cause of NALF and those who do not respond to established treatments.

DISCLOSURE

The authors have nothing to disclose.

Best Practices

What is the current practice for neonatal acute liver failure?

Best practice/guideline/care path objectives
- Begin antiinfectives without delay.
- Initiate diagnostic evaluation immediately.
- Provide supportive care while determining cause for specific treatment.
- Determine need for liver transplant.

What changes in current practice are likely to improve outcomes?

- Assess coagulation studies on any neonate who presents with lethargy, organomegaly, ascites, or peripheral edema.

- Begin empiric antibiotics and acyclovir without delay.

- Have a low threshold for treatment with IVIG (1 g/kg) any time GALD is suspected.

Major recommendations

- Obtain cultures and viral PCRs (especially HSV and enterovirus) and treat empirically with antibiotics and acyclovir until HSV is ruled out.

- Obtain transaminase levels; INR; and ferritin, alpha fetoprotein, and lactate levels at minimum to focus differential because most causes of NALF can be differentiated into 4 categories based on these tests, history, and physical examination.

- Collect urine succinylacetone to screen for tyrosinemia.

- Treat with IVIG (1 g/kg) as the diagnosis is being determined any time GALD is suspected.

- Eliminate lactose and galactose from the diet until galactosemia has been excluded.

- Supportive care should be provided to all patients to maintain euglycemia, avoid cerebral edema, provide adequate nutrition, manage encephalopathy, and control bleeding.

- Specific treatment should be provided once a cause is determined.

- Liver transplant should be considered in neonates with unknown cause or those not responding to specific therapy.

Data from Refs.[1,2,11,31,40]

REFERENCES

1. Squires RH Jr, Shneider BL, Bucuvalas J, et al. Acute liver failure in children: the first 348 patients in the pediatric acute liver failure study group. J Pediatr 2006; 148:652–8.

2. Sundaram SS, Alonso EM, Narkewicz MR, et al, for Pediatric Acute Liver Failure Study Group. Characterization and outcomes of young infants with acute liver failure. J Pediatr 2011;159:813–8.

3. Ng VL, Li R, Loomes KM, et al, for the Pediatric Acute Liver Failure Study Group. Outcomes of children with and without hepatic encephalopathy from the Pediatric Acute Liver Failure Study Group. Pediatr Gastroenterol Nutr 2016;63(3):357–64.

4. Washington K. Metabolic and toxic conditions of the liver, and inflammatory and infectious diseases of the liver. In: Iacobuzio-Donahue CA, Montgomery E, Goldblum JR, editors. Gastrointestinal and liver pathology. Philadelphia: Churchill Livingstone Elsevier; 2005. p. 519–52.

5. Pan X, Kelly S, Melin-Aldana H, et al. Novel mechanism of fetal hepatocyte injury in congenital alloimmune hepatitis involves the terminal complement cascade. Hepatology 2010;51(6):2061–8.

6. Durand P, Debray D, Mandel R, et al. Acute liver failure in infancy: a 14-year experience of a pediatric liver transplantation center. J Pediatr 2001;139(6):871–6.

7. Feldman AG, Whitington PF. Neonatal hemochromatosis. J Clin Exp Hepatol 2013;3(4):313–20.

8. Bonilla S, Prozialeck JD, Malladi P, et al. Neonatal iron overload and tissue siderosis due to gestational alloimmune liver disease. J Hepatol 2012;56(6):1351–5.

9. Heissat S, Collardeau-Frachon S, Baruteau J, et al. Neonatal hemochromatosis: diagnostic work-up based on a series of 56 cases of fetal death and neonatal liver failure. J Pediatr 2015;166(1):66–73.

10. Rand EB, Karpen SJ, Kelly S, et al. Treatment of neonatal hemochromatosis with exchange transfusion and intravenous immunoglobulin. J Pediatr 2009;155(4):566–71.

11. Taylor SA, Whitington PF. Neonatal acute liver failure. Liver Transpl 2016;22(5):677–85.

12. Whitington PF, Kelly S. Outcome of pregnancies at risk for neonatal hemochromatosis is improved by treatment with high-dose intravenous immunoglobulin. Pediatrics 2008;121(6):e1615–21.

13. Verma A, Dhawan A, Zuckerman M, et al. Neonatal herpes simplex virus infection presenting as acute liver failure: prevalent role of herpes simplex virus type 1. J Pediatr Gastroenterol Nutr 2006;42:282–6.

14. Lv XQ, Qian LH, Wu T, et al. Enterovirus infection in febrile neonates: a hospital-based prospective cohort study. J Paediatr Child Health 2016;52(8):837–41.

15. Coggins SA, Wynn JL, Weitkamp JH. Infectious causes of necrotizing enterocolitis. Clin Perinatol 2015;42(1):133–54.

16. Isselbacher KJ, Anderson EP, Kurahashi K, et al. Congenital galactosemia a single enzymatic block in galactose metabolism. Science 1956;123:625.

17. Karadag N, Zenciroglu A, Eminoglu FT, et al. Literature review and outcome of classic galactosemia diagnosed in the neonatal period. Clin Lab 2013;59(9–10):1139–46.

18. Demirbas D, Brucker WJ, Berry GT. Inborn errors of metabolism with hepatopathy: metabolism defects of galactose, fructose, and tyrosine. Pediatr Clin North Am 2018;65(2):337–52.

19. Yuzyuk T, Viau K, Andrews A, et al. Biochemical changes and clinical outcomes in 34 patients with classic galactosemia. J Inherit Metab Dis 2018;41(2):197–208.

20. Rubio-Gozalbo ME, Haskovic M, Bosch AM, et al. The natural history of classic galactosemia: lessons from the GalNet registry. Orphanet J Rare Dis 2019;14:86.

21. Welling L, Bernstein LE, Berry GT, et al. International clinical guideline for the management of classical galactosemia: diagnosis, treatment, and follow-up. J Inherit Metab Dis 2017;40(2):171–6.

22. Krooth R, Winberg AN. Studies on cell lines developed from the tissues of patients with galactosemia. J Exp Med 1961;113:1155.

23. Lak R, Yazdizadeh B, Davari M, et al. Newborn screening for galactosaemia. Cochrane Database Syst Rev 2017;(12):CD012272.

24. Kvittingen EA, Brodtkorb E. The pre- and post-natal diagnosis of tyrosinemia type 1 and the detection of the carrier state by assay of fumarylacetoacetase. Scand J Clin Lab Invest Suppl 1986;184:35.

25. Scott CR. The genetic tyrosinemias. Am J Med Genet C Semin Med Genet 2006;142C:121–6.

26. van Spronsen FJ, Thomasse Y, Smit GP, et al. Hereditary tyrosinemia Type I: a new clinical classification with difference in prognosis on dietary treatment. Hepatology 1994;20:1187–91.

27. Bartlett DC, Lloyd C, McKiernan PJ, et al. Early nitisinone treatment reduces the need for liver transplantation in children with tyrosinaemia type 1 and improves post-transplant renal function. J Inherit Metab Dis 2014;37:745–52.

28. Mayorandan S, Meyer U, Gokcay G, et al. Cross-sectional study of 168 patients with hepatorenal tyrosinaemia and implications for clinical practice. Orphanet J Rare Dis 2014;9:107.

29. Tran C. Inborn errors of fructose metabolism. what can we learn from them? Nutrients 2017;9(4):356.

30. Li H1, Byers HM, Diaz-Kuan A, et al. Acute liver failure in neonates with undiagnosed hereditary fructose intolerance due to exposure from widely available infant formulas. Mol Genet Metab 2018;123(4):428–32.

31. Bitar R, Thwaites R, Davison S, et al. Liver failure in early infancy. J Pediatr Gastroenterol Nutr 2017;64(1):70–5.

32. Fellman V, Kotarsky H. Mitochondrial hepatopathies in the newborn period. Semin Fetal Neonatal Med 2011;16(4):222–8.

33. Wieser T. Carnitine palmitoyltransferase II deficiency. In: Adam MP, Ardinger HH, Pagon RA, et al, editors. GeneReviews®. Seattle (WA): University of Washington, Seattle; 2019. Available at: http://www.ncbi.nlm.nih.gov/books/NBK1253/.

34. Strauss A, Andersen B, Bennett M. Mitochondrial fatty oxidation defects. In: Sarafoglou K, editor. Pediatric endocrinology and inborn errors of metabolism. 1st edition. New York: McGraw-Hill Companies; 2009. p. 51–70.

35. El-Hattab AW, Scaglia F, Wong L-J. Deoxyguanosine kinase deficiency. In: Adam MP, Ardinger HH, Pagon RA, et al, editors. GeneReviews®. Seattle (WA): University of Washington, Seattle; 2016. Available at: http://www.ncbi. nlm.nih.gov/books/NBK7040/.

36. Dimmock DP, Zhang Q, Dionisi-Vici C, et al. Clinical and molecular features of mitochondrial DNA depletion due to mutations in deoxyguanosine kinase. Hum Mutat 2008;29(2):330–1.

37. Wong L-JC, Brunetti-Pierri N, Zhang Q, et al. Mutations in the MPV17 gene are responsible for rapidly progressive liver failure in infancy. Hepatology 2007; 46(4):1218–27.

38. Visapää I, Fellman V, Vesa J, et al. GRACILE syndrome, a lethal metabolic disorder with iron overload, is caused by a point mutation in BCS1L. Am J Hum Genet 2002;71(4):863–76.

39. Risma K, Jordan MB. Hemophagocytic lymphohistiocytosis: updates and evolving concepts. Curr Opin Pediatr 2012;24(1):9–15.

40. Henter J-I, Horne A, Aricó M, et al. HLH-2004: diagnostic and therapeutic guidelines for hemophagocytic lymphohistiocytosis. Pediatr Blood Cancer 2007;48(2): 124–31.

41. Garland JS, Werlin SL, Rice TB. Ischemic hepatitis in children: diagnosis and clinical course. Crit Care Med 1988;16(12):1209–12.

42. Zozaya Nieto C, Fernández Caamaño B, Muñoz Bartolo G, et al. Presenting features and prognosis of ischemic and nonischemic neonatal liver failure. J Pediatr Gastroenterol Nutr 2017;64(5):754–9.

43. Shi Q, Yang X, Greenhaw JJ, et al. Drug-induced liver injury in children: clinical observations, animal models, and regulatory status. Int J Toxicol 2017;36(5):365–79.

44. Squires J, McKiernan P, Squires RH. Acute liver failure. Clin Liver Dis 2018;22(4): 773–805.

45. Sundaram SS, Alonso EM, Anand R. Outcomes after liver transplantation in young infants. J Pediatr Gastroenterol Nutr 2008;47(5):486–92.

Autoinflammatory Disorders with Perinatal Onset

Nissim G. Stolberg, DO, James W. Verbsky, MD, PhD*

KEYWORDS

- Autoinflammatory disorders • Perinatal period • Genetic defects • Infant

KEY POINTS

- Autoinflammatory disorders are genetic defects leading to spontaneous inflammation.
- Autoinflammatory disorders can present in the perinatal period.
- Autoinflammatory disorders are rare, but should be considered in an infant with fevers, rash, or inflammation without obvious cause.
- Using modern sequencing, one can rapidly screen for these disorders, leading to effective, targeted therapies.

INTRODUCTION

Autoinflammatory disorders are genetic defects that result in spontaneous episodic or persistent inflammation. These disorders are thought to occur because of the inappropriate activation of the innate immune system. This component of the immune system acts as a first line of defense against pathogens and is particularly important in the perinatal period, because infants will not have developed an adaptive immune system (ie, antigen experienced T and B cells) and rely on maternal antibodies as their adaptive immune system. Autoinflammatory disorders lack features of autoimmune disorders (ie, autoreactive T cells and/or autoantibodies), which are exceedingly rare in the newborn or perinatal period because it takes time for the adaptive immune response to develop. There are exceptions to this because there are now genetic defects that cause early-onset autoimmunity, such as the disorder IPEX (immune dyregulation, polyendocrinopathy, enteropathy, X-linked) cased by variants in *FOXP3*.

The age of onset of autoinflammatory disorders varies considerably, with appearance as early as the perinatal or infantile period. Most autoinflammatory disorders present with rash and fevers, which are not uncommon symptoms during this period, and often lead to an infectious workup. Rashes alone may not spur further investigation, because many neonatal rashes are benign and present early in life, and although similarities exist between innocuous neonatal rashes and autoinflammatory disorders,

Division of Rheumatology, Department of Pediatrics, Medical College of Wisconsin, 8701 Watertown Plank Road, Milwaukee, WI 53226, USA
* Corresponding author.
E-mail address: jverbsky@mcw.edu

Clin Perinatol 47 (2020) 41–52
https://doi.org/10.1016/j.clp.2019.10.007
0095-5108/20/© 2019 Elsevier Inc. All rights reserved.

most physicians will not recognize their unique aspects. Autoinflammatory diseases, rare as they may be, can be severe, and one should be aware of their presentations, how they are diagnosed, and the steps required for further evaluation.

Innate immunity is essential to the initial detection of invading pathogens as well as damaged tissues and has a wide variety of receptors available to recognize these products and initiate inflammation. These receptors include pathogen recognition receptors, which recognize pathogen-associated molecular patterns (PAMPs) and include Toll-like receptors, nucleotide-binding oligomerization domain-like receptors (NODs), and RIG-1 like receptors. In addition, tissue damage leads to the production of damage-associated molecular patterns (DAMPs), which are altered metabolic products of damaged and stressed cells, such as uric acid or extracellular adenosine triphosphate, and immune pathways may detect these patterns.[1,2] Genetic defects in any of these receptors may lead to spontaneous activation of downstream signaling pathways and production of proinflammatory cytokines leading to autoinflammatory disease. Because different receptors produce different inflammatory cytokines, it is clinically useful to classify these diseases based on their mechanism of inflammation.

INFLAMMASOMOPATHIES: INTERLEUKIN-1β-MEDIATED DISEASES

Some of the first autoinflammatory disorders in which the molecular mechanisms were elucidated involved the inflammasome, an intracellular macromolecule of 5 different proteins.[2,3] When stimulated by specific ligands, such as PAMPS (eg, intracellular DNA, microbial peptides) and DAMPS (eg, uric acid crystals), the complex assembles, leading to activation of the protease caspase-1, resulting in conversion of pro-interleukin-1β (IL-1β) and pro-IL-18 into their active forms, IL-1β and IL-18, and inflammation.[2,4] Spontaneous production of IL-1β leads to fevers, rashes, and markers of acute inflammation (**Table 1**).

Cryopyrin-Associated Periodic Syndrome

Genetic defects in cryopyrin, a component of the inflammasome encoded by *NLRP3*, cause the cryopyrin-associated periodic syndromes (CAPS), a clinical spectrum of 3 autosomal dominant disorders; familial cold autoinflammatory syndrome (FCAS), Muckle-Wells syndrome (MWS), and neonatal onset multisystem inflammatory disorder (NOMID). Symptoms begin in the neonatal period and vary in severity with FCAS being the mildest and NOMID being the most severe. All are due to gain-of-function mutations of the *NLRP3* gene on the short arm of chromosome 1.[5–7] These variants cluster in an autoinhibitory domain of cryopyrin, leading to spontaneous inflammasome assembly, activation of caspase-1, and increased conversion of biologically active IL-1β.[8] Cold appears to help stabilize the complex in its activated form, and thus, symptoms can be cold induced. The clinical presentation varies, but rash is universal, presents soon after birth, and is described as hivelike, because it tends to appear and resolve spontaneously. However, angioedema is not present, and pathology has shown the rash to be a neutrophilic infiltrate. Clinical indicators of chronic inflammation, including neutrophilia, thrombocytosis, anemia, and elevated inflammatory markers, are present to varying degrees depending on the severity of the amino acid substitution. Other features include fevers, arthralgia/arthritis, and conjunctivitis. In more severe cases, spontaneous aseptic meningitis can occur, leading to hearing and vision loss, meningeal signs, seizures, and intellectual disability over time. Amyloidosis may also occur. In patients with FCAS, cold exposure leads to episodes of fevers, conjunctivitis, joint pain, and rash. MWS is more severe, and patients will have daily symptoms, and if not treated, may progress to hearing loss and

Table 1
Clinical characteristics of IL-1β-mediated diseases

IL-1-Related Diseases	Presentation	Inheritance Pattern	Gene/Protein	Treatment
FMF	Episodic fevers, serositis, arthritis, abdominal pain, rash	Autosomal recessive	MEFV/Pyrin	Colchicine, IL-1 blocking agents
CAPS-FCAS	Recurrent episodes of fever and rash after cold exposure, arthralgias, conjunctivitis	Autosomal dominant	CIAS1/Cryopyrin	NSAIDs, IL-1 blocking agents, limiting cold exposure
CAPS-MWS	Fevers, daily rash, conjunctivitis arthralgia, aseptic meningitis, hearing loss, cartilage overgrowth	Autosomal dominant	CIAS1/Cryopyrin	IL-1 blocking agents
CAPS-NOMID	Fevers, daily rash, conjunctivitis arthralgia, aspectic meningitis, hearing loss, cartilage overgrowth manifestations, frontal bossing	Autosomal dominant	CIAS1/Cryopyrin	IL-1 blocking agents
DIRA	Erythroderma with pustulosis, multifocal osteomyelitis, osteopenia/periostitis, respiratory distress, venous thrombi, and joint pain with periarticular swelling	Autosomal recessive	IL1RN/IL-1 receptor antagonist	IL-1 blocking agents
Hyper IgD	Episodic fever sometimes triggered by illness/vaccination, lymphadenopathy, rash, vomiting, arthritis/arthralgia, elevated IgD/IgA	Autosomal recessive	MVK/MVK	IL-1 blocking agents, etanercept, hematopoietic stem cell transplants
Majeed syndrome	Episodic fever, nonbacterial multifocal osteomyelitis, neutrophilic dermatosis, dyserythropoietic anemia	Autosomal recessive	LPIN2/Lipin 2	IL-1 blocking agents, others (steroids, methotrexate, NSAIDs, TNF inhibitors)
AFEC	Fevers, vomiting, secretory diarrhea, duodenitis, splenomegaly, and rash	Autosomal dominant	NLRC4/NLRC4	IL-1 and IL-18 blocking agents

amyloidosis. NOMID is the most severe and will have significant rash, fevers, and elevated inflammatory markers. Patients with NOMID have the most significant central nervous system inflammation, including seizures, aseptic meningitis, hearing loss, vision changes, increased intracranial pressure, and intellectual disability.[8,9] Diagnosis is based on a history of a newborn urticarial-like rash, elevated inflammatory markers in the absence of infection, and genetic testing demonstrating variants in *NLRP3*. Somatic mosaicism resulting in CAPS has been reported.[10,11] Treatment with IL-1 blockers (eg, IL-1 receptor antagonist or IL-1 blocking monoclonal antibodies) leads to rapid resolution of symptoms and can be diagnostic.[12,13]

Deficiency in Interleukin-1 Receptor Antagonist

In addition to disorders of excessive production of IL-1β, there are disorders in inhibitory molecules that help regulate inflammation due to IL-1β. Deficiency of IL-1 receptor antagonist (DIRA) is an autoinflammatory disorder presenting in the neonatal period with erythroderma with pustulosis, multifocal osteomyelitis, periostitis, and osteopenia. The disease may further progress to include respiratory distress with interstitial lung disease, venous thrombi, and joint pain with periarticular swelling and may progress to death without treatment.[14,15] DIRA is caused by autosomal recessive loss-of-function mutations in the *IL1RN* gene, leading to lack of production of serum IL-1 receptor antagonist, a competitive inhibitor that binds and blocks the IL-1 receptor.[15,16] Constitutive IL-1 signaling leads to systemic inflammation. The profound osteopenia and osteomyelitis highlight the importance of IL-1 in osteoclast activation.[17,18] Diagnosis is with clinical history, laboratory evidence of inflammation, characteristic skin findings, and imaging demonstrating osteopenia, osteolytic lesions, and widened ribs.[14,18] Genetic testing of the IL1RN gene will confirm the diagnosis. Treatment with IL-1 receptor antagonist leads to immediate resolution of symptoms and laboratory test abnormalities.[15]

Familial Mediterranean Fever, Hyper Immunoglobulinemia D Syndrome, and Autoinflammation with Infantile Enterocolitis

A variety of other proteins interact with and modulate the inflammasome, and genetic variants in these genes can also lead to autoinflammatory disorders. Familial Mediterranean fever (FMF) is caused by variants in the *MEFV* gene that encode the protein pyrin, a pathogen recognition receptor expressed in monocytes, neutrophils, and dendritic cells.[19] Pyrin is kept in an inhibited state when bound to the 14-3-3e protein, but when a cell is invaded, alterations in the intracellular cytoskeleton occur, resulting in decreased function of the RhoA GTPase-dependent protein kinases, dephosphorylation of pyrin, and dissociation from the 14-3-3e protein. The pyrin inflammasome assembles with resultant caspase-1 activation and conversion of IL-1β and IL-18 into active forms. This mechanism of inflammasome activation highlights another recognition system, whereby metabolic changes in cells owing to pathogen invasion are sensed by cells leading to inflammation. Patients classically present with episodic fevers (1–3 days), serositis (pericarditis or peritonitis), arthritis, and an erysipelas-like rash.[2,4,20,21] It can present in early childhood, but may not exhibit all of the classic features. It has been reported to begin as early as the first week of life with recurrent fevers, episodic vomiting, and elevated inflammatory markers.[22] Untreated patients can develop amyloidosis after many years of untreated symptoms, although this is highly dependent on which genetic variant is present. Diagnosis is made by genetic testing. Treatment is classically with colchicine, which augments the function of RhoA GTPase. Recently, there has been increased use of IL-1 blocking agents with success.[19,21]

Hyper immunoglobulinemia D (IgD) syndrome, caused by hypomorphic variants in mevalonate kinase (*MVK*),[7] is an autoinflammatory syndrome whose pathophysiology is similar to FMF. MVK is involved in sterol and isoprenoid biosynthesis, and low levels of MVK result in low levels of geranylgeranylated proteins, including RhoA leading to disinhibition of the pyrin molecule and inflammasome activation.[23,24] Patients were initially noted to have elevated IgD levels,[23] and thus, its initial naming, although these can be normal. Patients present with recurrent febrile attacks every 4 to 8 weeks[25] and typically present before 1 year of age. These attacks are triggered by stress, infection, and vaccination.[26] Presentation is with fevers lasting from 2 to 7 days, maculopapular rashes, arthralgia/myalgias, a range of gastrointestinal (GI) complaints, splenomegaly, cervical lymphadenopathy, and aphthous ulcers. This disorder is autosomal recessive with hypomorphic, loss-of-function variants, which produce a partial deficiency in MVK.[26,27] Laboratory testing demonstrates elevated or normal IgD and elevated urinary mevalonic acid and is confirmed by genetic testing.[28,29] Complete deficiency in MVK results in mevalonic aciduria, an inborn error of metabolism that can exhibit fevers.[30] Previously treatment was with nonsteroidal anti-inflammatory drugs (NSAIDs), steroids, and colchicine. More recently, IL-1 blocking agents and etanercept have been shown to be effective, with hematopoietic stem cell transplants used for severe disease or possibly to treat the neurologic symptoms in mevalonic aciduria.[5,6]

Autoinflammation with infantile enterocolitis (AFEC) is a recently recognized inflammasome-mediated disease. It is reported to present in the neonatal and infantile period with vomiting, secretory diarrhea, fever, splenomegaly, elevated inflammatory markers, anemia, rash, and duodenitis.[31,32] This disease can progress to macrophage activation syndrome, a life-threatening complication of excessive inflammation characterized by pancytopenia, hepatitis, hyperferritinemia/hypertriglyceridemia, and disseminated intravascular coagulation and bleeding. AFEC is due to gain-of-function missense mutations in *NLRC4*, an NOD-like receptor with an autoinhibitory domain, and variants in this protein occur in this highly conserved nucleotide-binding domain (ie, Thr337Ser and Val341Ala). These variants lead to poor autoinhibition of NLRC4, spontaneous oligomerization of NLRC4 with the apoptosis-associated specklike protein, and procaspase 1, constitutive caspase 1 activation, and conversion of pro-IL-1β and pro-IL-18 to active IL-1β and IL-18.[31,32] The enterocolitis is thought to be due to the higher expression of NLRC4 in intestinal macrophages, which is thought to detect pathogenic bacteria in the gut.[33] Diagnosis is confirmed with genetic testing of pathogenic variants in *NLRC4*. Treatment is with IL-1 and IL-18 antagonists.[34]

INTERFERONOPATHIES

Type 1 interferons (eg, IFN-α and IFN-β) are innate immune system molecules that are produced in response to viral infections and are important in fighting these infections.[35] Interferonopathies are genetic defects that result in the spontaneous production of type 1 interferons and autoinflammation. Many of these disorders affect pathways that process or detect intracellular nucleic acids, a sign of viral infections, resulting in the production of type 1 interferon. Both monogenic and polygenic defects have been elucidated, leading to disease as early as the neonatal period.[36] Some of these disorders can be confused with autoimmune diseases, such as systemic lupus erythematosus, which interestingly exhibits a dysregulated interferon signature.[35,36] Interferons activate interferon receptors that require Janus kinase (JAK) proteins to signal, and relatively new JAK inhibitors have shown promise in the treatment of these disorders (**Table 2**).

Table 2
Clinical characteristics of interferon-related diseases

Interferon-Related Diseases	Presentation	Inheritance	Gene/Protein	Treatment
AGS	Leukoencephalopathy with calcifications, cerebral atrophy, hepatosplenomegaly, anemia	Autosomal recessive or dominant negative	TREX1/3' repair exonuclease	JAK inhibitors
SAVI	Fever, vasculitic rash with infarction on fingers, face, ears, nose, pulmonary disease	Autosomal dominant	TMEM173/STING	JAK inhibitors
CANDLE	Fevers, purpuric skin rash, neutrophilic dermatosis, lipodystrophy, developmental delay, basal ganglion calcification	Autosomal recessive loss of function	PSMB8/ proteasome subunit β8	JAK inhibitors

Aicardi Goutieres Syndrome

Aicardi Goutieres syndrome (AGS) is the earliest interferonopathy to be described. In the perinatal period, it presents as a leukoencephalopathy with calcifications, neurologic deficits (eg, jitteriness and seizures), poor feeding, hepatosplenomegaly, elevated aminotransferases, thrombocytopenia, and anemia that may require transfusions.[37] These symptoms may be misinterpreted as congenital infection (toxoplasma gondii, other viruses, rubella, cytomegalovirus, and herpes simplex). Although several genetic forms of AGS have been described, it is classically due to a recessive or dominant-negative loss of function variants in the *TREX1* gene. *TREX1* encodes a cytosolic DNA exonuclease, and defective function of this exonuclease results in the accumulation of nucleic acids and activation of the type I IFN pathway.[36] Cerebrospinal fluid studies will be significant for a lymphocytosis, elevated IFN-α, and elevated neopterin levels.[38] Imaging may demonstrate basal ganglia calcifications and progressive cerebral atrophy, and genetic testing shows *TREX1* genetic variants. Treatment has been largely symptomatic, but JAK inhibitors have recently shown promise.[39]

Stimulator of Interferon Genes-Associated Vasculopathy

STimulator of INterferon Genes (STING)-associated vasculopathy of infancy (SAVI) is an autoinflammatory disease presenting in the neonatal period.[40,41] Clinical features are variable and include intermittent low-grade fevers, a telangiectatic, pustular, or blistering rash on the cheeks, nose, or digits, myositis, arthritis, and evidence of interstitial lung disease.[40,41] Ulceration of the distal extremities with tissue infarcts, oral ulcers, Raynaud phenomenon, telangiectasias, livedo reticularis, and nailfold capillary changes have all been described.[40,41] It is autosomal dominantly inherited because of heterozygous gain-of-function mutations in the Transmembrane protein 173 (TMEM173).[7] TMEM173 codes for the key adapter signaling molecule STING, which binds cyclic guanosine monophosphate–adenosine monophosphate in response to altered intracytoplasmic double-stranded DNA levels and leads to the production of IFN-β.[7,42] Constitutive activation of STING leads to elevated interferon levels and systemic inflammation. Lesional biopsies demonstrate leukocytoclastic vasculitis, and they may exhibit low-titer antineutrophil cytoplasmic antibody and antiphospholipid antibodies.[42,43] Currently, there is no treatment, although JAK inhibitors are available based on in vitro studies and case reports.[41,44,45]

Chronic Atypical Neutrophilic Dermatosis with Lipodystrophy and Elevated Temperature

Appropriate cell function requires removal of misfolded or damaged proteins by the proteasome. The proteasome functions to degrade, remove, and assist in antigen presentation of ubiquitinated or damaged intracellular proteins as well as phagocytosed extracellular products.[46] Defects in disposal by the proteasome leads to build up of dysfunctional or misfolded proteins, which are sensed by the cell with resultant interferon production. Proteasome defects occurs in the syndrome known as chronic atypical neutrophilic dermatosis with lipodystrophy and elevated temperature (CANDLE). Mild infections, cold, or stress affect metabolic demands, which can precipitate episodes of inflammation in this disorder. Patients present in the first month of life with recurrent fevers and rash. The skin lesions can appear as pernio on the fingers, toes, face, and ears, and erythematous or violaceous periorbital and perioral edema. Erythematous nodules or plaques can occur and will progress to purpuric lesions. Biopsies show recruitment of monocytes, neutrophils, and plasmacytoid dendritic cells.[47] Leukocytoclastic vasculitis occurs with fibrinoid necrosis, and panniculitis also occurs. Laboratory tests are significant for elevated inflammatory markers, chronic anemia, thrombocytosis, and hypergammaglobulinemia. Over time, lipodystrophy, aseptic meningitis, and synovitis develop, and if untreated, a variety of end-organ damage may occur.[41] It classically results from autosomal recessive loss-of-function mutations in the *PSMB8* gene, which codes for the proteasome subunit β5i.[36] Since its initial description, genetic variants in the other subunits of the proteasome have been discovered in patients with similar characteristics. Imaging may show basal ganglia calcifications on computed tomography and MRI. Diagnosis is with clinical history and genetic testing.[47] Treatment in the past has included a variety of immunosuppressive drugs and biologic therapies with limited clinical effectiveness. Type 1 interferons are elevated in this disorder, and these bind interferon receptors and activate the JAK/STAT pathway.[46] In limited case reports, JAK inhibitors have shown promise.[48]

NUCLEAR FACTOR-κB-RELATED DISORDERS

A variety of cytokine receptors and immune signal transduction pathways lead to the activation of a nuclear factor-κB (NF-κB), which transcribes a variety of inflammatory cytokines. NF-κB family members are sequestered in the cytoplasm bound to inhibitory proteins (eg, IκBα, NEMO), and when activated, these proteins are degraded via the ubiquitin pathway allowing for the nuclear translocation of NF-κB and gene transcription.[49,50] Deubiquitinating enzymes inhibit this process, and genetic variants in 2 of these proteins, otulin and A20, lead to autoinflammatory disorders that can present early in life. Otulipenia, because of homozygous loss-of-function mutations in the *FAM105B* gene that encode otulin, inhibits deubiquitination of this pathway, and thus, there is constitutive activation of NF-κB.[49,51] Otulipenia, although very rare, has been reported to present in the neonatal period with episodes of recurrent fevers, joint swelling, painful nodular red rash, GI inflammation with diarrhea, and failure to

Table 3
Clinical characteristics of nuclear factor-κB-related diseases

NF-κB-Mediated Diseases	Presentation	Inheritance Pattern	Gene/Protein	Treatment
A20	Oral and genital ulcerations, uveitis, fevers. Mimics familial Behcet disease	Autosomal dominant	CARD14/CARD14	Steroids, colchicine, anti-TNF, or anti-IL-1 agents
Blau syndrome	Intermittent fevers, erythematous granulomatous rash, uveitis, and arthritis develop over time	Autosomal dominant	NOD2/nucleotide-binding oligomerization domain-containing protein 2	Oral steroids ± methotrexate, cyclosporin, mycophenolate mofetil, anti-IL-1, and anti-TNF therapy
Otulipenia	Recurrent fevers, joint swelling, painful nodular red rash, GI inflammation/diarrhea, and failure to thrive	Autosomal recessive	FAM105B/Otulin	Some success with anti-TNF therapy
Tumor necrosis factor receptor-associated periodic syndrome	Fevers lasting more than 7 d, migratory rash, periorbital edema, conjunctivitis, arthralgia, GI tract inflammation, myositis with cardiac involvement	Autosomal dominant	TNFRSF1A/TNFRSF1A	Steroids during acute attacks, anti-TNF agents, IL-1 agents

thrive.[49,51] Biopsies of the rash will show a neutrophilic dermatosis and small/medium vessel vasculitis. Laboratory tests demonstrate normal immune cell numbers, immunoglobulin levels, and vaccine titers. Treatment of the few cases reported has shown success with anti-TNF-α therapy, with less success with other agents.[52,53] A20 haploinsufficiency is an autosomal dominantly inherited autoinflammatory disorder caused by genetic variants in the *TNFAIP3* gene. Patients present with systemic inflammation, oral and genital ulcers, uveitis, and fevers similar to familial Behcet disease. There are several other disorders of NF-κB activation that present later in life (**Table 3**).

SUMMARY

Autoinflammatory disorders can occur in the newborn or infantile period and present with fevers, rash, and systemic inflammation in the absence of infections. These disorders are rare but should be considered in infants with unusual inflammatory features in the absence of another explanation. Studies have begun to delineate the mechanisms of action of these disorders, and activation of IL-1β, interferons, and cytokine signaling pathways is central to these disorders. Given the number of autoinflammatory disorders and their overlapping symptoms, it can be difficult to differentiate these disorders based on clinical features alone. Fortunately, next-generation sequencing technologies allow for the rapid genetic detection of these disorders with ever-decreasing costs. Gene panels are available to rapidly screen for all of these disorders. This rapid diagnosis can lead to personalized treatment plans and the best outcomes for infants affected by these disorders.

Best Practices

What is the current best practice?

Perinatal autoinflammatory diseases
  Best practice/guideline/care path objectives
  - Autoinflammatory disorders should be considered in an infant with unexplained fevers, rash, and evidence of systemic inflammation with a negative infectious workup
  - Early referral to subspecialist for evaluation and treatment is important
  - Early initiation of anti-inflammatory interventions to suppress systemic inflammation can prevent morbidity and mortality

What changes in current practice are likely to improve outcomes?

  - Advancing education for perinatal care clinicians on autoinflammatory disorders
  - Consideration of autoinflammatory disorders in infants with persistent inflammation in the setting of a negative sepsis and infectious workup
  - Incorporating next-generation sequencing panels into the perinatal evaluation of inflammation

Major recommendations

  - Consider genetic testing for autoinflammatory disorders in an infant with recurrent or persistent inflammation in the absence of infection
  - Referral to a specialist to interpret positive genetic testing and implement therapies
  - The type of autoinflammatory disorder can lead to personalized specific therapies
  - Long-term complications can occur and need to be monitored for the life of the patient

REFERENCES

1. Turvey SE, Broide DH. Innate immunity. J Allergy Clin Immunol 2010;125(2): S24–32.
2. Heilig R, Broz P. Function and mechanism of the pyrin inflammasome. Eur J Immunol 2018;48(2):230–8.
3. Martinon F, Burns K, Tschopp J. The inflammasome: a molecular platform triggering activation of inflammatory caspases and processing of proIL-beta. Mol Cell 2002;10(2):417–26.
4. Sharma D, Kanneganti T-D. The cell biology of inflammasomes: mechanisms of inflammasome activation and regulation. J Cell Biol 2016;213(6):617–29.
5. ter Haar N, Lachmann H, Özen S, et al. Treatment of autoinflammatory diseases: results from the Eurofever Registry and a literature review. Ann Rheum Dis 2013; 72(5):678–85.
6. Arkwright PD, Abinun M, Cant AJ. Mevalonic aciduria cured by bone marrow transplantation. N Engl J Med 2007;357(13):1350.
7. Martorana D, Bonatti F, Mozzoni P, et al. Monogenic autoinflammatory diseases with Mendelian inheritance: genes, mutations, and genotype/phenotype correlations. Front Immunol 2017;8:344.
8. Hoffman HM, Mueller JL, Broide DH, et al. Mutation of a new gene encoding a putative pyrin-like protein causes familial cold autoinflammatory syndrome and Muckle–Wells syndrome. Nat Genet 2001;29(3):301–5.
9. Aksentijevich I, Putnam CD, Remmers EF, et al. The clinical continuum of cryopyrinopathies: novel CIAS1 mutations in North American patients and a new cryopyrin model. Arthritis Rheum 2007;56(4):1273–85.
10. Walker UA, Hoffman HM, Williams R, et al. Brief report: severe inflammation following vaccination against streptococcus pneumoniae in patients with cryopyrin-associated periodic syndromes. Arthritis Rheumatol 2016;68(2): 516–20.
11. Federici S, Gattorno M. A practical approach to the diagnosis of autoinflammatory diseases in childhood. Best Pract Res Clin Rheumatol 2014;28(2):263–76.
12. Hoffman HM, Rosengren S, Boyle DL, et al. Prevention of cold-associated acute inflammation in familial cold autoinflammatory syndrome by interleukin-1 receptor antagonist. Lancet 2004;364(9447):1779–85.
13. Matsubara T, Hasegawa M, Shiraishi M, et al. A severe case of chronic infantile neurologic, cutaneous, articular syndrome treated with biologic agents. Arthritis Rheum 2006;54(7):2314–20.
14. Almeida de Jesus AA, Goldbach-Mansky R. Monogenic autoinflammatory diseases: concept and clinical manifestations. Clin Immunol 2013;147(3):155–74.
15. Reddy S, Jia S, Geoffrey R, et al. An autoinflammatory disease due to homozygous deletion of the IL1RN locus. N Engl J Med 2009;360(23):2438–44.
16. Dripps DJ, Brandhuber BJ, Thompson RC, et al. Interleukin-1 (IL-1) receptor antagonist binds to the 80-kDa IL-1 receptor but does not initiate IL-1 signal transduction. J Biol Chem 1991;266(16):10331–6.
17. Lorenzo JA, Sousa SL, Alander C, et al. Comparison of the bone-resorbing activity in the supernatants from phytohemagglutinin-stimulated human peripheral blood mononuclear cells with that of cytokines through the use of an antiserum to interleukin 1. Endocrinology 1987;121(3):1164–70.
18. Jimi E, Nakamura I, Duong LT, et al. Interleukin 1 induces multinucleation and bone-resorbing activity of osteoclasts in the absence of osteoblasts/stromal cells. Exp Cell Res 1999;247(1):84–93.

19. Cekin N, Akyurek ME, Pinarbasi E, et al. MEFV mutations and their relation to major clinical symptoms of familial mediterranean fever. Gene 2017;626:9–13.
20. Siegal S. Benign paroxysmal peritonitis. Ann Intern Med 1945;23(1):1.
21. Alghamdi M. Familial Mediterranean fever, review of the literature. Clin Rheumatol 2017;36(8):1707–13.
22. Keskindemirci G, Ayaz NA, Aldemir E, et al. Familial Mediterranean fever: diagnosing as early as 3 months of age. Case Rep Pediatr 2014;2014:1–3.
23. Verbsky JW. When to suspect autoinflammatory/recurrent fever syndromes. Pediatr Clin North Am 2017;64(1):111–25.
24. Manthiram K, Zhou Q, Aksentijevich I, et al. The monogenic autoinflammatory diseases define new pathways in human innate immunity and inflammation. Nat Immunol 2017;18(8):832–42.
25. Drenth JPH, Haagsma CJ, Van Der Meer JWM. Hyperimmunoglobulinemia D and periodic fever syndrome. Medicine 1994;73(3):133–44.
26. Sag E, Bilginer Y, Ozen S. Autoinflammatory diseases with periodic fevers. Curr Rheumatol Rep 2017;19(7):41.
27. D'Osualdo A, Picco P, Caroli F, et al. MVK mutations and associated clinical features in Italian patients affected with autoinflammatory disorders and recurrent fever. Eur J Hum Genet 2005;13(3):314–20.
28. ter Haar NM, Jeyaratnam J, Lachmann HJ, et al. The phenotype and genotype of mevalonate kinase deficiency: a series of 114 cases from the Eurofever Registry: phenotype and genotype of MKD. Arthritis Rheumatol 2016;68(11):2795–805.
29. Shinar Y, Obici L, Aksentijevich I, et al. Guidelines for the genetic diagnosis of hereditary recurrent fevers. Ann Rheum Dis 2012;71(10):1599–605.
30. Hoffmann GF, Charpentier C, Mayatepek E, et al. Clinical and biochemical phenotype in 11 patients with mevalonic aciduria. Pediatrics 1993;91(5):915–21.
31. Romberg N, Al Moussawi K, Nelson-Williams C, et al. Mutation of NLRC4 causes a syndrome of enterocolitis and autoinflammation. Nat Genet 2014;46(10):1135–9.
32. Canna SW, de Jesus AA, Gouni S, et al. An activating NLRC4 inflammasome mutation causes autoinflammation with recurrent macrophage activation syndrome. Nat Genet 2014;46(10):1140–6.
33. Franchi L, Kamada N, Nakamura Y, et al. NLRC4-driven production of IL-1β discriminates between pathogenic and commensal bacteria and promotes host intestinal defense. Nat Immunol 2012;13(5):449–56.
34. Canna SW, Girard C, Malle L, et al. Life-threatening NLRC4-associated hyperinflammation successfully treated with IL-18 inhibition. J Allergy Clin Immunol 2017;139(5):1698–701.
35. Volpi S, Picco P, Caorsi R, et al. Type I interferonopathies in pediatric rheumatology. Pediatr Rheumatol 2016;14(1). https://doi.org/10.1186/s12969-016-0094-4.
36. Lee-Kirsch MA. The type I interferonopathies. Annu Rev Med 2017;68(1):297–315.
37. Crow YJ. Chapter 166–Aicardi–Goutières syndrome. In: Dulac O, Lassonde M, Sarnat HB, editors. Handbook of clinical neurology, vol. 113. Amsterdam: Elsevier; 2013. p. 1629–35.
38. Website Crow YJ. Aicardi-Goutières syndrome. In: Adam MP, Ardinger HH, Pagon RA, et al, editors. GeneReviews® [Internet]. Seattle (WA): University of Washington, Seattle; 2016. p. 1993–2019. Available at: https://www.ncbi.nlm.nih.gov/books/NBK1475/. Accessed June 12, 2019.

39. Tüngler V, König N, Engel K, et al. Effects of Janus kinase inhibition in two children with Aicardi-Goutières syndrome. Neuropediatrics 2017;48(S 01):S1–45.
40. Liu Y, Jesus AA, Marrero B, et al. Activated STING in a vascular and pulmonary syndrome. N Engl J Med 2014;371(6):507–18.
41. Kim H, Sanchez GA, Goldbach-Mansky R. Insights from mendelian interferonopathies: comparison of CANDLE, SAVI with AGS, monogenic lupus. J Mol Med 2016;94(10):1111–27.
42. Wu J, Sun L, Chen X, et al. Cyclic GMP-AMP is an endogenous second messenger in innate immune signaling by cytosolic DNA. Science 2013; 339(6121):826–30.
43. Alghamdi M. Autoinflammatory disease-associated vasculitis/vasculopathy. Curr Rheumatol Rep 2018;20(12):87.
44. Damsky W, King BA. JAK inhibitors in dermatology: the promise of a new drug class. J Am Acad Dermatol 2017;76(4):736–44.
45. Frémond M-L, Rodero MP, Jeremiah N, et al. Efficacy of the Janus kinase 1/2 inhibitor ruxolitinib in the treatment of vasculopathy associated with TMEM173-activating mutations in 3 children. J Allergy Clin Immunol 2016;138(6):1752–5.
46. Torrelo A. CANDLE syndrome as a paradigm of proteasome-related autoinflammation. Front Immunol 2017;8:927.
47. Torrelo A, Patel S, Colmenero I, et al. Chronic atypical neutrophilic dermatosis with lipodystrophy and elevated temperature (CANDLE) syndrome. J Am Acad Dermatol 2010;62(3):489–95.
48. Boyadzhiev M, Marinov L, Boyadzhiev V, et al. Disease course and treatment effects of a JAK inhibitor in a patient with CANDLE syndrome. Pediatr Rheumatol 2019;17(1). https://doi.org/10.1186/s12969-019-0322-9.
49. Aksentijevich I, Zhou Q. NF-κB pathway in autoinflammatory diseases: dysregulation of protein modifications by ubiquitin defines a new category of autoinflammatory diseases. Front Immunol 2017;8:399.
50. Komander D, Clague MJ, Urbé S. Breaking the chains: structure and function of the deubiquitinases. Nat Rev Mol Cell Biol 2009;10(8):550–63.
51. Nabavi M, Shahrooei M, Rokni-Zadeh H, et al. Auto-inflammation in a patient with a novel homozygous OTULIN mutation. J Clin Immunol 2019;39(2):138–41.
52. Damgaard RB, Walker JA, Marco-Casanova P, et al. The deubiquitinase OTULIN is an essential negative regulator of inflammation and autoimmunity. Cell 2016; 166(5):1215–30.e20.
53. Zhou Q, Yu X, Demirkaya E, et al. Biallelic hypomorphic mutations in a linear deubiquitinase define otulipenia, an early-onset autoinflammatory disease. Proc Natl Acad Sci USA 2016;113(36):10127–32.

Rare Vesiculopustular Eruptions of the Neonatal Period

Leah E. Lalor, MD[a,b,*], Yvonne E. Chiu, MD[a,b]

KEYWORDS

- Blister • Vesicle • Bulla • Pustule • Erosion • Ulcer • Newborn • Neonate

KEY POINTS

- Blistering diseases of the neonatal period range from benign self-limited eruptions to potentially fatal disorders.
- Careful attention to the morphology of the skin lesions (either vesicles/bullae, pustules, or erosions/ulcers) will guide the clinician in developing an effective differential diagnosis.
- Best practices include a thorough history, careful skin examination, and other diagnostic procedures, including potentially microbiologic assays, laboratory testing, cutaneous biopsies, and genetic testing.

INTRODUCTION

Vesiculopustular eruptions are relatively common in the neonatal period. Most of these disorders are benign and self-limited, with erythema toxicum neonatorum as the single most common eruption in newborns.[1] Yet life-threatening infections, such as herpes simplex virus, genetic diseases with cutaneous manifestations, and other systemic illnesses can also present with vesicles and pustules. Accurate diagnosis of neonates with a vesiculopustular eruption is crucial to ensure proper management. A case series of 64 afebrile neonates with pustules and vesicles evaluated in a pediatric emergency department found that none of the 22 admitted infants had serious central nervous system or blood infections.[2] Unnecessary testing or treatment can expose a newborn to undue morbidity, although appropriate workup is also necessary to avoid missing serious illness.

A systematic approach is needed to evaluate the blistering newborn (**Fig. 1**). Using proper terminology for describing skin lesions is an important part of understanding these diseases and for communicating within the care team. A vesicle is a lesion

[a] Department of Dermatology (Pediatric Dermatology), Medical College of Wisconsin, 8701 Watertown Plank Road, Milwaukee, WI 53226, USA; [b] Department of Pediatrics, Medical College of Wisconsin, 8701 Watertown Plank Road, Milwaukee, WI 53226, USA
* Corresponding author. Department of Dermatology (Pediatric Dermatology), Medical College of Wisconsin, 8701 Watertown Plank Road, Milwaukee, WI 53226.
E-mail address: llalor@mcw.edu

Clin Perinatol 47 (2020) 53–75
https://doi.org/10.1016/j.clp.2019.09.005
0095-5108/20/© 2019 Elsevier Inc. All rights reserved.

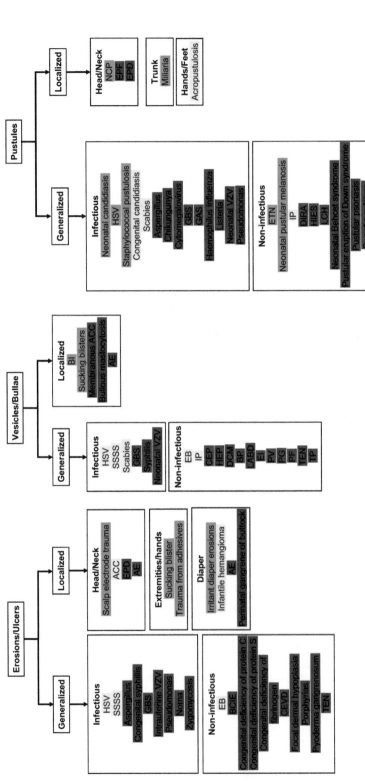

Fig. 1. Diagnostic algorithm for vesiculopustular eruptions in neonates based on primary lesion morphology and distribution. Conditions highlighted in green are common, yellow are uncommon, and red are rare. *Abbreviations:* ACC, Aplasia cutis congenita; AE, Acrodermatitis enteropathica; BCIE, Bullous congenital ichthyosiform erythroderma; BI, Bullous impetigo; BP, Bullous pemphigoid; CEP, Congenital erythropoietic porphyria; CEVD, Congenital erosive and vesicular dermatosis; DCM, Diffuse cutaneous mastocytosis; DIRA, Deficiency of IL-1 receptor antagonist; EB, Epidermolysis bullosa; EI, Epidermolytic ichthyosis; EPD, Erosive pustular dermatosis of the scalp; EPF, Eosinophilic pustular folliculitis; ETN, Erythema toxicum neonatorum; GAS, Group A streptococcus; GBS, Group B streptococcus; HEP, Hepatoerythropoietic porphyria; HIES, Hyper IgE syndrome; HSV, Herpes simplex virus; IP, Incontinentia pigmenti; LABD, Linear IgA bullous dermatosis; LCH, Langerhans cell histiocytosis; NCP, Neonatal cephalic pustulosis; PF, Pemphigus foliaceus; PG, Pemphigoid gestationis; PV, Pemphigus vulgaris; SSSS, Staphylococcal scalded skin syndrome; TEN, Toxic epidermal necrolysis; TP, Transient porphyrinemia; VZV, Varicella zoster virus.

containing clear fluid and measuring less than 1 cm in diameter, while a bulla is a lesion containing clear fluid and measuring ≥1 cm in diameter. A pustule is a fluid-filled lesion that contains purulent exudate. Any of these can rupture and lead to secondary changes, such as erosions (superficial and only partial loss of the epidermal layer of the skin), ulcers (deeper and full loss of the epidermal layer of the skin), or crust (dried blood, pus, or serum).

Table 1 summarizes the most common vesiculopustular eruptions that can present in the neonatal period. The following cases highlight several of the rare blistering disorders that may occur in a newborn.

CASE PRESENTATION 1

A 32-year-old G2P2 woman gives birth at 39 weeks gestation after an uncomplicated pregnancy. At birth, the neonate is noted to have areas of weeping, denuded skin on the trunk and extremities. At several hours of life, multiple blisters are seen forming at areas of trauma (**Fig. 2**).[3] The neonate is otherwise stable and without additional abnormal findings. Mother has no personal history of blistering, and there is no family history of blistering skin diseases or disorders. The most likely diagnosis in this case is which of the following:

A. Linear IgA bullous dermatosis
B. Epidermolysis bullosa
C. Aplasia cutis congenita
D. *TP63*-related ectodermal dysplasia
E. Bullous pemphigoid

Answer: B. Epidermolysis Bullosa

Epidermolysis bullosa (EB) is a group of genetic disorders whereby skin fragility is the predominant feature. Skin fragility in these conditions is caused by variations in genes encoding several proteins in the epidermis, basement membrane zone, and

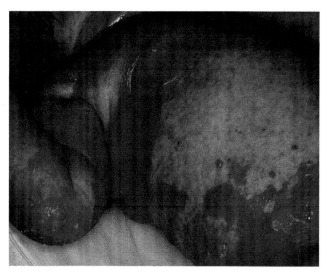

Fig. 2. Widespread blisters and erosions on a neonate. (Treatment of Skin Disease 5e, 2018, ISBN: 9780702069123, Lebwohl et al ed.)

Table 1
Common vesiculopustular eruptions in the neonatal period

Condition	Onset	Location	Morphology	Other Features	Diagnosis and Workup	Management	Duration
Neonatal cephalic pustulosis	Days to weeks	Cheeks, forehead, scalp, eyelids, neck, upper chest	Papules and pustules with surrounding redness	May have scaling in scalp, otherwise healthy	Clinical	Expectant management; topical ketoconazole and hydrocortisone	
Neonatal pustular melanosis	Birth	Anywhere; usually forehead, ears, back, fingers, toes	Pustules without redness, collarettes of scale, hyperpigmented macules	Term infants, more common in black infants	Clinical; can do Wright's stain to identify neutrophils	Expectant management	Pustular lesions: 1–2 d, hyperpigmented macules: weeks to months
Erythema toxicum neonatorum	24–48 h	Anywhere excluding palms and soles	Red macules, papules, pustules with surrounding wheals	Term infants >2500 g	Usually clinical; can do Wright's stain for eosinophils	Expectant management	Exacerbations and remissions over first 2 weeks of life
Miliaria crystallina	Birth, neonatal, later	Forehead, upper trunk, arms	Fragile vesicles without redness	Anywhere that was occluded; usually history of fever	Clinical	Remove occlusive clothing and swaddles	
Miliaria rubra	First few weeks of life	Upper trunk, proximal arms	Red papules, vesicles	Anywhere that was occluded	Clinical	Remove occlusive clothing and swaddles	

Neonatal herpes simplex virus infection	5–21 d of life	Anywhere, especially scalp and torso	Vesicles, pustules, erosions, crusts	May involve mucosa, may be septic	PCR, Tzanck smear, viral culture	
Neonatal candidiasis	First few days of life	Anywhere; upper torso, palms, and soles often involved	Erythema, small monomorphic papules, pustules; burn-like dermatitis and scaling in ELBW neonates		KOH preparation of lesion positive for hyphae and budding yeast; culture of lesion	
Staphylococcal pustulosis	Neonatal through infancy	Any site, often in diaper area in neonates	Pustules, red papules, bullae		Culture of a lesion	Topical and/or systemic anti-staphylococcal antibiotics

Abbreviations: ELBW, extremely low birthweight; KOH, potassium hydroxide; PCR, polymerase chain reaction.

dermis, causing splitting of the skin at different levels, resulting in blistering, erosions, and ulcerations of the skin and mucous membranes. It has an estimated incidence of 20 per 1,000,000 births in the United States.[4] There are 4 major types of EB, including EB simplex (EBS), junctional EB (JEB), dystrophic EB (DEB), and Kindler syndrome (KS), with many additional subtypes within each category.[5] The major types are classified based on the location of the abnormal protein in the skin, with EBS due to abnormal proteins in the epidermis, JEB due to abnormal proteins in the basement membrane zone, DEB due to abnormal proteins in the dermis, and KS due to abnormal proteins at various levels within the skin and a unique clinical phenotype (**Fig. 3**).[5]

At birth, it can be difficult or impossible to distinguish among the various types of EB. Typical findings include congenital absence of skin and blisters at sites of trauma that may be congenital or may develop several hours after birth. The differential diagnosis of EB may include autoimmune blistering conditions, infectious etiologies, ectodermal dysplasias, and diffuse cutaneous mastocytosis; histopathology of a blister can help distinguish among these conditions. Definitive diagnosis of specific EB subtypes has historically been accomplished via skin biopsy of an induced blister for electron microscopy or direct immunofluorescence; however, this process can be inexact and nondiagnostic. More recently, clinicians have been relying on DNA analysis to determine the genetic variation causing the skin fragility, resulting in more accurate diagnosis and prognostic information.[6]

There are many challenges in caring for a neonate with EB, including failure to thrive, thermal instability, fluid, protein, and electrolyte losses, increased risk of infection, pain management, wound care, and family bonding, among others. They are best cared for in a neonatal intensive care unit with experience in EB and a variety of subspecialist clinicians available. Prognosis depends on the subtype of EB: some forms (such as certain subtypes of EBS and dominant DEB) have normal life expectancies and few complications, while others (such as JEB, recessive DEB, and the more severe and generalized forms of EBS) may result in many critical complications and early death.

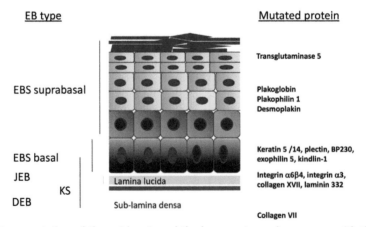

Fig. 3. Representation of the epidermis and the basement membrane zone with the locations of the mutated proteins in epidermolysis bullosa subtypes. DEB, dystrophic epidermolysis bullosa; EB, epidermolysis bullosa; EBS, epidermolysis bullosa simplex; JEB, junctional epidermolysis bullosa; KS, Kindler syndrome. (*From* Fine JD, Bruckner-Tuderman L, Eady RA, et al. Inherited epidermolysis bullosa: updated recommendations on diagnosis and classification. J Am Acad Dermatol 2014;70(6):1103-1126; with permission.)

Linear IgA Bullous Dermatosis

Linear IgA bullous dermatosis (LABD, also known as chronic bullous dermatosis of childhood) is the most common autoimmune blistering disorder of childhood and typically presents from age 6 months to 5 years, although neonatal presentations have been reported.[7–15] LABD is caused by autoantibodies directed against fragments of collagen XVII (also known as the 180-kDa bullous pemphigoid [BP] antigen or BP180), which resides in the basement membrane zone between the epidermis and dermis.[16] This results in poor adherence of the epidermis to the dermis, leading to mucocutaneous blistering. The typical presentation is abrupt onset of tense vesicles and bullae that may be clear or hemorrhagic on normal or erythematous skin.[17] New lesions typically arise around healing lesions, resulting in arciform or annular bullae surrounding a central crust, leading to the classic appearance of a string of pearls, cluster of jewels, or rosette pattern (**Fig. 4**). Younger children tend to have perioral and perineal involvement, while older children may have more generalized disease.[18] Neonates with LABD seem to have more severe mucosal involvement, including in the eyes, mouth, esophagus, and upper respiratory tract,[7–12,14] although there are rare reports of uncomplicated cases.[13,15]

The differential diagnosis of LABD in infants and young children includes other acquired blistering disorders, including autoimmune blistering disorders, such as BP, the pemphigus group, dermatitis herpetiformis, EB acquisita, and bullous systemic lupus erythematosus, as well as infectious etiologies, such as herpes simplex, varicella zoster virus, enterovirus, bullous impetigo due to *Staphylococcus aureus*, and staphylococcal scalded skin syndrome, in addition to idiopathic or medication reactions including toxic epidermal necrolysis, Stevens-Johnson syndrome, and erythema multiforme. The differential diagnosis of the neonatal presentation of LABD must include genetic etiologies of generalized blistering, including EB and diffuse cutaneous mastocytosis. Diagnosis is made via cutaneous biopsy for both histopathology and direct immunofluorescence. Histopathology of a blister will demonstrate a subepidermal split with neutrophils collecting at the dermoepidermal junction, and direct immunofluorescence of a perilesional skin biopsy will show linear deposition of IgA along the basement membrane zone.[19]

Treatment is aimed at suppressing the inflammatory response, and typically includes an initial course of systemic corticosteroids followed by long-term maintenance with dapsone. Other immunosuppressive medications have been used in

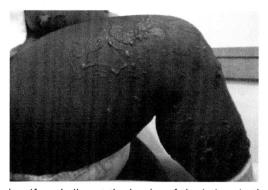

Fig. 4. Annular and arciform bullae at the border of the lesions in the classic "string of pearls" pattern.

treatment-resistant cases in older children.[20,21] In the neonatal period, supportive care is essential, particularly in those with severe mucosal involvement. Prognosis is usually good, with spontaneous resolution achieved in most patients within months to years,[17] although cases of resultant blindness and dysphagia have been reported.[7,9]

Aplasia Cutis Congenita

Aplasia cutis congenita (ACC) is an uncommon condition characterized by a localized area of absent skin noted at birth. It is usually not associated with any other anomalies.[22] The pathogenesis of ACC is unknown, and it is likely that all ACC cannot be attributed to a single cause.[23] Therefore, ACC should be considered a physical finding indicating that there has been a disruption of skin development in utero, and that the causes of these disruptions vary.[22] ACC may rarely be associated with various other malformations, specific genetic syndromes, and underlying cranial or spinal dysraphism.[22] The most common presentation is a single, round, crusted or weeping erosion or ulceration less than 1 cm in diameter located near the hair whorl on the scalp of a neonate. There may be multiple grouped lesions; rarely, lesions may appear bullous with a membrane overlying the area of absent skin.[22]

The differential diagnosis of ACC typically includes intrauterine or perinatal trauma, as well as intrauterine or perinatal infections. Diagnosis is usually clinical. Prognosis is excellent, as healing occurs within a few weeks with an alopecic scar.

TP63-Related Ectodermal Dysplasia

Ectodermal dysplasias caused by pathogenic variants in TP63 are a group of disorders with a combination of partially overlapping features, including ectodermal dysplasia, cleft lip and/or palate, and limb defects. Ectodermal dysplasia involves alterations in two or more structures derived from the embryonic ectoderm, including skin, hair, teeth, nails, sweat glands, and the lens of the eye. The TP63-related disorders are caused by genetic variations in a transcription factor that is a key regulator of ectodermal, orofacial, and limb development.[24,25] There are currently seven defined TP63-related syndromes, five of which have the feature of ectodermal dysplasia: ankyloblepharon-ectodermal defects-cleft lip/palate syndrome (AEC), Rapp-Hodgkin syndrome, ectodactyly-ectodermal dysplasia-cleft lip/palate syndrome, limb-mammary syndrome, and acro-dermato-ungual-lacrimal-tooth syndrome.[26] The clinical features of these conditions are wide-ranging, but in the context of the case presentation question, one of the major phenotypes involves severe and extensive congenital erosion of the crown of the scalp. This finding is most common in AEC and may be so severe as to be life-threatening.[26] Various other ectodermal structures show abnormalities in these syndromes, and clinical findings may include skin connections between upper and lower eyelids (ankyloblepharon); red and fissured skin in the neonatal period with subsequent development of thin, dry skin over time; recurrent scalp infections, erosions, and granulation tissue; sparse and coarse lightly colored hair; hypohidrosis; few and abnormal teeth; and nail dystrophy.[26] Cleft lip and/or palate is a nearly constant feature, and split hand-foot deformities are the typical limb malformations.[26]

The differential diagnosis of the various TP63-related ectodermal dysplasias includes other syndromes that fall under the same umbrella. The constellation of features is fairly unique and diagnosis tends to be self-evident and clinical. Confirmation of the diagnosis can be made via DNA analysis. Treatment is aimed at surgical management of the eyelid, orofacial, and limb malformations. Emollients may be used to help ameliorate skin dryness and excellent wound care should be performed for scalp manifestations. Prognosis is generally good, as the cutaneous manifestations tend to improve with age.[27]

Bullous Pemphigoid

Bullous pemphigoid is a rare autoimmune bullous disorder of childhood caused by autoantibodies directed against one of two proteins found in the basement membrane zone, termed antigens BP180 and BP230.[28] These autoantibodies lead to destruction of these structural proteins, resulting in urticarial plaques, generalized blistering on the skin and mucosal surfaces, and severe pruritus.[29] Blisters are tense and typically ungrouped and are found predominantly on flexural surfaces, palms, and soles.[29] There may or may not be mucosal involvement. There have been no reports of neonatal onset BP, although there are many reports of infantile and childhood BP.[30]

The differential diagnosis of infantile or childhood BP is the same as for LABD. Diagnosis is made via cutaneous biopsy for histopathology and direct immunofluorescence. Histopathology of a vesicle will demonstrate a subepidermal blister with predominantly eosinophils in the superficial dermis, while direct immunofluorescence of perilesional skin will show linear deposition of C3 and IgG along the basement membrane zone.[30] Similar to LABD, treatment is aimed at suppressing the immune response. Systemic corticosteroids are the typical initial therapy, while maintenance therapy may include topical corticosteroids and a variety of immunosuppressant medications and antibiotics used for their anti-inflammatory effects.[30] Prognosis is generally good, with remission achieved in most patients and uncommon relapses.[30]

CASE PRESENTATION 2

A previously healthy 6-week-old infant has been admitted several days after developing acute-onset generalized pustules and red nodules associated with high spiking fevers and leukocytosis (**Fig. 5**). Infectious workup thus far has been negative, and the infant has not improved after several days of broad-spectrum antibiotic coverage. You suspect this infant may have which of the following:

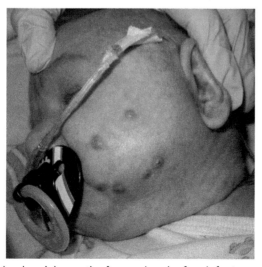

Fig. 5. Pustules and red nodules on the face and neck of an infant.

A. Eosinophilic pustular folliculitis
B. Pustular eruption of Down syndrome
C. Langerhans cell histiocytosis
D. Acute febrile neutrophilic dermatosis (Sweet syndrome)
E. Staphylococcal pyoderma

Answer: D. Acute Febrile Neutrophilic Dermatosis (Sweet Syndrome)

Acute febrile neutrophilic dermatosis (AFND) is an acquired disorder thought to be a reactive phenomenon secondary to infections, other inflammatory conditions, medications, vaccinations, or malignancies, in particular acute myeloid leukemia and myelomonocytic leukemia.[31–37] It is characterized by the rapid onset of tender, edematous, brightly erythematous papules, plaques, nodules, and sometimes pustules primarily on the face and extremities. New lesions frequently occur at sites of trauma. Patients frequently have high spiking fevers and leukocytosis and may have arthralgia, arthritis, conjunctivitis, iridocyclitis, proteinuria, hematuria, and lung infiltrates. Central nervous system involvement has rarely been reported.

AFND is quite rare in children, and even rarer in the neonatal period. Neonatal disease, defined by some as having onset before age 6 months, may be secondary to viral infection, primary immunodeficiency, neonatal lupus, gastrointestinal disease, HIV infection, and genetic etiologies.[38] Infants with symptoms before age 6 weeks tend to have a serious underlying illness or genetic problem (familial Sweet syndrome, chronic atypical neutrophilic dermatosis with lipodystrophy, and elevated temperature syndrome, neonatal onset multisystem inflammatory disease, or a primary immunodeficiency).[38] The differential diagnosis is broad and includes other neutrophilic dermatoses and infectious etiologies, and diagnosis is made via cutaneous biopsy demonstrating a diffuse dermal infiltrate of neutrophils without neutrophilic vasculitis. Prognosis of AFND is good, with rapid improvement after administration of systemic corticosteroids; however, a thorough investigation to determine potential inciting factors must be made.

Eosinophilic Pustular Folliculitis

Eosinophilic pustular folliculitis (EPF) is a rare condition of unknown etiology characterized by recurrent crops of papules and pustules in the scalp, although other areas of the skin may be involved (**Fig. 6**).[39] These lesions may be itchy and may be associated with peripheral eosinophilia. The average age of onset is around 6 months, with 95% of cases presenting before 14 months.[40] There is a male predominance with a male-to-female ratio of 4:1.[40] The differential diagnosis of EPF includes other pustular eruptions of neonates, including but not limited to erythema toxicum neonatorum, transient pustular melanosis, scabies infestation, incontinentia pigmenti, and Langerhans cell histiocytosis (LCH) , as well as bacterial, viral, and fungal infections. An important clinical mimicker is hyper-IgE syndrome, which is a rare primary immunodeficiency that may present initially with a pustular eruption in the scalp. Diagnosis of EPF may be confirmed via examination of a smear of pustular contents stained with Wright stain to demonstrate prominent eosinophils or via histopathological evaluation of a cutaneous biopsy demonstrating dense dermal eosinophilic infiltrates in a perifollicular, interfollicular, and/or periadnexal distribution.[40] Bacterial, viral, and fungal cultures are negative.

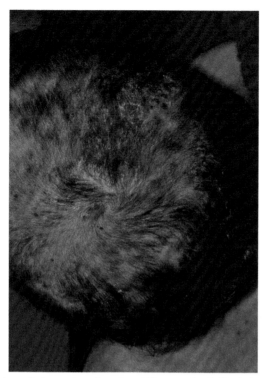

Fig. 6. Crusted and eroded papules of eosinophilic pustular folliculitis on the scalp. (*From* Eichenfield LF, Frieden IJ, Mathes EF, et al. Neonatal and infant dermatology, 3e. London: Elsevier Saunders; 2015; with permission.)

Flares of EPF respond well to topical corticosteroids but are also self-limited and may be managed expectantly. Both oral and topical antibiotics may also be effective. Prognosis is excellent with resolution generally seen by 3 years of age.[40]

Pustular Eruption in Myeloproliferative Disorder of Down Syndrome

Neonates with trisomy 21 may have a rare vesiculopustular eruption in association with a transient myeloproliferative disorder (TMD).[41–46] Typically, the eruption begins on the face within the first few days of life and may generalize to involve the entire cutaneous surface. It may also demonstrate pathergy, with lesions developing at sites of cutaneous trauma, such as venipunctures or biopsy sites. The eruption spontaneously resolves as the TMD resolves. Patients with this eruption in association with TMD may subsequently develop leukemia,[41,42] therefore long-term monitoring is required. It is usually associated with elevated peripheral white blood cell counts and may be associated with systemic symptoms related to the TMD. Differential diagnosis includes other pustular eruptions of infancy, particularly including infectious etiologies, such as herpes simplex virus, *S aureus*, and congenital or neonatal candidiasis. Diagnosis can be made with a cutaneous biopsy demonstrating intraepidermal spongiosis and inflammatory cell infiltrate with a perivascular infiltrate of immature myeloid cells in the clinical context of a child with trisomy 21 and a TMD. This condition has also been reported in patients with mosaic forms of trisomy 21.[43,47]

Langerhans Cell Histiocytosis

LCH presenting in the neonatal period is a polymorphous eruption caused by collections of mononuclear antigen-presenting Langerhans cells in the skin. The eruption may present at birth or early in the neonatal period and may be composed of generalized pustules, erosions, ulceration, or crusting; new lesions may continue to erupt over the first few weeks of life.[48] The lesions themselves can range from a few millimeters up to a few centimeters in size. The pathogenesis of LCH is unknown. The differential diagnosis of this condition is wide and includes intrauterine herpes simplex virus infection, neonatal varicella zoster virus infection, congenital candidiasis, and intrauterine graft-versus-host disease, among others, depending on the morphology of the primary lesions. Diagnosis can be made with a Tzanck preparation[49] or with a cutaneous biopsy, which will demonstrate an infiltrate of mononuclear cells in the upper dermis with irregularly shaped vesicular nuclei and eosinophilic cytoplasm that will stain positively with S100 and immunohistochemical markers specific for Langerhans cells.[50] Once diagnosed, patients with LCH must have a comprehensive physical examination with laboratory evaluation including complete blood count, liver function tests, and urine osmolality, as well as imaging including a skeletal survey and chest radiograph.[51] Evaluation by an oncologist is recommended.[51] When presenting congenitally or in the neonatal period, LCH has an excellent prognosis, with spontaneous remission the usual course. However, relapses of LCH and progression to systemic involvement have been reported, thus long-term follow-up is certainly required.[52–55] When presenting after the neonatal period, LCH is more likely to have systemic involvement and has a poorer prognosis.[51]

Staphylococcal Pyoderma

Pyoderma is a cutaneous bacterial infection due to *S aureus* and can be polymorphous in appearance. It is not present at birth but may develop in the first few days to weeks of life and typically presents with vesicles and pustules in a localized or generalized distribution.[56,57] Commonly, the condition is seen at sites of trauma, such as the umbilicus or in the diaper area, particularly in male neonates after circumcisions, as well as areas of skin-to-skin contact, such as the neck and axillae. Most neonates are otherwise well without fever or other systemic symptoms, and clear their infection with topical or oral antibiotics.[58,59] Differential diagnosis may be broad, depending on the morphology of the primary lesions, but diagnosis is generally made based on clinical suspicion in the typical clinical context with confirmation via bacterial culture from a lesion.

CASE PRESENTATION 3

A 3-day-old female neonate was evaluated in the neonatal intensive care unit for a widespread rash present since day 1 of life. The infant had also been having apneic episodes with desaturations and had been in a radiant warmer since birth. She was born at term via spontaneous vaginal delivery to a mother with a history of diet-controlled gestational diabetes. On dermatologic examination, there were innumerable, clear vesicles on an erythematous base in a linear and whorled distribution on the head, neck, trunk, and extremities (**Fig. 7**). Head ultrasound was normal, but magnetic resonance imaging of the brain showed multiple foci of restricted diffusion with rim enhancement in the subcortical white matter of the cerebral hemispheres, bilateral thalami, basal ganglia, cerebellum, and medulla. What is the diagnosis?

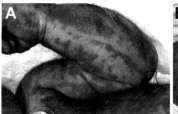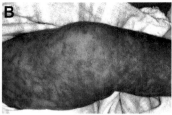

Fig. 7. (*A*) Linear erythematous plaques with superficial vesiculation on the arm. (*B*) Vesicles on an erythematous base on the leg. (*Courtesy of* R. Delahoussaye-Shields, MD, New Orleans, LA.)

A. Incontinentia pigmenti
B. Congenital erythropoietic porphyria
C. Scabies infestation
D. Transient porphyrinemia

Answer A. Incontinentia Pigmenti

Incontinentia pigmenti (IP) is a multisystem disease caused by pathogenic variants in the *IKBKG* gene, which encodes a modulator of the nuclear factor κB inflammatory pathway.[60] It is inherited in an X-linked dominant manner and is lethal in utero in most male infants; affected males have been reported in rare cases, usually because of an XXY genotype or low-level mosaicism.

Cutaneous findings occur in all IP cases and characteristically occur in 4 stages: vesicular, verrucous, hyperpigmented, and atrophic. The lesions are arranged within the lines of Blaschko, which are ectodermal cell migration pathways determined during embryogenesis, with involvement of some lines of Blaschko and sparing of others because of X chromosome inactivation. The vesicular stage appears within the first few weeks of life with clear-yellow vesicles on an erythematous base. As the first stage resolves around 4 to 6 months of age, the vesicles are replaced by the verrucous, hyperkeratotic papules of stage II that then last a few months to a few years. The hyperpigmented third stage lasts the longest, starting in the latter half of infancy and persisting into the adolescent and adult years. The brown and gray patches follow the linear and whorled pattern of the lines of Blaschko. Stage IV is variable and may not occur in all individuals. The linear hypopigmented patches are associated with alopecia and loss of eccrine glands, resulting in loss of sweating in those areas.

In addition to skin involvement, the hair (27%), teeth (44%), and nails (15%) can also be affected.[61] Alopecia is most characteristic in stage IV disease, but sparse scalp, eyebrow, and eyelash hair can occur in childhood. Woolly hair that is lusterless, wiry, and coarse can be an additional feature. Delayed dentition, hypodontia, microdontia, cone-shaped teeth, and impaction have been reported dental findings. Nail dystrophy resembles onychomycosis and occurs most commonly in stage II.

Central nervous system and ophthalmologic manifestations of IP are each present in approximately 30% of cases. Central nervous system vasculopathy, resulting in ischemic and hemorrhagic strokes are likely the cause of the neurologic manifestations, with seizures as the most commonly seen clinical manifestation.[62] Most seizures will present in infancy. Mild intellectual disability, primary brain anomalies, and spastic paresis may be additional neurologic features. Retinal vascular proliferation is the most common eye finding, which can cause bleeding, scarring, retinal detachment, and vision defects.[61]

Leukocytosis, eosinophilia, breast anomalies, and primary pulmonary hypertension are additional reported features. Life expectancy is generally normal although severe extracutaneous complications can cause morbidity or mortality.

Diagnostic criteria for IP have been proposed by multiple authors, most recently by Minić and colleagues[63] in 2014 (**Table 2**). Skin biopsy of a stage I vesicle is the most helpful and specific, where the main histologic findings include dyskeratotic keratinocytes and intraepidermal vesicles containing eosinophils, while biopsies of lesions in other stages are less specific.[63] Genetic testing of *IKBKG* can confirm the diagnosis of IP if the clinical features are inconclusive.

Management of IP requires multidisciplinary care, with coordination between the neonatologist, dermatologist, geneticist, neurologist, ophthalmologist, and dentist. There is no specific therapy for the syndrome, with treatment directed at each disease manifestation as it arises.

Congenital Erythropoietic Porphyria

The porphyrias are rare metabolic disorders resulting from enzymatic defects in the heme biosynthesis pathway, resulting in the accumulation of porphyrins (**Table 3**). The symptoms of porphyria can be acute neurovisceral manifestations, cutaneous photosensitivity, or a combination of both. Most childhood cases are inherited, while porphyria cutanea tarda in adults is commonly acquired. There are three porphyrias that present in infancy or early childhood: congenital erythropoietic porphyria (CEP), hepatoerythropoietic porphyria (HEP), and erythropoietic protoporphyria (EPP).

CEP is a very rare disorder caused by deficient uroporphyrinogen III synthase enzyme activity, most commonly due to autosomal recessively inherited pathogenic variants in *UROS* or rarely *GATA1*, which binds a promoter element of the

Table 2	
Diagnostic criteria for incontinentia pigmenti	
Major Criteria	**Minor Criteria**
Incontinentia pigmenti (IP)-type skin stages distributed along Blaschko lines	Dental anomalies
	Ocular anomalies
	CNS anomalies
	Alopecia
	Hair abnormalities
	Nail abnormalities
	Palate anomalies
	Breast anomalies
	Multiple male miscarriages
	Typical skin biopsy findings

If no evidence of IP in a first-degree female relative:
- At least 2 major criteria or 1 major and ≥1 minor criteria are necessary to make a diagnosis of sporadic IP in the absence of pathogenic variants in *IKBKG*.
- Any single major or minor criterion is satisfactory for IP diagnosis in the presence of *IKBKG* mutation.

If evidence of IP in a first-degree female relative:
- Any single major or ≥2 minor criteria

Data from Minic S, Trpinac D, Obradovic M. Incontinentia pigmenti diagnostic criteria update. Clin Genet 2014;85(6):536-542.

Table 3
Characteristics of the porphyrias

Disorder	Enzyme Defect (Gene)	Inheritance	Typical Age of Onset	Clinical Features
Acute intermittent porphyria (AIP)	Porphobilinogen deaminase (*PBGD*)	AD	Adulthood	Acute neurologic attacks but no photosensitivity/cutaneous manifestations
Variegate porphyria (VP)	Protoporphyrinogen oxidase (*PPOX*)	AD	Adulthood	Acute neurologic attacks similar to AIP and cutaneous manifestations similar to PCT
Hereditary coproporphyria (HCP)	Coproporphyrinogen oxidase (*CPO*)	AD	Adulthood	Acute neurologic attacks Photosensitivity and blistering can occur
ALA-D deficiency porphyria (ADP)	δ-Aminolevulinic acid dehydratase (*ALAD*)	AR	Variable	Acute neurologic attacks but no photosensitivity/cutaneous manifestations
Porphyria cutanea tarda (PCT)	Uroporphyrinogen decarboxylase (*UROD*)	Acquired in 75% AD in 25%	Adulthood	Photosensitivity Vesicles, bullae, crusted erosions, and scarring on sun-exposed areas Hypertrichosis
Erythropoietic protoporphyria (EPP)	Ferrochelatase (*FECH*)	Semi-dominant	Early childhood	Photosensitivity Pain, erythema, and edema with sun exposure but no blistering Skin thickening and waxy scars with time Cholelithiasis

(continued on next page)

Table 3
(continued)

Disorder	Enzyme Defect (Gene)	Inheritance	Typical Age of Onset	Clinical Features
Congenital erythropoietic porphyria (CEP)	Uroporphyrinogen III synthase (*UROS*)	AR	Infancy	Very severe course Photosensitivity Vesicles, bullae, crusted erosions, and scarring on sun-exposed areas Hypertrichosis Red urine and teeth Hemolytic anemia
Hepatoerythropoietic porphyria (HEP)	*UROD*	AR	Infancy	Similar to CEP but milder and fewer extracutaneous manifestations Photosensitivity Vesicles, bullae, crusted erosions, and scarring on sun-exposed areas Hypertrichosis Red urine and teeth
X-Linked dominant protoporphyria (XLP)	δ-Aminolevulinic acid synthase 2 (*ALAS2*)	XLD	Early childhood	Cutaneous manifestations similar to EPP

Abbreviations: AD, autosomal dominant; AR, autosomal recessive; XLS, X-linked dominant.

UROS gene.[64,65] The enzyme defect causes accumulation of porphyrins in erythrocytes, skin, bones, teeth, and eyes. Red urine that fluoresces under a Woods lamp is often the first sign of the disease at birth. The cutaneous manifestations present at a median age of 1.75 years, although there is wide variability in age of onset, from in utero hydrops fetalis to mild cases arising in adulthood.[66] The hallmark feature is blistering in photo-exposed areas, which in neonates may be precipitated by phototherapy for neonatal hyperbilirubinemia or placement in a radiant warmer.[67,68] Disease sequelae include crusted erosions, scarring, dyspigmentation, hypertrichosis, and onycholysis (**Fig. 8**). Severely affected patients may progress to scarring disfigurement of the face and fingers. In addition to red urine, erythrodontia (red teeth) may develop.

Hemolytic anemia, ranging from mild to severe transfusion-dependent, is the main extracutaneous manifestation and important predictor of disease morbidity. Secondary hepatosplenomegaly may develop, leading to abnormal transaminases, leukopenia, and thrombocytopenia. Porphyrin deposition in the eyes may cause corneal ulcers, scarring, and blindness, and osteoporosis can develop from porphyrin deposition in the bones.

HEP is even less common than CEP but is very similar in its clinical manifestations; however, HEP tends to present later in childhood and with fewer extracutaneous manifestations. HEP is caused by autosomal recessively inherited pathogenic variants in *UROD*, resulting in decreased uroporphyrinogen decarboxylase activity.[69]

EPP presents in childhood with pain on sun exposure without vesicles or bullae. Extracutaneous manifestations of EPP include cholelithiasis and microcytic anemia. Also inherited in an autosomal recessive manner due to pathogenic variants in *FECH*, ferrochelatase enzyme activity is compromised in EPP.[70]

The diagnosis of porphyria is made through biochemical testing showing porphyrin elevations in plasma, erythrocytes, urine, and/or feces. Samples must be protected from light during collection and transport to prevent porphyrin degradation. Urine porphyrin testing, either via random spot testing or 24-h collections, is the

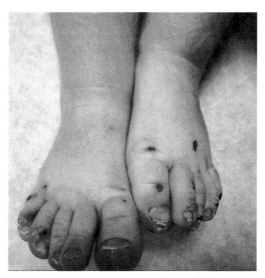

Fig. 8. 18-month-old with onset of CEP in the second year of life. She had crusted erosions, a vesicle on the left second toe, and hypertrichosis of the shins.

screening test of choice for CEP, HEP, and the blistering cutaneous porphyrias. CEP will show elevated urine levels of uroporphyrin I and coproporphyrin I, while HEP will have elevated urine levels of uroporphyrin and heptacarboxyl porphyrin. The diagnosis can be confirmed by genetic testing. Skin biopsy is usually not necessary for the diagnosis.

There are no specific therapies for the porphyrias, and treatment is supportive. Strict photoprotection is the mainstay of therapy for CEP and HEP, and children should be protected from ultraviolet light as well as visible light in the shorter blue wavelengths. Sun-protective clothing and window films for the car and home may be required. Zinc- and titanium-containing sunscreens are preferred over chemical sunscreens, but they are usually not sufficiently effective in isolation. Fluorescent lights in schools and hospitals may trigger blistering in some susceptible children. For children with severe hemolytic anemia, chronic blood transfusions can suppress erythropoiesis and porphyrin synthesis but splenectomy may be required.[71] Bone marrow transplant is curative for patients with extremely severe disease.[72]

Scabies Infestation

Neonatal scabies infestation is uncommon and often misdiagnosed because of its atypical appearance. Neonates present within the first few weeks of life with crusted papules, nodules, and vesicles (**Fig. 9**).[73] In contrast to older children and adults who have lesions clustering in the axillae, groin, and wrists, neonatal cases are more generalized with a predilection for the scalp, palms, and soles. Family members may also have a pruritic eruption on careful questioning. There have been reports of neonatal scabies misdiagnosed as LCH, so accurate diagnosis of this entity is important.[74,75] Treatment with sulfur preparations is generally recommended for infants less than 2 months of age, although permethrin 5% cream has also been used.[73,76]

Transient Porphyrinemia

Transient porphyrinemia is an extremely rare acquired porphyrin elevation seen in neonates. The infants usually have hemolytic disease of the newborn and develop a cutaneous eruption when treated with phototherapy for hyperbilirubinemia. Erythema and purpura are the typical reaction, but blisters have been reported.[77,78] Elevated urine, plasma, and erythrocyte porphyrins are present on testing. Porphyrin levels normalize spontaneously within the first few months of life.

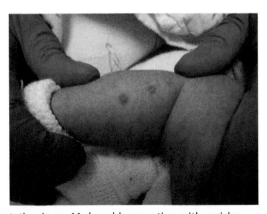

Fig. 9. Scabies infestation in an 11-day-old presenting with vesicles.

SUMMARY

A variety of disorders can present with blistering in the neonatal period. Targeted questioning of the prenatal, maternal, and family history and a thorough examination of the skin, mucosae, hair, and nails are important to elicit subtle findings and guide the diagnostic evaluation. Unroofing the vesicle or pustule is necessary to obtain ample fluid for viral polymerase chain reaction or bacterial cultures. Skin biopsies may be necessary in certain cases. Although unlikely to be encountered by many clinicians over the course of their career, having an index of suspicion will ensure prompt and accurate diagnosis of these rare vesiculopustular eruptions of the neonatal period.

DISCLOSURE

The authors have nothing to disclose.

REFERENCES

1. Kanada KN, Merin MR, Munden A, et al. A prospective study of cutaneous findings in newborns in the United States: correlation with race, ethnicity, and gestational status using updated classification and nomenclature. J Pediatr 2012; 161(2):240–5.
2. Manice CS, Planet PJ, Chase HS, et al. Management of afebrile neonates with pustules and vesicles in a pediatric emergency department. Pediatr Dermatol 2018;35(5):660–5.
3. Bolognia J, Jorizzo JL, Schaffer JV. Dermatology. 3rd edition. Philadelphia: Elsevier Saunders; 2012.
4. Fine JD. Epidemiology of inherited epidermolysis bullosa based on incidence and prevalence estimates from the National Epidermolysis Bullosa Registry. JAMA Dermatol 2016;152(11):1231–8.
5. Fine JD, Bruckner-Tuderman L, Eady RA, et al. Inherited epidermolysis bullosa: updated recommendations on diagnosis and classification. J Am Acad Dermatol 2014;70(6):1103–26.
6. Lucky AW, Dagaonkar N, Lammers K, et al. A comprehensive next-generation sequencing assay for the diagnosis of epidermolysis bullosa. Pediatr Dermatol 2018;35(2):188–97.
7. Hruza LL, Mallory SB, Fitzgibbons J, et al. Linear IgA bullous dermatosis in a neonate. Pediatr Dermatol 1993;10(2):171–6.
8. Gluth MB, Witman PM, Thompson DM. Upper aerodigestive tract complications in a neonate with linear IgA bullous dermatosis. Int J Pediatr Otorhinolaryngol 2004;68(7):965–70.
9. Kishida Y, Kameyama J, Nei M, et al. Linear IgA bullous dermatosis of neonatal onset: case report and review of the literature. Acta Paediatr 2004;93(6):850–2.
10. Lee SY, Leung CY, Leung CW, et al. Linear IgA bullous dermatosis in a neonate. Arch Dis Child Fetal Neonatal Ed 2004;89(3):F280.
11. Akin MA, Gunes T, Akýn L, et al. A newborn with bullous pemphigoid associated with linear IgA bullous dermatosis. Acta Dermatovenerol Alp Pannonica Adriat 2009;18(2):66–70.
12. Salud CM, Nicolas ME. Chronic bullous disease of childhood and pneumonia in a neonate with VATERL association and hypoplastic paranasal sinuses. J Am Acad Dermatol 2010;62(5):895–6.

13. Julapalli MR, Brandon KL, Rosales CM, et al. Neonatal linear immunoglobulin a bullous dermatosis: a rare presentation. Pediatr Dermatol 2012;29(5):610–3.

14. Romani L, Diociaiuti A, D'Argenio P, et al. A case of neonatal linear IgA bullous dermatosis with severe eye involvement. Acta Derm Venereol 2015;95(8):1015–7.

15. Mazurek MT, Banihani R, Wong J, et al. Uncomplicated neonatal linear IgA bullous dermatosis: a case report. J Cutan Med Surg 2018;22(4):431–4.

16. Wojnarowska F, Collier PM, Allen J, et al. The localization of the target antigens and antibodies in linear IgA disease is heterogeneous, and dependent on the methods used. Br J Dermatol 1995;132(5):750–7.

17. Mintz EM, Morel KD. Clinical features, diagnosis, and pathogenesis of chronic bullous disease of childhood. Dermatol Clin 2011;29(3):459–62, ix.

18. Wojnarowska F, Marsden RA, Bhogal B, et al. Chronic bullous disease of childhood, childhood cicatricial pemphigoid, and linear IgA disease of adults. A comparative study demonstrating clinical and immunopathologic overlap. J Am Acad Dermatol 1988;19(5 Pt 1):792–805.

19. Collier PM, Wojnarowska F, Millard PR. Variation in the deposition of the antibodies at different anatomical sites in linear IgA disease of adults and chronic bullous disease of childhood. Br J Dermatol 1992;127(5):482–4.

20. Eskin-Schwartz M, David M, Mimouni D. Mycophenolate mofetil for the management of autoimmune bullous diseases. Dermatol Clin 2011;29(4):555–9.

21. Eskin-Schwartz M, David M, Mimouni D. Mycophenolate mofetil for the management of autoimmune bullous diseases. Immunol Allergy Clin North Am 2012; 32(2):309–15, vii.

22. Frieden IJ. Aplasia cutis congenita: a clinical review and proposal for classification. J Am Acad Dermatol 1986;14(4):646–60.

23. Demmel U. Clinical aspects of congenital skin defects. I. Congenital skin defects on the head of the newborn. Eur J Pediatr 1975;121(1):21–50.

24. Yang A, Schweitzer R, Sun D, et al. p63 is essential for regenerative proliferation in limb, craniofacial and epithelial development. Nature 1999;398(6729):714–8.

25. Mills AA, Zheng B, Wang XJ, et al. p63 is a p53 homologue required for limb and epidermal morphogenesis. Nature 1999;398(6729):708–13.

26. Rinne T, Brunner HG, van Bokhoven H. p63-associated disorders. Cell Cycle 2007;6(3):262–8.

27. Zhang Z, Cheng R, Liang J, et al. Ankyloblepharon-ectodermal dysplasia-clefting syndrome misdiagnosed as epidermolysis bullosa and congenital ichthyosiform erythroderma: case report and review of published work. J Dermatol 2019; 46(5):422–5.

28. Chimanovitch I, Hamm H, Georgi M, et al. Bullous pemphigoid of childhood: autoantibodies target the same epitopes within the NC16A domain of BP180 as autoantibodies in bullous pemphigoid of adulthood. Arch Dermatol 2000;136(4): 527–32.

29. Nemeth AJ, Klein AD, Gould EW, et al. Childhood bullous pemphigoid. Clinical and immunologic features, treatment, and prognosis. Arch Dermatol 1991; 127(3):378–86.

30. Schwieger-Briel A, Moellmann C, Mattulat B, et al. Bullous pemphigoid in infants: characteristics, diagnosis and treatment. Orphanet J Rare Dis 2014;9:185.

31. Cohen PR, Kurzrock R. Sweet's syndrome and cancer. Clin Dermatol 1993;11(1): 149–57.

32. Uihlein LC, Brandling-Bennett HA, Lio PA, et al. Sweet syndrome in children. Pediatr Dermatol 2012;29(1):38–44.

33. Jain KK. Sweet's syndrome associated with granulocyte colony-stimulating factor. Cutis 1996;57(2):107–10.
34. Walker DC, Cohen PR. Trimethoprim-sulfamethoxazole-associated acute febrile neutrophilic dermatosis: case report and review of drug-induced Sweet's syndrome. J Am Acad Dermatol 1996;34(5 Pt 2):918–23.
35. Govindarajan G, Bashir Q, Kuppuswamy S, et al. Sweet syndrome associated with furosemide. South Med J 2005;98(5):570–2.
36. Khan Durani B, Jappe U. Drug-induced Sweet's syndrome in acne caused by different tetracyclines: case report and review of the literature. Br J Dermatol 2002;147(3):558–62.
37. Jovanović M, Poljacki M, Vujanović L, et al. Acute febrile neutrophilic dermatosis (Sweet's syndrome) after influenza vaccination. J Am Acad Dermatol 2005;52(2):367–9.
38. Gray PE, Bock V, Ziegler DS, et al. Neonatal Sweet syndrome: a potential marker of serious systemic illness. Pediatrics 2012;129(5):e1353–9.
39. Eichenfield LF, Frieden IJ, Mathes EF, et al. Neonatal and infant dermatology. 3rd edition. London: Elsevier Saunders; 2015.
40. Hernández-Martín Á, Nuño-González A, Colmenero I, et al. Eosinophilic pustular folliculitis of infancy: a series of 15 cases and review of the literature. J Am Acad Dermatol 2013;68(1):150–5.
41. Lerner LH, Wiss K, Gellis S, et al. An unusual pustular eruption in an infant with Down syndrome and a congenital leukemoid reaction. J Am Acad Dermatol 1996;35(2 Pt 2):330–3.
42. Nijhawan A, Baselga E, Gonzalez-Ensenat MA, et al. Vesiculopustular eruptions in Down syndrome neonates with myeloproliferative disorders. Arch Dermatol 2001;137(6):760–3.
43. Burch JM, Weston WL, Rogers M, et al. Cutaneous pustular leukemoid reactions in trisomy 21. Pediatr Dermatol 2003;20(3):232–7.
44. Uhara H, Shiohara M, Baba A, et al. Transient myeloproliferative disorder with vesiculopustular eruption: early smear is useful for quick diagnosis. J Am Acad Dermatol 2009;60(5):869–71.
45. Narvaez-Rosales V, de-Ocariz MS, Carrasco-Daza D, et al. Neonatal vesiculopustular eruption associated with transient myeloproliferative disorder: report of four cases. Int J Dermatol 2013;52(10):1202–9.
46. Nar I, Surmeli-Onay O, Aytac S, et al. Vesiculopustular eruption in neonatal transient myeloproliferative disorder. Indian J Pediatr 2014;81(4):391–3.
47. Solky BA, Yang FC, Xu X, et al. Transient myeloproliferative disorder causing a vesiculopustular eruption in a phenotypically normal neonate. Pediatr Dermatol 2004;21(5):551–4.
48. Herman LE, Rothman KF, Harawi S, et al. Congenital self-healing reticulohistiocytosis. A new entity in the differential diagnosis of neonatal papulovesicular eruptions. Arch Dermatol 1990;126(2):210–2.
49. Colon-Fontanez F, Eichenfield LE, Krous HF, et al. Congenital Langerhans cell histiocytosis: the utility of the Tzanck test as a diagnostic screening tool. Arch Dermatol 1998;134(8):1039–40.
50. Rowden G, Connelly EM, Winkelmann RK. Cutaneous histiocytosis X. The presence of S-100 protein and its use in diagnosis. Arch Dermatol 1983;119(7):553–9.
51. Satter EK, High WA. Langerhans cell histiocytosis: a review of the current recommendations of the Histiocyte Society. Pediatr Dermatol 2008;25(3):291–5.
52. Zaenglein AL, Steele MA, Kamino H, et al. Congenital self-healing reticulohistiocytosis with eye involvement. Pediatr Dermatol 2001;18(2):135–7.

53. Chunharas A, Pabunruang W, Hongeng S. Congenital self-healing Langerhans cell histiocytosis with pulmonary involvement: spontaneous regression. J Med Assoc Thai 2002;85(Suppl 4):S1309–13.
54. Larsen L, Merin MR, Konia T, et al. Congenital self-healing reticulohistiocytosis: concern for a poor prognosis. Dermatol Online J 2012;18(10):2.
55. Mandel VD, Ferrari C, Cesinaro AM, et al. Congenital "self-healing" Langerhans cell histiocytosis (Hashimoto-Pritzker disease): a report of two cases with the same cutaneous manifestations but different clinical course. J Dermatol 2014; 41(12):1098–101.
56. Hebert AA, Esterly NB. Bacterial and candidal cutaneous infections in the neonate. Dermatol Clin 1986;4(1):3–21.
57. Sandhu K, Kanwar AJ. Generalized bullous impetigo in a neonate. Pediatr Dermatol 2004;21(6):667–9.
58. James L, Gorwitz RJ, Jones RC, et al. Methicillin-resistant *Staphylococcus aureus* infections among healthy full-term newborns. Arch Dis Child Fetal Neonatal Ed 2008;93(1):F40–4.
59. Alsubaie S, Bahkali K, Somily AM, et al. Nosocomial transmission of community-acquired methicillin-resistant *Staphylococcus aureus* in a well-infant nursery of a teaching hospital. Pediatr Int 2012;54(6):786–92.
60. Smahi A, Courtois G, Vabres P, et al. Genomic rearrangement in NEMO impairs NF-kappaB activation and is a cause of incontinentia pigmenti. The International Incontinentia Pigmenti (IP) Consortium. Nature 2000;405(6785):466–72.
61. Fusco F, Paciolla M, Conte MI, et al. Incontinentia pigmenti: report on data from 2000 to 2013. Orphanet J Rare Dis 2014;9:93.
62. Meuwissen ME, Mancini GM. Neurological findings in incontinentia pigmenti; a review. Eur J Med Genet 2012;55(5):323–31.
63. Minić S, Trpinac D, Obradovic M. Incontinentia pigmenti diagnostic criteria update. Clin Genet 2014;85(6):536–42.
64. Deybach JC, de Verneuil H, Boulechfar S, et al. Point mutations in the uroporphyrinogen III synthase gene in congenital erythropoietic porphyria (Gunther's disease). Blood 1990;75(9):1763–5.
65. Phillips JD, Steensma DP, Pulsipher MA, et al. Congenital erythropoietic porphyria due to a mutation in GATA1: the first trans-acting mutation causative for a human porphyria. Blood 2007;109(6):2618–21.
66. Katugampola RP, Badminton MN, Finlay AY, et al. Congenital erythropoietic porphyria: a single-observer clinical study of 29 cases. Br J Dermatol 2012; 167(4):901–13.
67. Baran M, Eliacik K, Kurt I, et al. Bullous skin lesions in a jaundiced infant after phototherapy: a case of congenital erythropoietic porphyria. Turk J Pediatr 2013;55(2):218–21.
68. Hogeling M, Nakano T, Dvorak CC, et al. Severe neonatal congenital erythropoietic porphyria. Pediatr Dermatol 2011;28(4):416–20.
69. Garey JR, Hansen JL, Harrison LM, et al. A point mutation in the coding region of uroporphyrinogen decarboxylase associated with familial porphyria cutanea tarda. Blood 1989;73(4):892–5.
70. Lamoril J, Boulechfar S, de Verneuil H, et al. Human erythropoietic protoporphyria: two point mutations in the ferrochelatase gene. Biochem Biophys Res Commun 1991;181(2):594–9.
71. Piomelli S, Poh-Fitzpatrick MB, Seaman C, et al. Complete suppression of the symptoms of congenital erythropoietic porphyria by long-term treatment with high-level transfusions. N Engl J Med 1986;314(16):1029–31.

72. Katugampola RP, Anstey AV, Finlay AY, et al. A management algorithm for congenital erythropoietic porphyria derived from a study of 29 cases. Br J Dermatol 2012;167(4):888–900.
73. Kim D, Teng J. Scabies infection in a neonate. J Pediatr 2014;165(6): 1266–1266.e1.
74. Talanin NY, Smith SS, Shelley ED, et al. Cutaneous histiocytosis with Langerhans cell features induced by scabies: a case report. Pediatr Dermatol 1994;11(4): 327–30.
75. Burch JM, Krol A, Weston WL. *Sarcoptes scabiei* infestation misdiagnosed and treated as Langerhans cell histiocytosis. Pediatr Dermatol 2004;21(1):58–62.
76. Quarterman MJ, Lesher JL Jr. Neonatal scabies treated with permethrin 5% cream. Pediatr Dermatol 1994;11(3):264–6.
77. Mallon E, Wojnarowska F, Hope P, et al. Neonatal bullous eruption as a result of transient porphyrinemia in a premature infant with hemolytic disease of the newborn. J Am Acad Dermatol 1995;33(2 Pt 2):333–6.
78. Karg E, Kovacs L, Ignacz F, et al. Phototherapy-induced blistering reaction and eruptive melanocytic nevi in a child with transient neonatal porphyrinemia. Pediatr Dermatol 2018;35(5):e272–5.

Omenn Syndrome Identified by Newborn Screening

Matthew Tallar, MD*, John Routes, MD

KEYWORDS

- Neonatal • Severe combined immunodeficiency • SCID • Omenn syndrome • RAG1
- Newborn screen

KEY POINTS

- Diffuse erythematous/eczematous rash at birth should raise the question of immunodeficiency, especially Omenn syndrome versus maternal engraftment.
- Abnormal TREC assay must be followed-up with flow cytometry for lymphocyte enumeration including evaluation of B, T, NK, and naive/memory T cells.
- Omenn syndrome, a form of "Leaky" SCID, is due to hypomorphic mutations in any potential SCID-causing gene. Genetic sequencing is critical in evaluating the underlying case and may alter conditioning regimens for bone marrow transplantation.

INTRODUCTION

Severe combined immunodeficiency (SCID) is a group of diseases with several genetic causes, but all forms of SCID are characterized by a lack of naive T cells. SCID is universally fatal if not diagnosed and treated in infancy. Clinically, infants with SCID present with recurrent infections, failure to thrive, and chronic diarrhea. SCID is diagnosed by the absence or very low number of naive T cells ($<300/\mu L$ CD3 T cells) and reduced T cell function ($<10\%$ of the lower limit of normal) following response to T cell mitogens *in vitro* in infants that do not have a secondary cause for T cell lymphopenia.[1]

Newborn screening for SCID was begun in Wisconsin in 2008 and, as of 2018, all infants in the United States are screened at birth for SCID using the T cell receptor excision circle (TREC) assay. The T cell receptor is a heterodimer composed of either $\alpha\beta$ or $\gamma\delta$ chains. Approximately 95% of human T cells express the $\alpha\beta$ T cell receptor in peripheral blood. During T cell receptor rearrangement in the thymus, small, non-replicating pieces of DNA are formed known as TRECs. Using DNA extracted from dried blood spots on the newborn screening (NBS) card, the TREC assay enumerates a specific TREC that is generated by the formation of $\alpha\beta$ T cells by quantitative real-time polymerase chain reaction. TRECs do not replicate during cell division. Therefore,

Pediatrics, Medical College of Wisconsin, 9000 West Wisconsin Avenue Suite 440, Milwaukee, WI 53226, USA
* Corresponding author.
E-mail address: mtallar@mcw.edu

Clin Perinatol 47 (2020) 77–86
https://doi.org/10.1016/j.clp.2019.09.004
0095-5108/20/© 2019 Elsevier Inc. All rights reserved.
perinatology.theclinics.com

the TREC assay is a biomarker of the number of naive $\alpha\beta$ T cells (also known as recent thymic emigrants). The TREC assay has been shown to have a 100% sensitivity in detecting SCID.[2]

As an example, we describe a patient who had zero TRECs at NBS and who presented with diffuse erythroderma and flow cytometry consistent with T-B-NK$^+$ SCID. Using high-throughput (HT) DNA sequencing, the infant was subsequently diagnosed with Omenn syndrome because of biallelic mutations in the RAG1 gene. This case illustrates the utility of combining NBS for SCID using the TREC assay and HT DNA sequencing to determine the genetic cause of SCID and thereby optimizing Rx. This case also highlights the clinical problems associated with the diagnosis of T-B-NK$^+$ SCID.

CASE REPORT

A 5-day-old boy was urgently admitted with diffuse erythroderma, pustular rash on extremities, and zero TRECs on NBS. He was born at 38w3d gestational age to a group B streptococcus-negative mother. Rash was noted previous to discharge from the hospital incorrectly diagnosed as erythema toxicum versus transient neonatal pustular melanosis. Following discharge, the rash had progressively worsened with development of crusting in the periocular, perioral, and periauricular areas. Shotty cervical lymphadenopathy was present, but without hepatosplenomegaly. Because of his rash and zero TRECs on NBS he was urgently admitted to the hospital. He was evaluated by multiple subspecialists including dermatology, immunodeficiency, bone marrow transplant, and infectious disease specialists. Initial complete blood count demonstrated significant eosinophilia (**Table 1**). Subsequent flow cytometry showed marked CD3$^+$ lymphopenia with profound decrease in the number and percentage of naive CD4$^+$CD45RA$^+$ T cells, and a marked reduction B cells and normal numbers of natural killer (NK) cells (**Table 2**). In immunologically normal infants, greater than 90% of T cells are naive. Therefore, based on the presence of diffuse erythroderma in the setting of a severe decrease in the number of naive T cells, the diagnosis of T-B-NK$^+$ SCID was made with either Omenn syndrome or maternal engraftment. Chimerism testing in the infant showed that all the T cells were from the infant ruling

Table 1 Miscellaneous labs		
	Patient	**Normal**
WBC (/μL)	17,800	9100–34,000
Segs (%)	21	32–62
Lymphs (%)	17	26–36
Eos (%)	59	0–4
Abs Segs (/μL)	3700	2900–21,100
Abs Lymphs (/μL)	3000	2400–13,000
Abs Eos (/μL)	10,500	0–700
Unconjugated bilirubin (mg/dL)	14.9	0.6–10.5
Conjugated bilirubin (mg/dL)	0.0	0.0–0.6
IgG (mg/dL)	793	139–725
IgM (mg/dL)	5	11–68
IgA (mg/dL)	<6	1–40
IgE (mg/dL)	6	24–85

Table 2
Lymphocyte subset enumeration

Cell Type	Patient (/mm^3)	Normal (/mm^3)
CD3+	666	2500–5000
CD3+CD4+	484	1600–4000
CD3+CD8+	182	560–1700
CD56+	1785	170–1100
CD19+	30	300–2000

out maternal engraftment and establishing the diagnosis of Omenn syndrome. Empiric antimicrobial prophylaxis was initiated with ampicillin, cefepime, acyclovir, and fluconazole. Skin cultures were obtained showing few enterococcus and mixed cutaneous flora susceptible to ampicillin. Treatment with systemic corticosteroids and tacrolimus was started and the erythematous rash resolved.

Mutations in one of several genes are known to cause T-B-NK$^+$ SCID (**Table 3**). In terms of clinical management in this case, it is important to determine if the genetic cause of SCID (radiation-sensitive SCID) rendered the infant more sensitive to ionizing radiation or immunosuppressive drugs used in conditioning for hematopoietic stem cell transplantation (HSCT). Examples of T-B-NK$^+$ SCID radiation-sensitive SCID include damaging mutations in *LIG4*, *DCLRE1C*, *NHEJ1*, *PRKDC*, and *NBS1*. Targeted HT DNA sequencing that included all genes known to cause primary immunodeficiency was ordered and 1-week post-admission biallelic damaging mutations in the *RAG1* gene were found frame shift mutation (c.256_257del, p.(Lys86Valfs*33)) and missense (c.1186C>T, p.(Arg396Cys) mutation) thereby excluding radiation-sensitive SCID. Both *RAG1* mutations have been described previously in patients with Omenn syndrome.[3] HLA studies demonstrated that the proband's sister was a full HLA match and he subsequently underwent HLA matched HSCT and is currently fully engrafted without significant problems.

Table 3
Classification of SCID based on lymphocyte subsets

Type	Gene Mutations
T-B + NK$^-$	*IL2RG* *JAK3*
T-B-NK$^+$	*RAG1* *RAG2* *DCLRE1C* *PRKDC* *LIG4* *NHEJ1* *NBS1*
T-B + NK$^+$	*IL7R* *CD3D(δ)* *CD3E(ε)* *CD247(ζ)*
T-B-NK$^-$	ADA PNP AK2

DISCUSSION
Overview of Newborn Screening for Severe Combined Immunodeficiency

SCID is a heterogenous group of disorders owing to absence or low presence of T cells and no or low T cell function. They are traditionally classified into 4 different groups based on the presence of absence of NK and B cells (see **Table 3**). SCID is further subdivided into 2 categories based on the number and function of T cells. "Typical" SCID is defined as the absence or extremely low number of CD3$^+$ T cells (<300/μL) with no or very low T cell function (<10% of the lower limit of normal) measured by the proliferative response to the T cell mitogen, phytohemagglutinin (PHA). In contrast, in "leaky" SCID, T cell counts are higher and range from 300 to 1500/μL with a reduction of between 10% and 50% of the normal response to PHA. Leaky SCID is due to hypo-morphic mutations (mutations in genes in which the protein product has residual function) in a gene that causes typical SCID. The residual function of the protein production of the gene leads to an increased number of T cells in the periphery and increased T cell function compared with typical SCID. In both typical and leaky SCID, the infants have a profound deficiency in naive T cells.[4] Therefore, it is of critical importance to measure the number of naive (CD45RA$^+$) and memory (CD45RO$^+$) T cells in the evaluation of infants with an abnormal NBS for SCID.

Newborn screening through the TREC assay has improved the early detection and outcomes of infants with SCID. In the largest study to date over 3 million newborn infants from 10 states (CA, CO, CT, DE, MA, MI, MS, NY, TX, and WI) and the Navajo Nation were screened for SCID using the TREC assay between January of 2008 and July of 2013. Fifty-two infants were found to have SCID, with a frequency of 1 in 58,000 newborns, significantly higher than the previously reported rate of 1 in 100,000 live births. Importantly, no cases of SCID were missed by the TREC assay.

Mutations in *IL2RG* (IL-2 receptor γ), which is X-linked, was found to be the most common genetic cause of typical SCID followed by mutations in *ADA* and *RAG1* (**Fig. 1**). In contrast, mutations in *RAG1* were the most common cause of "leaky SCID" (see **Fig. 1**). The percentage of patients with either typical or leaky SCID that were ultimately found to have mutations in *IL2RG* was much lower than reported before NBS for SCID, whereas the number of patients with mutations in *RAG1* was higher.

A very small percentage of infants was found to have low T cell counts, did not have secondary causes of T cell lymphopenia (**Table 4**), and did not fit the definition of either typical or leaky SCID. These infants had idiopathic T cell lymphopenia. The cause, clinical course, and frequency of idiopathic T cell lymphopenia detected in newborns remains to be defined. However, the T cell counts normalize in approximately one-third of patients.[5]

The TREC assay that is performed in NBS for SCID is a biomarker for naive T cells. Therefore, it is not surprising that secondary causes of T cell lymphopenia account for the vast majority of positive TREC results on NBS (**Fig. 2**). Excluding prematurity, congenital syndromes such as 22q11.2 deletion syndrome and other secondary causes leading to T cell loss from the intravascular compartment (cardiac abnormalities or multiple congenital abnormalities) are the most common cause of a positive TREC assay on NBS (see **Fig. 2**). Importantly, the TREC assay only detects a minority of patients with 22q11.2 deletion syndrome because T cell lymphopenia is not severe enough to be detected.

HSCT is currently the most commonly used treatment for SCID and leaky SCID and results in a long-term survival of greater than 90%.[6] As expected, long-term outcomes of HSCT for SCID is improved if the transplant is performed before infection.[6]

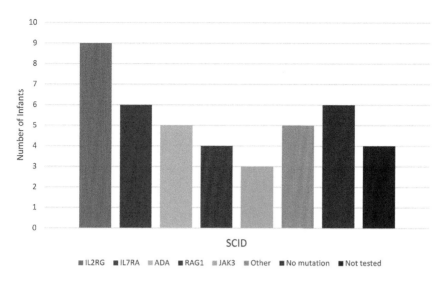

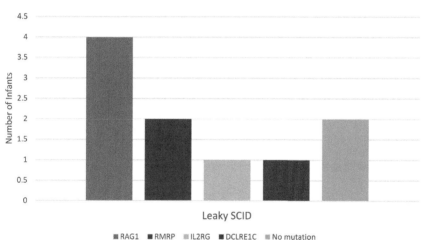

Fig. 1. Genetic etiology of SCID or leaky SCID in infants detected by NBS for SCID. (*Data from* Kwan A, Abraham RS, Currier R, et al. Newborn screening for severe combined immunodeficiency in 11 screening programs in the United States. JAMA 2014;312(7):729-38 https://doi.org/10.1001/jama.2014.9132[published Online First: Epub Date].)

Alternative forms of treatment include gene therapy and adenosine deaminase enzyme replacement therapy in ADA SCID.

T-B-NK⁺ severe combined immunodeficiency/Omenn syndrome

Typical SCID traditionally has been divided into 4 discrete phenotypes based on the presence or absence of NK and B cells (see **Table 3**). Our discussion focusses on T-B-NK⁺ SCID, which was present in the current case.

Molecular mutations in the recombinase activating genes (*RAG*) are the most common cause of T-B-NK⁺ SCID (see **Fig. 1**). *RAG1* and *RAG2* are essential in the V(D)J recombination of B and T cell receptors. Expression of *RAG1* and *RAG2* is limited to lymphocytes, and mutations in these genes do not lead to radiation-sensitive SCID.

Table 4
Secondary causes of T cell lymphopenia

Type	Disorder
Genetic syndromes	22q11.2 deletion
	Trisomy 21
	Ataxia telangiectasia
	Trisomy 18
	CHARGE
	Jacobsen
	CLOVES
	ECC
	Fryns
	Nijmegen breakage
	Noonan syndrome
	Rac2 defect
	Renpenning
	TAR
	Cytogenetic
Medial conditions	Congenital heart vascular leakage
	Hydrops
	GI anomalies
	Leukemia
Idiopathic	

Abbreviations: CHARGE, coloboma, heart defects, atresia choanae (choanal atresia), growth retardation, genital abnormalities, and ear abnormalities; CLOVES, congenital lipomatous (fatty) overgrowth, vascular malformations, epidermal nevi and scoliosis/skeletal/spinal anomalies; ECC, ectrodactyly, ectodermal, dysplasia, cleft lip/palate; Rac2, Rac family small GTPase 2; TAR, thrombocytopenia absent radius.

Recombinase activating gene defects account for approximately 50% of T-B-NK$^+$ SCID with phenotypes ranging from typical SCID to Omenn syndrome. Null mutations in the *RAG* genes cause typical SCID, whereas hypomorphic mutations lead to Omenn syndrome.[7] In contrast, genes involved in the non-homologous end-joining pathway (NHEJ) of DNA repair (*DCLRE1C* [Artemis], *PRKDC*, *NEHJ1*, *NBS1*, and *LIG4*) are ubiquitously expressed and mutations in these genes lead to radiation-sensitive SCID.

The clinical presentation of infants with T-B-NK$^+$ Omenn syndrome is distinct from typical T-B-NK$^+$ SCID. Infants with Omenn usually present with diffuse erythroderma and eosinophilia. Gastrointestinal tract involvement with diarrhea and hepatosplenomegaly are frequently present and Omenn syndrome is clinically similar to graft versus host disease (GVHD). The clinical manifestations of Omenn syndrome are secondary to the infiltration of activated, anergic, oligoclonal T cells that migrate into and damage organs such as skin, liver, spleen, and intestine.[8] Hypomorphic mutations of *RAG1* or *RAG2* are the most common cause of Omenn syndrome. However, hypomorphic mutations in any gene that can cause SCID may be responsible.[9]

Maternal T cells can be transmitted to infants during the birthing process, engraft, and proliferate. In infants with SCID, maternally engrafted lymphocytes may result in a similar clinical phenotype as Omenn syndrome. In both maternal engraftment and Omenn syndrome, the number of T cells in the peripheral blood is higher than that found in typical SCID. Nearly all of the T cells in both Omenn syndrome and maternal engraftment are memory (CD3$^+$CD45RO$^+$) and not naive T cells (CD3$^+$CD45RA$^+$). The vast majority of T cells in immunologically normal infants are naive T cells. To distinguish between maternal engraftment and Omenn syndrome chimerism studies

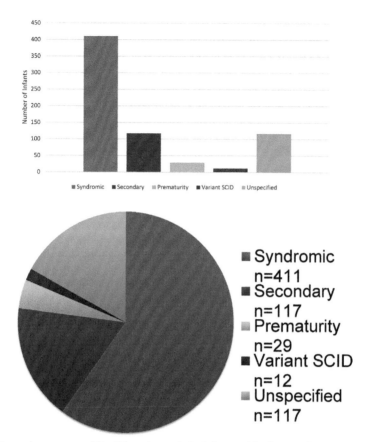

Fig. 2. Secondary causes of T cell lymphopenia in infants with abnormal NBS assay for SCID. (*Data from* Kwan A, Abraham RS, Currier R, et al. Newborn screening for severe combined immunodeficiency in 11 screening programs in the United States. JAMA 2014;312(7):729-38 https://doi.org/10.1001/jama.2014.9132[published Online First: Epub Date].)

must be performed to determine if the T cells are host- or maternally derived. It is important to rule out maternal engraftment syndrome before HSCT because its presence increases the risk of post-transplant GVHD.[10] Treatment of Omenn syndrome involves the use of immunosuppressive medications, usually corticosteroids and tacrolimus or cyclosporin and supportive care before HSCT.

Omenn syndrome was first described in 1965 by Gilbert S. Omenn MD. Before universal newborn screening Omenn syndrome patients would commonly present in the first year of life with chronic diarrhea, *Pneumocystis jiroveci* pneumonitis, and failure to thrive.[9] In contrast to SCID, Omenn syndrome by definition includes the presence of oligoclonal T cells, a reduction of between 10% and 50% of the normal response to PHA, eosinophilia, elevated IgE, erythroderma, and hepatosplenomegaly.[1] Typical symptoms, as noted above, develop within the first few weeks of live and were universally fatal, usually by 2 to 6 months of age.[11]

Infants with leaky SCID have reduced numbers of CD3[+] T cells (300–1500/μL) with decreased but not absent T cell proliferation to mitogens. T cells in leaky SCID are of host, not maternal, origin. Lymphoproliferation leading to hepatosplenomegaly and lymphadenopathy and progressive erythroderma are not common features of leaky

SCID.[4] Similar to Omenn syndrome and maternal engraftment, in leaky SCID the T cells present are all of the memory phenotype. In Omenn syndrome, maternal engraftment and leaky SCID TRECs are low or absent in the TREC assay despite having a significant number of T cells in the peripheral blood. TRECs do not replicate and are diluted out with the multiple rounds of T cell division that occur in Omenn syndrome or maternal engraftment.

Radiation sensitivity and severe combined immunodeficiency

Disorders with defects in the NHEJ pathway of DNA repair such as DCLRE1C (Artemis) and NHEJ1 are causes of radiation-sensitive T-B-NK+ SCID. Genes in the NHEJ pathways of DNA repair are expressed in all nucleated cells including stem cells. Consequently, defects in NHEJ pathway generally, but not always, lead to phenotypic abnormalities such as microcephaly, developmental delay, and impaired growth. Patients with defects in the NHEJ pathway are more susceptible to damage from alkylating agents and ionizing radiation, which leads to alterations in the pre-conditioning regimens before HSCT.[12] Diagnostic studies using radiation are typically restricted, if even possible, making these infants challenging to clinically manage. Overall survival with HSCT of patients with SCID due to mutations in DCLRE1C has been shown to be equivalent to HSCT with defects in RAG.[13] However, patients with mutations in DCLRE1C developed more late-term complications such as growth delay, endocrine abnormalities, and dental issues.[13] The optimal pre-conditioning regimens for patients with defects in NHEJ pathway is an area of active research.

High-throughput DNA sequencing

The ability to quickly analyze the human genome has dramatically increased since the introduction of Sanger sequencing in 1986.[14] In 2008 the first genomic sequence generated from HT DNA sequencing was published.[15] Since that time the technology of HT DNA sequencing has continued to rapidly advance allowing for diagnosis of known and previously genetic causes of human disease. Whole-exome DNA sequencing (sequencing the entire exomes of all genes) and targeted DNA sequencing (sequencing a panel of genes) are increasingly used in medical practice. For many diseases such as SCID, metabolic disorders, and other genetic diseases early diagnosis is tantamount to treatment and the long-term survival in patients.

HT DNA sequencing is increasingly used to aid in the genetic diagnosis and treatment of infants with SCID. HT DNA sequencing provides a rapid and cost-effective approach to evaluate the multiple genes that can lead to T cell lymphopenia and SCID. For example, Yu and colleagues[16] published a series of 20 patients with low TRECs on newborn screening or a positive family history or clinical suspicion of SCID or other primary immunodeficiency disease. Genetic causes of disease were identified in 70% of these infants. In our patient, a genetic diagnosis of Omenn syndrome due to biallelic mutations in RAG1 were found within a week through HT DNA sequencing. The genetic etiology of SCID simplified the management of the patient and led to optimization of the treatment plan for HSCT.

SUMMARY

Omenn syndrome is a form of leaky SCID due to hypomorphic mutations in any potential SCID-causing gene, which significantly reduces, but does not completely eliminate, T cell development.[9] Before NBS for SCID, these infants presented with diffuse, severe erythroderma, hepatosplenomegaly, failure to thrive, chronic diarrhea, and infectious complications. Chimerism studies are necessary to demonstrate that the T cells are not of maternal origin. Enumeration of the numbers of NK, B, and

T cells, including memory and naive T cells, is also essential in the evaluation of these patients. HT DNA sequencing can aid in the management of these patients by defining genetic etiology and determining if the form of SCID is radiation sensitive. Immunosuppressive therapy can improve the clinical manifestations of Omenn syndrome (eg, skin, GI manifestations) and allow for successful HSCT.

Best Practices

What is the current practice?

Omenn syndrome

Best practice/guideline/care path objectives
- Promptly enumerate the number of naive and memory T, NK, and B cells in an infant with zero TRECs on NBS and a diffuse erythematous rash.
- In a newborn infant with a diffuse erythematous rash and a large number of memory T cells in the peripheral blood, determine the origin of the T cells (maternal or infant) by ordering chimerism studies.
- Prompt immunosuppressive therapy is needed to treat the erythroderma and lymphoproliferation in Omenn syndrome.
- Defining the genetic etiology of Omenn syndrome can optimize the treatment.

What changes in current practice are likely to improve outcomes?

- NBS for SCID combined with HT DNA sequencing to define the genetic etiology will improve outcomes for infants with SCID.

Major recommendation

- Enumerate the number of naive and memory T, NK, and B cells in an infant with an abnormal NBS for SCID.

- Define the genetic etiology to facilitate the treatment and improve the outcome of infants with SCID.

- *Summary statement.* The diagnosis of infants with SCID by NBS will lead to decreased mortality.

- Defining the genetic etiology of SCID can facilitate the treatment and improve the outcome of such infants.

A high index of suspicion for Omenn syndrome/leaky SCID in any patient born with diffuse erythroderma and zero TRECs on NBC is essential for early diagnosis and treatment in these infants.

DISCLOSURE

The authors have nothing to disclose.

REFERENCES

1. Kwan A, Abraham RS, Currier R, et al. Newborn screening for severe combined immunodeficiency in 11 screening programs in the United States. JAMA 2014; 312(7):729–38.

2. Routes J, Verbsky J. Newborn screening for severe combined immunodeficiency. Curr Allergy Asthma Rep 2018;18(6):34.

3. Matthews AG, Briggs CE, Yamanaka K, et al. Compound heterozygous mutation of Rag1 leading to Omenn syndrome. PLoS One 2015;10(4):e0121489.

4. Delmonte OM, Schuetz C, Notarangelo LD. RAG deficiency: two genes, many diseases. J Clin Immunol 2018;38(6):646–55.

5. Albin-Leeds S, Ochoa J, Mehta H, et al. Idiopathic T cell lymphopenia identified in New York state newborn screening. Clin Immunol 2017;183:36–40.

6. Heimall J, Logan BR, Cowan MJ, et al. Immune reconstitution and survival of 100 SCID patients post-hematopoietic cell transplant: a PIDTC natural history study. Blood 2017;130(25):2718–27.

7. Notarangelo LD, Kim MS, Walter JE, et al. Human RAG mutations: biochemistry and clinical implications. Nat Rev Immunol 2016;16(4):234–46.

8. Gruber TA, Shah AJ, Hernandez M, et al. Clinical and genetic heterogeneity in Omenn syndrome and severe combined immune deficiency. Pediatr Transplant 2009;13(2):244–50.

9. Villa A, Notarangelo LD, Roifman CM. Omenn syndrome: inflammation in leaky severe combined immunodeficiency. J Allergy Clin Immunol 2008;122(6):1082–6.

10. Wahlstrom J, Patel K, Eckhert E, et al. Transplacental maternal engraftment and posttransplantation graft-versus-host disease in children with severe combined immunodeficiency. J Allergy Clin Immunol 2017;139(2):628–33.e10.

11. Omenn GS. Familial reticuloendotheliosis with eosinophilia. N Engl J Med 1965; 273:427–32.

12. Cowan MJ, Gennery AR. Radiation-sensitive severe combined immunodeficiency: the arguments for and against conditioning before hematopoietic cell transplantation–what to do? J Allergy Clin Immunol 2015;136(5):1178–85.

13. Schuetz C, Neven B, Dvorak CC, et al. SCID patients with ARTEMIS vs RAG deficiencies following HCT: increased risk of late toxicity in ARTEMIS-deficient SCID. Blood 2014;123(2):281–9.

14. Picard C, Fischer A. Contribution of high-throughput DNA sequencing to the study of primary immunodeficiencies. Eur J Immunol 2014;44(10):2854–61.

15. Wheeler DA, Srinivasan M, Egholm M, et al. The complete genome of an individual by massively parallel DNA sequencing. Nature 2008;452(7189):872–6.

16. Yu H, Zhang VW, Stray-Pedersen A, et al. Rapid molecular diagnostics of severe primary immunodeficiency determined by using targeted next-generation sequencing. J Allergy Clin Immunol 2016;138(4):1142–11451.e2.

Congenital Diarrheal Syndromes

Abdul Aziz Elkadri, MD

KEYWORDS

- Congenital diarrhea • VEOIBD • Enteropathy

KEY POINTS

- Congenital diarrheal disorders constitute a heterogeneous group of conditions that range from simple cow's milk protein intolerance to life-threatening defects of membrane polarization requiring intestinal transplantation.
- Advances in genomics has improved our understanding of the genotypic and phenotypic correlations, leading to a changing classification of the underlying defects of congenital diarrheal disorders.
- Understanding these underlying defects led to targeted and novel therapies, and guided providers away from potentially detrimental therapies for specific defects.

Congenital diarrheal disorders are a heterogeneous group of conditions characterized by watery diarrhea that can potentially lead to massive life-threatening fluid and electrolyte shifts within the first few months of life. As a broad range of illnesses can present similarly in infants, establishing the cause of neonatal- or infantile-onset diarrhea is challenging, with causes ranging from simple cow's milk protein intolerance to membrane polarization defects that require long-term total parental nutrition and possibly intestinal transplantation. Subtle forms of these disorders may go unnoticed during the early months of life and may present later with irreversible complications and significant morbidity and mortality; timely diagnosis is essential in preventing these complications and in identifying disorders that may have extraintestinal manifestations.

Advances in genomic medicine have led to improved understanding of congenital diarrheal disorders, increasing the list of identified causative genes, and the spectrum of genotype-phenotype correlations. Infantile diarrheal disorders are grouped into 5 categories based on pathophysiologic mechanisms and functional defects:[1]

1. Epithelial nutrient and electrolyte transport defects
2. Epithelial enzyme and metabolism defects
3. Epithelial trafficking and polarity defects

Medical College of Wisconsin, 8701 Watertown Plank Road, Milwaukee, WI, USA

E-mail address: aelkadri@mcw.edu

Clin Perinatol 47 (2020) 87–104
https://doi.org/10.1016/j.clp.2019.10.010

4. Enteroendocrine cell dysfunction
5. Immune dysregulation-associated enteropathy

Other similar classification schemes propose combining epithelial enzyme defects with nutrient and electrolyte transport defects.[2] As the understanding of these disorders improves, and as the implementation of molecular genetic testing increases, this current classification system will expand rather than contract. For example, the disorder associated with pathogenic variants in *PLVAP*, the gene encoding plasmalemma vesicle-associated protein, is related to a physical defect in endothelial fenestrated diaphragms that allows for the unregulated passage of specifically sized serum proteins and subsequent loss of barrier function,[3] and would not cleanly fall into any of the above categories of pathophysiology. Regardless of the underlying pathophysiologic mechanism, the diagnostic approach to congenital diarrheal disorders consists of establishing the presence of diarrhea by history, ascertaining the composition of the stool, determining the response to fasting, and pursuing specialized testing as indicated.

CLASSIFICATION OF DIARRHEA

Diarrhea is generally defined as 3 or more loose watery bowel movements per day, with distinct episodes of diarrhea defined as being separated by at least 2 days of non-diarrheal stooling between episodes.[4] Diarrhea lasting longer than 2 weeks is classified as chronic diarrhea, with acute diarrhea mostly being caused by infections. With respect to acute, infectious diarrhea, invasive organisms tend to be associated with the presence of fecal leukocytes and blood within the stool, whereas toxin-producing organisms activate or inhibit electrolyte transport mechanisms, producing more voluminous, watery diarrhea. Chronic diarrhea may have a variety of compositions, depending on the cause.

As increased stool output is due to a change in stool composition; examining the composition of the stool is vital in determining the cause of chronic diarrhea. The primary distinction is between osmotic and secretory diarrhea (**Table 1**); diarrhea that does not fit either category is classified as mixed. Further refinements to this classification system have been suggested[1]: diet-induced diarrhea has been suggested in the place of osmotic diarrhea to describe stools driven by unabsorbed components of the diet, with examples including lactose intolerance and hereditary fructose intolerance. Electrolyte transport-related diarrhea has been suggested in the place of secretory diarrhea, because the term secretory, although adequately capturing the notion that the pathophysiology is secondary to an active process, does not capture

Table 1		
Differentiating osmotic diarrhea from secretory diarrhea		
Characteristic	Diet-Induced Diarrhea (Osmotic Diarrhea)	Electrolyte Transport-Related Diarrhea (Secretory Diarrhea)
Volume	Typically <200 mL/24 h	Typically >200 mL/24 h
Response to 24–48 h of fasting	Dramatic improvement of diarrhea	Continued diarrhea
Stool osmotic gap	>100 mOsm	<50 mOsm
Stool pH	<5	>6
Stool sodium	<50 mmol/L	Typically >50 mmol/L, but variability has been noted

when diarrhea is caused by the loss of electrolytes or reduced absorption related to a congenital defect in a cellular channel. Examples of electrolyte transport-related diarrhea include congenital sodium-losing diarrhea and *Salmonella* enteritis.

History

Certain historical features may assist in determining the extent of diagnostic evaluation required. Because infectious and allergic causes are high on the differential diagnosis of congenital diarrhea, determining the timing of onset of symptoms is essential. A preceding introduction of formula may indicate an allergic cause, and the presence of other family members with similar symptoms may suggest infections. A detailed prenatal history is also helpful, with some congenital channelopathies resulting in polyhydramnios due to increased intestinal output in the fetus; prenatally identified dilated bowel loops are found in a variety of congenital gastrointestinal disorders. As a large number of congenital diarrheal syndromes are inherited in an autosomal recessive manner, a history of consanguinity may add greater import to pursuing genetic testing. Similarly, as there is a higher incidence of congenital diarrhea within some ethnic groups, specifically Middle Eastern, South Asian, Japanese, and Finnish groups, genetic testing may have a higher yield under these circumstances.

History should also delineate the consistency of stool. Oily stools suggest disorders of fat metabolism and transport, whereas an inability to distinguish stool from urine suggests an enteropathy or channelopathy. Foul-smelling stools generally suggest fermentation of components within the stool, as is the case with carbohydrate malabsorption. Diarrhea during daytime suggests toddler's diarrhea. A nutritional assessment, focusing on the growth and development of the infant, will suggest whether there is malnutrition secondary to malabsorption of nutrients.

Response to Fasting

One of the first steps in determining the cause of diarrhea is a simple fast. As the presence of unabsorbed dietary components within the intestinal lumen may be the ultimate cause, a period of fasting will allow for differentiating between diet-induced diarrhea and electrolyte transport-related diarrhea. Fasts should be 24 to 48 hours in duration,[5] as shorter intervals may result in subjective although transient and incomplete improvement in stool output, with resulting diagnostic confusion. Fasting in the setting of mixed diarrhea may still result in relative improvement, although fasting in the setting of diet-induced diarrhea should lead to definite improvement in stool output, allowing for better differentiation.

Stool Osmolality

Stool is up to 75% water; bacterial biomass comprises up to half of the solid components, and the remainder consists of undigested material.[6] As water makes up such a large part of stool, any increase in water content results in a great increase in stool volume. The normal stool volume in infants is around 10 mL/kg/d; 20 mL/kg/d or greater is generally considered diarrhea.[7]

The stool osmotic gap allows for the calculation of the contribution of electrolytes to the stool osmolality and is determined via the following formula:

$$\text{Osmotic gap} = 290 - [2 \times ([\text{Stool Na}^+] + [\text{Stool K}^+])]$$

Electrolyte transport-related diarrhea will contain a large amount of sodium and chloride, resulting in a lower stool osmotic gap of less than 50 mOsm. Diet-induced diarrhea will contain additional osmotically active components, resulting in a higher stool osmotic gap of greater than 100 mOsm.

Stool pH

Carbohydrates that fail to be absorbed in the small intestine are metabolized by bacteria on reaching the colon, undergoing anaerobic fermentation and producing C2-C6 short-chain fatty acids.[8] The presence of these fatty acids causes the pH of the stool to change from its typical neutral-to-increased value to a pH below 5. However, stool pH should not be used in isolation when assessing for carbohydrate malabsorption, because variations in diet can produce transient decreases in stool pH, and healthy neonates can often have relative carbohydrate malabsorption during the early development of the intestinal tract.[9]

Stool-Reducing Substances

Carbohydrate malabsorption can be demonstrated more directly by identifying reducing sugars in the stool, rather than by measuring the presence of fermented byproducts.[10] Stool-reducing substance assays detect the presence of an aldehyde or ketone group, effectively revealing the presence of carbohydrates within the stools, because all unabsorbed monosaccharides, as well as some disaccharides and oligosaccharides, contain aldehyde or ketone groups. Sucrose, however, is a nonreducing sugar, and will not be detected. Specimens must be liquid and should be submitted to the laboratory or frozen immediately to avoid further fermentation of the reducing sugars within the stool. A result of greater than 0.5% indicates malabsorption of a reducing sugar.

Stool Electrolytes

In addition to allowing for the calculation of the stool osmotic gap, stool electrolyte measurement can provide insight into particular electrolyte transport defects. Normal values for stool sodium range from 20 to 50 mmol/L. Interestingly, 1 patient with a confirmed congenital sodium-losing diarrhea was found to have a stool sodium of 30 mmol/L on 1 measurement,[11] suggesting that repeat stool studies may be necessary in cases with a high index of suspicion. Potassium absorption within the small bowel is typically high,[12] and as such it is highly atypical to find an increased stool potassium-level. Normal values are 83 to 95 mmol/L.[12] Increased stool potassium levels may be seen in neuroblastoma,[13] colonic pseudo-obstruction,[14,15] severe hemorrhagic shock,[11] and end-stage renal disease.[16] The normal range for stool chloride is 5 to 25 mmol/L; increases beyond this normal range can be associated with congenital chloride diarrhea, with values greater than 90 mmol/L being highly suggestive of this disorder.

Fecal Fat

The digestion of dietary fat requires the presence of lipase and bile acids, as well as the ability of the mucosa to absorb and the lymphatics to transport fat. Failure of any of these components may result in an increased fecal fat level and produce steatorrhea. Also, any condition decreasing bowel transit time will generally result in an increased stool fat due to the decreased time available to process fat. Reliably demonstrating abnormal fecal fat excretion requires quantifying the fat content of all stool output collected over a 72-hour period,[17,18] and is difficult to perform: in addition to collecting, storing, and transporting this potentially large volume of stool, dietary fat intake must remain consistent throughout the 72 hours. Normal levels are not definitively established, although they range from 5 to 15 g of fat per 100 g of stool.

Alternatively, stool microscopy for fat globules may provide a qualitative assessment as to the presence of fecal fat and can be performed in most laboratories using Sudan III or Carmine Red stain.[19,20] If there is sufficient clinical concern for fat malabsorption, or if fecal fat assays suggest fat malabsorption, fat-soluble vitamins should be assayed as well.

Fecal Elastase

Pancreatic sufficiency can be determined by testing fecal elastase-1 levels in stool. Levels are invariably low in meconium in all neonates, although term neonates with sufficient exocrine pancreatic function attain normal levels by 3 days of life once stools have transitioned. Premature infants born before 28 weeks of gestation attain normal levels by 14 days.[21] Fecal elastase-1 levels below 100 μg per gram of feces are indicative of exocrine pancreatic insufficiency; values between 100 and 200 μg per gram of feces are indeterminate. Supplementation with oral pancreatic enzymes does not affect testing, as porcine supplemental enzymes do not cross-react.[22] Fecal elastase testing is most sensitive when performed on formed stools, and, hence, a higher index of suspicion is required for infants and neonates due to their relatively unformed stools, as looser stools may sometimes result in falsely negative results.

Sweat Testing

The cystic fibrosis transmembrane conductance regulator (CFTR) is an ion channel for the transmembrane movement of chloride. Within the epithelial lining of the bowels, this channel is involved in the movement of fluid into mucus and is the target of enterotoxin, which results in an acute, infectious, and severe watery diarrhea. Although vital in chloride transport in the intestine, the diarrhea in patients with cystic fibrosis is typically secondary to pancreatic insufficiency, and not to dysfunction of the ion channel. Sweat chloride testing is the gold standard for diagnosing cystic fibrosis and CFTR-related metabolic syndrome.

Endoscopic Evaluation

In patients for whom evaluation does not clearly suggest diet-induced diarrhea, endoscopic evaluation with retrieval of tissue for further analysis is vital. Both upper endoscopy and colonoscopy are essential and identify the cause in the vast majority of cases.[23] Biopsies should be obtained, even when endoscopy appears grossly normal, as some autoimmune forms of enterocolitis may only be evident on pathology review.[24] Hematoxylin and eosin staining will delineate the immune activity and level of infiltration of the mucosa and can distinguish acute from chronic processes. Specimens for electron microscopy should also be obtained because polarization and enterocyte differentiation defects may not be evident on light microscopy. Disaccharidase testing[25] can determine the absence of lactase, sucrase, or isomaltase, but interpretation can sometimes be technically challenging and may show absence of activity in processes that cause villous blunting of the small bowel.

Molecular Genetic Testing

Given the increased appreciation of the genetic heterogeneity of inherited diarrheal disorders, single-gene testing has largely been supplanted with multigene panels and exome or genome sequencing, particularly in light of the increasing cost-effectiveness of these modalities. Molecular genetic testing has also supplanted less-specific functional assays, such as antienterocyte antibody testing in patients with autoimmune enteropathy, specifically when occurring within the context of additional syndromic features of immune dysregulation, polyendocrinopathy, enteropathy, and X-linked inheritance (IPEX). Genetic testing was able to demonstrate that most patients with this phenotypic constellation had a pathogenic variant within the *FOXP3* gene. Subsequently, in a large cohort of 173 patients with an IPEX phenotype,[26] 85 (49.1%) had no identifiable variant within the *FOXP3* gene; pathogenic variants within 9 other genes were found to result in a *FOXP3*-negative IPEX-like disorder.

Determining a genetic causality can allow for specific therapy, such as antiinterleukin-1 therapy in patients with mevalonate kinase deficiency,[27] or the avoidance of potentially life-threatening and ineffective therapies, such as hematopoietic stem cell transplantation in patients with epithelial barrier defects that were previously presumed to be immune-mediated, as the underlying defect remains despite transplantation.

Known genetic causes of infantile diarrhea

An overview of congenital diarrheal disorders is provided in **Table 2**. Specific disorders are discussed in greater detail below.

DEFECTS IN EPITHELIAL NUTRIENT AND ELECTROLYTE TRANSPORT
Congenital Chloride Diarrhea

Inherited in an autosomal recessive fashion and associated with pathogenic variants in *SLC26A3*, the gene that encodes for a coupled chloride-bicarbonate exchanger, this form of diarrhea is characterized by distal ileal chloride loss and bicarbonate retention, leading to a hypochloremic metabolic alkalosis. Stools are acidic, mainly secondary to activation of the sodium/hydrogen exchanger (NHE2 and NHE3); activation of the renin/angiotensin/aldosterone system results in hypokalemia. Multiple patient cohorts have been described, but genotype-phenotype correlations are still being defined.[16,28–30] In general, infants are noted to have distended loops of bowel, and most present with large-volume acidic diarrhea from birth. Meconium is typically absent, likely due to the large volume of watery diarrhea. Many patients manifest enamel defects, and in some patients of Finnish ancestry, intestinal inflammation may develop. The presentation may mimic Bartter or Gitelman syndromes,[31] particularly with respect to hypokalemia and metabolic alkalosis. The treatment is lifelong chloride supplementation in the form of either sodium or potassium chloride, and aggressive fluid supplementation when stool output increases. Oral butyrate has been suggested as a treatment, with mixed results.[29,32]

Congenital Sodium Diarrhea

Pathogenic variants in several genes have been associated with congenital sodium diarrhea; despite this genetic heterogeneity, the disorder itself is rare. Underlying all forms is an intrauterine-onset high-volume stool output with a high sodium content. A syndromic form is associated with pathogenic variants in *SPINT2*[33] and is characterized by a defect similar to that of congenital tufting enteropathy, but with other phenotypic defects, specifically facial features. Pathogenic variants in *SLC9A3* are associated with a sodium-losing diarrhea, which seems to be more significant during infancy, requiring enteral or parenteral sodium supplementation.[11,34] It is also associated with the development of inflammatory bowel disease, presumed to be secondary to changes in the microbiome related to sodium/hydrogen exchanger-induced changes in stool pH. Pathogenic variants in *GUCY2C* have been associated with a variable phenotype of small bowel obstruction, inflammatory bowel disease, and esophagitis.[35] These variants result in increased cyclic GMP production with resultant CFTR activation and chloride excretion. Interestingly, in a Bedouin cohort, autosomal recessive-inherited pathogenic variants resulting in deactivation of the *GUCY2C* gene produced a meconium ileus phenotype via inactivation of the CFTR gene.[36]

Glucose-Galactose Malabsorption

The absorption of glucose and galactose in the intestine is facilitated by the SGLT1 sodium/glucose cotransporter in the intestine, a protein encoded by the *SLC5A1* gene. Pathogenic variants in *SLC5A1* result in malabsorption of glucose and galactose[37–40] and a resulting osmotic diarrhea. Avoidance of both glucose and galactose is necessary, as well as avoidance of maltose, sucrose, and lactose, which are disaccharides broken down into glucose and, respectively, glucose, fructose, and galactose. As fructose is transported via a distinct transporter, it is used as the carbohydrate of choice in the diets of affected children to avoid the development of diarrhea.

Primary Bile Acid Diarrhea

Bile acids are necessary in the digestion of lipids within the intestinal tract. Enterohepatic circulation requires reuptake within the distal ileum using 2 transporters: SLC10A2 and SLC51B.[41] Pathogenic variants in the genes encoding these transporters have been associated with a fat malabsorption-related diarrhea secondary to the absence of bile acids[37,42]; patients with this disorder typically are deficient in fat-soluble vitamins as well.

Acrodermatitis Enteropathica

Zinc is absorbed within the duodenum and jejunum; defects in absorption result in a triad of symptoms: a scaly rash around the mouth and on the extremities, alopecia, and diarrhea. Affected patients are also at risk for immune dysfunction and recurrent infections. Defects within the transporter for zinc, SLC39A4, have been found in many affected Mediterranean families.[43] Treatment with oral zinc supplementation improves symptoms.

DEFECTS IN EPITHELIAL ENZYMES AND METABOLISM
Congenital Lactase Deficiency

Although primary lactase deficiency, colloquially known as lactose intolerance, is found in up to 75% of adults, and transient lactose intolerance is a common finding after infections,[44] congenital lactase deficiency is rare, described mainly in Finnish populations,[45] although in other populations as well.[46–48] Avoidance of lactose in formula or breast milk is required to prevent severe, potentially life-threatening dehydration from profuse diarrhea.

Congenital Sucrase-Isomaltase Deficiency

Congenital sucrase-isomaltase deficiency is rare, although the prevalence is as high as 5% among indigenous populations in Greenland and Canada.[49] With the relative ease of obtaining disaccharidase testing on intestinal biopsies and the advent of enzyme replacement therapy,[50] diagnosis and management have improved greatly, also showing the wide phenotypic variability inherent to this disorder, mainly due to the variability in the remaining enzyme activity. Isolated failure to thrive is a rare manifestation, whereas more severely affected individuals develop hypercalcemia, nephrocalcinosis, metabolic acidosis, and renal calculi.[51]

Table 2
Disorders leading to early-onset chronic diarrhea

Category	Disorder	Gene(s) Involved	Inheritance	Features
Defects in epithelial nutrient and electrolyte transport	Congenital chloride diarrhea	SLC26A3	AR	• High chloride in stools • Founder effect from Saudi Arabia (Taif region) and Finland • Premature with IUGR • Absence of meconium • Polyhydramnios and dilated loops of bowel on prenatal imaging, abdominal distension after birth • 24% had renal involvement (chronic kidney disease) • Dental carries • Some overlap with Bartter and Gitelman syndrome
	Congenital sodium diarrhea	SLC9A3 GUCY2C	AR AD	• Increased risk of development of IBD • Polyhydramnios and dilated loops of bowel on prenatal imaging • High sodium in stools • Diarrhea may improve with time
	Glucose-galactose malabsorption	SLC5A1	AR	• Treatment requires avoidance of all sugars other than fructose
	Primary bile acid diarrhea	SLC10A2 SLC51B	AR AR	• Associated with cholestasis, increased gamma-glutamyl transferase level, and fat-soluble vitamin deficiency
	Acrodermatitis enteropathica	SLC39A4	AR	• Perioral and extremity lesions, alopecia, and diarrhea • Recurrent infection from immune dysfunction

Category	Disease	Gene	Inheritance	Notes
Defects in epithelial enzymes and metabolism	Congenital lactase deficiency	LCT	AR	• Rare form of inherited diarrhea
	Congenital sucrase-isomaltase deficiency	SI	AR	• Bloating, diarrhea, and rarely associated with failure to thrive • High prevalence in Greenland and Inuit (5%), with 0.2% prevalence in Europeans • Variable phenotype
	Trehalase deficiency	TREH	AR	• Up to 8% of Greenland population • Similar to lactase deficiency
	Enterokinase deficiency	TMPRSS15	AR	• Deficiency of activator of pancreatic enzymes
	DGAT1 deficiency	DGAT1	AR	• Fat-soluble vitamin deficiency • Avoidance of enteral lipids seems to help
	Sieving protein-losing enteropathy	PLVAP	AR	• Protein loss of specific sizes • Syndromic with hydrops, dysmorphic facies, cardiac, and renal abnormalities
	Abetalipoproteinemia	MTTP	AR	• Enterocytes note lipid filled vacuoles
	Hypobetalipoproteinemia	APOB	AR	• Steatorrhea and failure to thrive
	Chylomicron retention disease	SAR1B	AR	• Later noted to have fat-soluble vitamin deficiency and bleeding issues
	Dyskeratosis congenita	DKC1 RTEL1	X AR	• Nail pitting, leukoplakia and immune defects
	Kabuki syndrome	KMT2D	AD	• Multiple congenital anomalies with varying phenotype
Defects in epithelial trafficking and polarity	Microvillous inclusion disease	MYO5B	AR	• Microvilli seen on electron microscopy are periodic acid Schiff positive • May be associated with Fanconi syndrome
		STX3	AR	• Rare form. May be associated with neurologic findings
	Tufting enteropathy	EPCAM	AR	• Teardrop-shaped tufts of enterocytes throughout the intestine
	Syndromic sodium-losing diarrhea	SPINT2	AR	• Phenotype similar to tufting enteropathy, but with sodium-losing diarrhea
	Trichohepatoenteric syndrome	TTC37 SKIV2L	AR AR	• Woolly hair, SCID-like phenotype and hepatic defects
	Familial hemophagocytic lymphohistiocytosis type 5	STXBP2	AR	• Recurrence after HSCT, villous blunting
	Multiple intestinal atresia	TTC7A	AR	• Variable phenotype with multiple intestinal atresia, SCID-like phenotype, and enterocolitis

(continued on next page)

Table 2 (continued)				
Category	Disorder	Gene(s) Involved	Inheritance	Features
Enteroendocrine cell dysfunction	Enteric anendocrinosis	NEUROG3	AR	• Severe malabsorptive diarrhea, neonatal-onset diabetes mellitus, and normal intestinal biopsies
	Proprotein convertase 1/3 deficiency	PCSK1	AR	• Age-dependent phenotype. Infants have TPN-dependent diarrhea and failure to thrive. Later appear to lose intestinal phenotype and develop multiple endocrine abnormalities
	X-linked lissencephaly with abnormal genitalia	ARX	X	• Seizures, abnormal genitalia, survival between 6 d to 6 y
	Mitchell-Riley syndrome	RFX6	AR	• Lack of enteroendocrine cells
	Intractable congenital diarrhea in infants	ICR	AR	• Secretory diarrhea caused by a noncoding variant with wide ranging effects on multiple intestinal genes
Immune dysregulation-associated enteropathy	Immune dysregulation, polyendocrinopathy, enteropathy X-linked	FOXP3	X	• Polyendocrinopathy
	Common variable immune deficiency (CVID) type 1	ICOS	AR	• Variable presentation. May have dietary-induced diarrhea
	CVID type 8	LRBA	AR	
	ADAM17 deficiency	ADAM17	AR	• Fatal in most patients
	EGFR deficiency	EGFR	AR	• Described in 3 patients
	CTLA-4	CTLA-4	AD	• Similar to LRBA. May respond to abatacept
	CD55 deficiency	CD55	AR	• Protein-losing enteropathy and thrombosis
	X-linked inhibitor of apoptosis	XIAP	X	• Responsive to HSCT

Abbreviations: AD, autosomal dominant; AR, autosomal recessive; EGFR, epidermal growth factor receptor; HSCT, hematopoietic stem cell transplantation; IBD, inflammatory bowel disease; IUGR intrauterine growth restriction; SCID, severe combined immunodeficiency; TPN, total parenteral nutrition; X, X-linked.

Trehalase Deficiency

Trehalose is an $\alpha(1,1)$-linked glucose dimer synthesized by certain bacteria, fungi, plants, and invertebrates, which is also used by the food industry to lower the freezing point of frozen foods. Deficiency of the disaccharidase trehalase is prevalent in up to 8% of the indigenous population in Greenland,[52] although is exceedingly rare outside of that population.[53] Symptoms are similar to those of lactose intolerance.

Enterokinase Deficiency

Within the duodenum, enterokinase activates pancreatic trypsinogen, which in turn activates the cascade of pancreatic enzymes. Deficiency is rare, but has been associated with failure to thrive, chronic diarrhea, and hypoalbuminemia.[54]

DGAT1 Deficiency

Patients with deficiency of the enzyme diacylglycerol-acyltransferase 1 secondary to pathogenic variants in the DGAT1 gene present with protein-losing enteropathy and fat-soluble vitamin deficiency. The mechanism has not been completely determined, but has been linked to aberrant lipid metabolism and increased susceptibility to lipid-induced cell death.[55] Treatment is the avoidance of enteral lipids and, if needed, parenteral lipid use. Also, fat-soluble vitamin supplementation is often necessary.

Sieving Protein-Losing Enteropathy

Pathogenic variants in PLVAP, the gene encoding the plasmalemma vesicle-associated protein, result in a rare syndromic form of protein-losing enteropathy due to the absence of a filter-type protein over fenestrae in the endothelia of the intestinal tract.[3] Syndromic features include hydrops, dysmorphic facial features, and cardiac and renal abnormalities.

Abetalipoproteinemia, Hypobetalipoproteinemia, and Chylomicron Retention Disease

The absorption and transport of dietary fat requires the proper structure, function, and interplay of apolipoprotein B, microsomal triglyceride transfer protein, very low-density lipoprotein, and chylomicrons. Defects within any of these components results in a phenotype of steatorrhea, failure to thrive, and, subsequently, fat-soluble vitamin deficiency.[56–58] Duodenal villi are characteristically white in color due to the presence of lipids within vacuoles. A low-fat diet with parenteral supplementation of fat-soluble vitamins seems to help patients with these disorders.

Dyskeratosis Congenita

Many telomere defects cause a severe syndrome associated with diarrhea and immune dysregulation and dysfunction.[59,60] Associated features include a characteristic nail dystrophy, leukoplakia, and failure to thrive. Immune defects are similar to those seen in severe combined immunodeficiency.

Kabuki Syndrome

A syndrome of multiple congenital anomalies with a defect in lysine specific methyltransferase has been noted in many patients to be associated with severe diarrhea of unclear cause.[61] The phenotype varies from a celiac disease-like disorder to intestinal failure.

DEFECTS IN EPITHELIAL TRAFFICKING AND POLARITY
Microvillus Inclusion Disease

Microvillus inclusion disease (MVID) is caused by defects in cellular trafficking within the microvilli, resulting in characteristic inclusion bodies within brush border cells on electron microscopy,[62] and a striking diarrhea that typically results in metabolic acidosis. Electrolyte derangements can be similar to those seen in Fanconi syndrome.[63] Patients with MVID due to pathogenic variants in STX3 may have associated neurologic findings of unclear significance.[64]

Tufting Enteropathy and Syndromic Sodium-Losing Diarrhea

The epithelial cell adhesion molecule (EpCAM) is an essential protein involved in cell-to-cell signaling, differentiation, migration, and proliferation, as well as calcium-independent cell adhesion. Defects in EpCAM result in dysplasia of the intestinal epithelium, producing "tufts" of enterocytes along with varying degrees of villous atrophy.[65] The resulting intestinal failure may require intestinal transplantation if long-term parenteral nutrition is not possible. Syndromic sodium-losing diarrhea is similar in morphology to congenital tufting enteropathy but is also associated with a sodium-losing diarrhea.[66]

Trichohepatoenteric Syndrome

Patients with pathogenic variants in TTC37 and SKIV2L present with wooly thickened hair that is prone to breakage (trichorrhexis nodosa), failure to thrive, hepatic defects, and immune dysfunction,[67–69] and may also present with colitis. The precise pathophysiologic mechanism is incompletely understood although is assumed to be epithelial.[70]

Familial Hemophagocytic Lymphohistiocytosis Type 5

In addition to manifesting the severe immune dysregulation of familial hemophagocytic lymphohistiocytosis, patients with certain pathogenic variants in STXBP2 may also demonstrate early-onset severe diarrhea and villous blunting that can reoccur even following allogeneic hematopoietic stem cell transplantation.[71–73]

Multiple Intestinal Atresia

Pathogenic variants in TTC7A have been associated with a spectrum of severe intestinal failure, ranging from multiple areas of intestinal atresia to a phenotype similar to severe combined immunodeficiency.[74] Although the immune defects resolve with allogeneic hematopoietic stem cell transplantation, the intestinal epithelial defects and associated diarrhea persist.[75]

ENTEROENDOCRINE CELL DYSFUNCTION

Enteroendocrine cells are located throughout the pancreas and gastrointestinal tract and produce hormones that regulate a variety of digestive and endocrine functions; pathogenic variants in a variety of genes can result in enteroendocrine cell dysfunction. The differentiation of pancreatic islet cells is directed by the transcription factor NEUROG3; pathogenic variants within the NEUROG3 gene result in enteric anendocrinosis, with variable phenotypes that typically include severe malabsorptive diarrhea and neonatal-onset diabetes mellitus.[76–79] Intestinal biopsies are typically normal. RFX6 encodes a transcription factor that regulates NEUROG3 expression; pathogenic variants render NEUROG3 unable to activate upstream and downstream targets, resulting in a lack of enteroendocrine cells and a malabsorptive diarrhea.[79] Pathogenic variants in *ARX* result in a severe phenotype that can result in neonatal death; most affected children die before the age of 6 years and have syndromic features that include lissencephaly, seizures, and abnormal genitalia.[80,81] Patients with pathogenic variants in *PCSK1* develop age-dependent manifestations, with failure to thrive, malabsorptive diarrhea, and total parenteral nutrition dependence in infancy, and multiple endocrine abnormalities and obesity with no intestinal manifestations later in life.[82,83] It has been theorized that *PCSK1* is involved in the processing of enteric hormone(s) involved in nutrient absorption. Proinsulin levels are typically significantly increased, up to 150 times the upper limit of normal, and may be a useful diagnostically. A pathogenic variant in a recently discovered noncoding region dubbed the intestine critical region underlies a disorder described in a cohort of individuals of Iraqi Jewish ancestry that have severe secretory diarrhea. The variants seem to result in up- and downregulation of a wide range of intestinal-specific genes.[84,85]

IMMUNE DYSREGULATION-ASSOCIATED ENTEROPATHY

Pathogenic variants in over 50 genes have been associated with neonatal, infantile, and very early-onset inflammatory bowel disease.[86,87] Associated phenotypic features vary according to the underlying genetic abnormality and often include immune dysregulation, although the hallmark is intestinal inflammation consistent with inflammatory bowel disease in children under 6 years. Identification of specific pathogenic variants allows for individualized treatment, which may include allogeneic hematopoietic stem cell transplantation or monoclonal antibody therapies.

SUMMARY

Congenital diarrheal disorders are genetically and phenotypically heterogeneous, and often mimic acquired forms of acute and chronic diarrhea in neonates and infants. The systematic evaluation of early-onset chronic diarrhea involves establishing the presence of diarrhea, ascertaining the composition of the stool, determining the response to fasting, and pursuing specialized testing as indicated. The phenotype produced via this process provides invaluable information, whether in establishing the diagnosis based on clinical, laboratory, imaging, and histopathologic criteria, or in informing the interpretation of molecular genetic assays. The increased implementation of exome and genome sequencing will allow for prompt and specific diagnosis of many congenital diarrheal disorders and can guide diagnosis-directed therapy. Future incorporation of stem cell-derived organoid models, RNA expression, and microbiome analyses will further enhance the diagnosis and management of congenital diarrheal disorders.

DISCLOSURE

The authors have nothing to disclose.

REFERENCES

1. Thiagarajah JR, Kamin DS, Acra S, et al. Advances in evaluation of chronic diarrhea in infants. Gastroenterology 2018;154:2045–59.e6.
2. Berni Canani R, Terrin G, Cardillo G, et al. Congenital diarrheal disorders: improved understanding of gene defects is leading to advances in intestinal physiology and clinical management. J Pediatr Gastroenterol Nutr 2010;50: 360–6.

3. Elkadri A, Thoeni C, Deharvengt SJ, et al. Mutations in plasmalemma vesicle associated protein result in sieving protein-losing enteropathy characterized by hypoproteinemia, hypoalbuminemia, and hypertriglyceridemia. Cell Mol Gastroenterol Hepatol 2015;1:381–94.e7.

4. Persistent diarrhoea in children in developing countries: memorandum from a WHO meeting. Bull World Health Organ 1988;66:709–17.

5. Farthing MJ. Chronic diarrhoea: current concepts on mechanisms and management. Eur J Gastroenterol Hepatol 1996;8:157–67.

6. Rose C, Parker A, Jefferson B, et al. The characterization of feces and urine: a review of the literature to inform advanced treatment technology. Crit Rev Environ Sci Technol 2015;45:1827–79.

7. Weaver LT. Bowel habit from birth to old age. J Pediatr Gastroenterol Nutr 1988;7: 637–40.

8. Holtug K, Clausen MR, Hove H, et al. The colon in carbohydrate malabsorption: short-chain fatty acids, pH, and osmotic diarrhoea. Scand J Gastroenterol 1992; 27:545–52.

9. Douwes AC, Oosterkamp RF, Fernandes J, et al. Sugar malabsorption in healthy neonates estimated by breath hydrogen. Arch Dis Child 1980;55:512–5.

10. Hammer HF, Fine KD, Santa Ana CA, et al. Carbohydrate malabsorption. Its measurement and its contribution to diarrhea. J Clin Invest 1990;86:1936–44.

11. Janecke AR, Heinz-Erian P, Yin J, et al. Reduced sodium/proton exchanger NHE3 activity causes congenital sodium diarrhea. Hum Mol Genet 2015;24:6614–23.

12. Agarwal R, Afzalpurkar R, Fordtran JS. Pathophysiology of potassium absorption and secretion by the human intestine. Gastroenterology 1994;107:548–71.

13. Wildhaber B, Niggli F, Bergstrasser E, et al. Paraneoplastic syndromes in ganglioneuroblastoma: contrasting symptoms of constipation and diarrhoea. Eur J Pediatr 2003;162:511–3.

14. van Dinter TG Jr, Fuerst FC, Richardson CT, et al. Stimulated active potassium secretion in a patient with colonic pseudo-obstruction: a new mechanism of secretory diarrhea. Gastroenterology 2005;129:1268–73.

15. Blondon H, Bechade D, Desrame J, et al. Secretory diarrhoea with high faecal potassium concentrations: a new mechanism of diarrhoea associated with colonic pseudo-obstruction? Report of five patients. Gastroenterol Clin Biol 2008;32:401–4.

16. Mathialahan T, Maclennan KA, Sandle LN, et al. Enhanced large intestinal potassium permeability in end-stage renal disease. J Pathol 2005;206:46–51.

17. Van De Kamer JH, Ten Bokkel Huinink H, Weyers HA. Rapid method for the determination of fat in feces. J Biol Chem 1949;177:347–55.

18. Raffensperger EC, D'Agostino F, Manfredo H, et al. Fecal fat excretion. An analysis of four years' experience. Arch Intern Med 1967;119:573–6.

19. Khouri MR, Huang G, Shiau YF. Sudan stain of fecal fat: new insight into an old test. Gastroenterology 1989;96:421–7.

20. Ghosh SK, Littlewood JM, Goddard D, et al. Stool microscopy in screening for steatorrhoea. J Clin Pathol 1977;30:749–53.

21. Kori M, Maayan-Metzger A, Shamir R, et al. Faecal elastase 1 levels in premature and full term infants. Arch Dis Child Fetal Neonatal Ed 2003;88:F106–8.

22. Struyvenberg MR, Martin CR, Freedman SD. Practical guide to exocrine pancreatic insufficiency—breaking the myths. BMC Med 2017;15:29.

23. Thomas AG, Phillips AD, Walker-Smith JA. The value of proximal small intestinal biopsy in the differential diagnosis of chronic diarrhoea. Arch Dis Child 1992;67: 741–3 [discussion: 743–4].

24. Avitzur Y, Guo C, Mastropaolo LA, et al. Mutations in tetratricopeptide repeat domain 7A result in a severe form of very early onset inflammatory bowel disease. Gastroenterology 2014;146:1028–39.
25. Dahlqvist A. Method for assay of intestinal disaccharidases. Anal Biochem 1964; 7:18–25.
26. Gambineri E, Ciullini Mannurita S, Hagin D, et al. Clinical, immunological, and molecular heterogeneity of 173 patients with the phenotype of immune dysregulation, polyendocrinopathy, enteropathy, X-linked (IPEX) syndrome. Front Immunol 2018;9:2411.
27. Bader-Meunier B, Florkin B, Sibilia J, et al. Mevalonate kinase deficiency: a survey of 50 patients. Pediatrics 2011;128:e152–9.
28. Kamal NM, Khan HY, El-Shabrawi MHF, et al. Congenital chloride losing diarrhea: a single center experience in a highly consanguineous population. Medicine (Baltimore) 2019;98:e15928.
29. Wedenoja S, Hoglund P, Holmberg C. Review article: the clinical management of congenital chloride diarrhoea. Aliment Pharmacol Ther 2010;31:477–85.
30. Amato F, Cardillo G, Liguori R, et al. Twelve novel mutations in the SLC26A3 gene in 17 sporadic cases of congenital chloride diarrhea. J Pediatr Gastroenterol Nutr 2017;65:26–30.
31. Matsunoshita N, Nozu K, Yoshikane M, et al. Congenital chloride diarrhea needs to be distinguished from Bartter and Gitelman syndrome. J Hum Genet 2018;63: 887–92.
32. Wedenoja S, Holmberg C, Hoglund P. Oral butyrate in treatment of congenital chloride diarrhea. Am J Gastroenterol 2008;103:252–4.
33. Heinz-Erian P, Muller T, Krabichler B, et al. Mutations in SPINT2 cause a syndromic form of congenital sodium diarrhea. Am J Hum Genet 2009;84:188–96.
34. Dimitrov G, Bamberger S, Navard C, et al. Congenital sodium diarrhea by mutation of the SLC9A3 gene. Eur J Med Genet 2019;62(10):103712.
35. Fiskerstrand T, Arshad N, Haukanes BI, et al. Familial diarrhea syndrome caused by an activating GUCY2C mutation. N Engl J Med 2012;366:1586–95.
36. Romi H, Cohen I, Landau D, et al. Meconium ileus caused by mutations in GUCY2C, encoding the CFTR-activating guanylate cyclase 2C. Am J Hum Genet 2012;90:893–9.
37. Al-Suyufi Y, ALSaleem K, Al-Mehaidib A, et al. SLC5A1 mutations in Saudi Arabian patients with congenital glucose-galactose malabsorption. J Pediatr Gastroenterol Nutr 2018;66:250–2.
38. Pode-Shakked B, Reish O, Aktuglu-Zeybek C, et al. Bitterness of glucose/galactose: novel mutations in the SLC5A1 gene. J Pediatr Gastroenterol Nutr 2014;58: 57–60.
39. Xin B, Wang H. Multiple sequence variations in SLC5A1 gene are associated with glucose-galactose malabsorption in a large cohort of Old Order Amish. Clin Genet 2011;79:86–91.
40. Martin MG, Turk E, Lostao MP, et al. Defects in Na$^+$/glucose cotransporter (SGLT1) trafficking and function cause glucose-galactose malabsorption. Nat Genet 1996;12:216–20.
41. Shneider BL. Intestinal bile acid transport: biology, physiology, and pathophysiology. J Pediatr Gastroenterol Nutr 2001;32:407–17.
42. Oelkers P, Kirby LC, Heubi JE, et al. Primary bile acid malabsorption caused by mutations in the ileal sodium-dependent bile acid transporter gene (SLC10A2). J Clin Invest 1997;99:1880–7.

43. Schmitt S, Kury S, Giraud M, et al. An update on mutations of the SLC39A4 gene in acrodermatitis enteropathica. Hum Mutat 2009;30:926–33.
44. Mattar R, de Campos Mazo DF, Carrilho FJ. Lactose intolerance: diagnosis, genetic, and clinical factors. Clin Exp Gastroenterol 2012;5:113–21.
45. Kuokkanen M, Kokkonen J, Enattah NS, et al. Mutations in the translated region of the lactase gene (LCT) underlie congenital lactase deficiency. Am J Hum Genet 2006;78:339–44.
46. Fazeli W, Kaczmarek S, Kirschstein M, et al. A novel mutation within the lactase gene (LCT): the first report of congenital lactase deficiency diagnosed in Central Europe. BMC Gastroenterol 2015;15:90.
47. Uchida N, Sakamoto O, Irie M, et al. Two novel mutations in the lactase gene in a Japanese infant with congenital lactase deficiency. Tohoku J Exp Med 2012;227: 69–72.
48. Torniainen S, Freddara R, Routi T, et al. Four novel mutations in the lactase gene (LCT) underlying congenital lactase deficiency (CLD). BMC Gastroenterol 2009; 9:8.
49. Gudmand-Hoyer E, Fenger HJ, Kern-Hansen P, et al. Sucrase deficiency in Greenland. Incidence and genetic aspects. Scand J Gastroenterol 1987;22:24–8.
50. Lucke T, Keiser M, Illsinger S, et al. Congenital and putatively acquired forms of sucrase-isomaltase deficiency in infancy: effects of sacrosidase therapy. J Pediatr Gastroenterol Nutr 2009;49:485–7.
51. Naim HY, Heine M, Zimmer KP. Congenital sucrase-isomaltase deficiency: heterogeneity of inheritance, trafficking, and function of an intestinal enzyme complex. J Pediatr Gastroenterol Nutr 2012;55(Suppl 2):S13–20.
52. Gudmand-Hoyer E, Fenger HJ, Skovbjerg H, et al. Trehalase deficiency in Greenland. Scand J Gastroenterol 1988;23:775–8.
53. Murray IA, Coupland K, Smith JA, et al. Intestinal trehalase activity in a UK population: establishing a normal range and the effect of disease. Br J Nutr 2000;83: 241–5.
54. Holzinger A, Maier EM, Buck C, et al. Mutations in the proenteropeptidase gene are the molecular cause of congenital enteropeptidase deficiency. Am J Hum Genet 2002;70:20–5.
55. van Rijn JM, Ardy RC, Kuloglu Z, et al. Intestinal failure and aberrant lipid metabolism in patients with DGAT1 deficiency. Gastroenterology 2018;155: 130–43.e15.
56. Pons V, Rolland C, Nauze M, et al. A severe form of abetalipoproteinemia caused by new splicing mutations of microsomal triglyceride transfer protein (MTTP). Hum Mutat 2011;32:751–9.
57. Di Leo E, Magnolo L, Bertolotti M, et al. Variable phenotypic expression of homozygous familial hypobetalipoproteinaemia due to novel APOB gene mutations. Clin Genet 2008;74:267–73.
58. Silvain M, Bligny D, Aparicio T, et al. Anderson's disease (chylomicron retention disease): a new mutation in the SARA2 gene associated with muscular and cardiac abnormalities. Clin Genet 2008;74:546–52.
59. Knight SW, Heiss NS, Vulliamy TJ, et al. Unexplained aplastic anaemia, immunodeficiency, and cerebellar hypoplasia (Hoyeraal-Hreidarsson syndrome) due to mutations in the dyskeratosis congenita gene, DKC1. Br J Haematol 1999;107: 335–9.
60. Ballew BJ, Joseph V, De S, et al. A recessive founder mutation in regulator of telomere elongation helicase 1, RTEL1, underlies severe immunodeficiency and features of Hoyeraal Hreidarsson syndrome. PLoS Genet 2013;9:e1003695.

61. Genevieve D, Amiel J, Viot G, et al. Atypical findings in Kabuki syndrome: report of 8 patients in a series of 20 and review of the literature. Am J Med Genet A 2004; 129A:64–8.
62. Ruemmele FM, Muller T, Schiefermeier N, et al. Loss-of-function of MYO5B is the main cause of microvillus inclusion disease: 15 novel mutations and a CaCo-2 RNAi cell model. Hum Mutat 2010;31:544–51.
63. Golachowska MR, van Dael CM, Keuning H, et al. MYO5B mutations in patients with microvillus inclusion disease presenting with transient renal Fanconi syndrome. J Pediatr Gastroenterol Nutr 2012;54:491–8.
64. Julia J, Shui V, Naveen M, et al. Microvillus inclusion disease, a diagnosis to consider when abnormal stools and neurological impairments run together due to a rare syntaxin 3 gene mutation. J Neonatal Perinatal Med 2019;12(3):313–9.
65. Goulet O, Salomon J, Ruemmele F, et al. Intestinal epithelial dysplasia (tufting enteropathy). Orphanet J Rare Dis 2007;2:20.
66. Salomon J, Goulet O, Canioni D, et al. Genetic characterization of congenital tufting enteropathy: epcam associated phenotype and involvement of SPINT2 in the syndromic form. Hum Genet 2014;133:299–310.
67. Egritas O, Dalgic B, Onder M. Tricho-hepato-enteric syndrome presenting with mild colitis. Eur J Pediatr 2009;168:933–5.
68. Fabre A, Charroux B, Martinez-Vinson C, et al. SKIV2L mutations cause syndromic diarrhea, or trichohepatoenteric syndrome. Am J Hum Genet 2012;90: 689–92.
69. Hartley JL, Zachos NC, Dawood B, et al. Mutations in TTC37 cause trichohepatoenteric syndrome (phenotypic diarrhea of infancy). Gastroenterology 2010;138: 2388–98, 2398.e1-2.
70. Overeem AW, Posovszky C, Rings EH, et al. The role of enterocyte defects in the pathogenesis of congenital diarrheal disorders. Dis Model Mech 2016;9:1–12.
71. Meeths M, Entesarian M, Al-Herz W, et al. Spectrum of clinical presentations in familial hemophagocytic lymphohistiocytosis type 5 patients with mutations in STXBP2. Blood 2010;116:2635–43.
72. Pagel J, Beutel K, Lehmberg K, et al. Distinct mutations in STXBP2 are associated with variable clinical presentations in patients with familial hemophagocytic lymphohistiocytosis type 5 (FHL5). Blood 2012;119:6016–24.
73. Stepensky P, Bartram J, Barth TF, et al. Persistent defective membrane trafficking in epithelial cells of patients with familial hemophagocytic lymphohistiocytosis type 5 due to STXBP2/MUNC18-2 mutations. Pediatr Blood Cancer 2013;60: 1215–22.
74. Jardine S, Dhingani N, Muise AM. TTC7A: steward of intestinal health. Cell Mol Gastroenterol Hepatol 2019;7:555–70.
75. Lien R, Lin YF, Lai MW, et al. Novel mutations of the tetratricopeptide repeat domain 7A gene and phenotype/genotype comparison. Front Immunol 2017;8: 1066.
76. Hancili S, Bonnefond A, Philippe J, et al. A novel NEUROG3 mutation in neonatal diabetes associated with a neuro-intestinal syndrome. Pediatr Diabetes 2018;19: 381–7.
77. Pinney SE, Oliver-Krasinski J, Ernst L, et al. Neonatal diabetes and congenital malabsorptive diarrhea attributable to a novel mutation in the human neurogenin-3 gene coding sequence. J Clin Endocrinol Metab 2011;96:1960–5.
78. Sayar E, Islek A, Yilmaz A, et al. Extremely rare cause of congenital diarrhea: enteric anendocrinosis. Pediatr Int 2013;55:661–3.

79. Wang J, Cortina G, Wu SV, et al. Mutant neurogenin-3 in congenital malabsorptive diarrhea. N Engl J Med 2006;355:270–80.
80. Kato M, Dobyns WB. X-linked lissencephaly with abnormal genitalia as a tangential migration disorder causing intractable epilepsy: proposal for a new term, "interneuronopathy". J Child Neurol 2005;20:392–7.
81. Terry NA, Lee RA, Walp ER, et al. Dysgenesis of enteroendocrine cells in aristaless-related homeobox polyalanine expansion mutations. J Pediatr Gastroenterol Nutr 2015;60:192–9.
82. Martin MG, Lindberg I, Solorzano-Vargas RS, et al. Congenital proprotein convertase 1/3 deficiency causes malabsorptive diarrhea and other endocrinopathies in a pediatric cohort. Gastroenterology 2013;145:138–48.
83. Pepin L, Colin E, Tessarech M, et al. A new case of PCSK1 pathogenic variant with congenital proprotein convertase 1/3 deficiency and literature review. J Clin Endocrinol Metab 2019;104:985–93.
84. Straussberg R, Shapiro R, Amir J, et al. Congenital intractable diarrhea of infancy in Iraqi Jews. Clin Genet 1997;51:98–101.
85. Oz-Levi D, Olender T, Bar-Joseph I, et al. Noncoding deletions reveal a gene that is critical for intestinal function. Nature 2019;571:107–11.
86. Uhlig HH, Schwerd T, Koletzko S, et al. The diagnostic approach to monogenic very early onset inflammatory bowel disease. Gastroenterology 2014;147:990–1007.e3.
87. Alruwaithi M, Sherlock M. Neonatal inflammatory skin and bowel disease caused by a homozygous EGFR mutation: a case report and review of the medical literature. J Can Assoc Gastroenterol 2018;1:367–8.

Nonimmune Hydrops Fetalis

Corinne Swearingen, MD[a], Zachary A. Colvin, DO[b],
Steven R. Leuthner, MD, MA[a],*

KEYWORDS

- Nonimmune hydrops • Prenatal diagnosis • Pleural effusions • Ascites
- Cystic hygroma • Fetal anemia • Fetal congestive heart failure • Palliative care

KEY POINTS

- Nonimmune hydrops fetalis (NIHF) should be thought of as a symptom or an end-stage status of a variety of diseases.
- There are 4 pathophysiologic mechanisms.
- Multidisciplinary counseling and shared decision making are needed.
- Mortality from NIHF depends on whether there is therapy for the underlying cause.

DEFINITION

The term hydrops fetalis describes excessive, pathologic fluid accumulation within the fetal soft tissues and body cavities.[1,2] It is defined by the presence of 2 or more abnormal fluid collections in the fetus on ultrasonography imaging. These fluid collections include ascites, pleural effusions, pericardial effusion, and generalized skin edema (with skin thickness >5 mm).[3] Other associated findings include placental edema and polyhydramnios.[4]

There are 2 categories of hydrops fetalis: immune and nonimmune. Nonimmune hydrops fetalis (NIHF) refers specifically to cases not caused by red cell alloimmunization.[4] With the widespread use of Rhesus (Rh) D immune globulin, the incidence of immune hydrops fetalis has significantly decreased in recent years.[1,4] As a result, NIHF now accounts for up to 90% of cases of fetal hydrops.[5]

EPIDEMIOLOGY

The incidence of NIHF is estimated to be 1 per 1700 to 3000 pregnancies, whereas the incidence in live-born infants is reported to be 1 per 4000.[1,4] The lower incidence in live-born infants is related to intrauterine death and elective termination of pregnancy.

---

[a] Department of Pediatrics, Medical College of Wisconsin, 999 North 92nd Street, Suite C410, Wauwatosa, WI 53226, USA; [b] Department of Obstetrics and Gynecology, Medical College of Wisconsin, 9200 West Wisconsin Avenue, Milwaukee, WI 53226, USA
* Corresponding author.
E-mail address: sleuthne@mcw.edu

Clin Perinatol 47 (2020) 105–121
https://doi.org/10.1016/j.clp.2019.10.001
0095-5108/20/© 2019 Elsevier Inc. All rights reserved.
perinatology.theclinics.com

CAUSE

NIHF should be thought of as a symptom or an end-stage status of a variety of diseases. Previous meta-analyses conducted by Bellini and colleagues[5,6] divided causes of NIHF into 14 categories. **Fig. 1** shows the relative frequency of each cause based on the most recent meta-analysis.[6] There is no identifiable primary cause in about 20% of cases of NIHF.

FLUID REGULATION IN THE FETUS

Normally, fluid extravasates from the capillaries into the interstitial space, and then is reabsorbed by the lymphatics and returned to the vasculature. Until recently, fluid movement was thought to be governed by the Starling equation, which stresses opposing hydrostatic and oncotic forces in the vascular and interstitial spaces.[7] This theory has been modified with the discovery of the glycocalyx layer.

The glycocalyx layer is a semipermeable layer composed of capillary endothelium and overlying glycocalyx.[8] When intact, it forms a molecular filter that limits water and protein flux into the cell-cell junction, regulating plasma/interstitial fluid balance and solute exchange.[9] Newly formed vessels during angiogenesis have a thinner glycocalyx layer, which is more permeable, allowing more fluid flux.[9] Abnormal glycocalyx is also induced by inflammatory cytokines and ischemia-reperfusion, leading to increased capillary permeability. The fetus is therefore at risk for interstitial fluid accumulation because of a thinner glycocalyx layer, highly

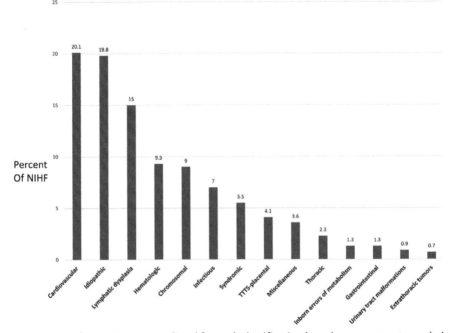

Fig. 1. Cause of NIHF. Percentages listed for each classification based on recent meta-analysis conducted by Bellini and colleagues[6] 2015. TTTS, twin-twin transfusion syndrome. (*Data from* Bellini C, Donarini G, Paladini D, et al. Etiology of non-immune hydrops fetalis: an update. Am J Med Genet A 2015;167A:1082-1088.)

compliant interstitial compartment, and marked sensitivity of lymphatic return by venous pressure.[7]

PATHOPHYSIOLOGY

Four main mechanisms have been proposed to explain the distribution of body fluids in NIHF: (1) increase in hydrostatic capillary pressure; (2) reduction in plasma oncotic pressure; (3) obstruction of lymphatic flow; and (4) damage to peripheral capillary integrity. NIHF may result from 1 or more of these mechanisms depending on the cause.[7,10,11]

Increase in Hydrostatic Capillary Pressure

Increased hydrostatic pressure occurs when there is increased central venous pressure (CVP). Increased CVP may result from (1) congestive heart failure (CHF) or (2) increased intrathoracic pressure.

Causes of congestive heart failure

CHF can develop in many fetal conditions, including cardiovascular, hematologic, urinary/renal, and placental/umbilical cord disorders and twin-twin transfusion syndrome (TTTS).

   CHF causes increased CVP that obstructs venous return from the placenta and fetal tissues. This obstruction leads to increased hydrostatic back pressure and sets up a cascade of events resulting in other mechanisms of hydrops. Placental edema leads to impaired maternal-fetal gas exchange and hypoxic damage of the fetal capillary membrane with plasma protein loss.[10] Lymphatic uptake is also compromised because of increased CVP, resulting in worsening interstitial fluid accumulation.

Cardiovascular disorders Cardiovascular disorders leading to NIHF can be divided into 4 categories: (1) structural heart disease; (2) cardiomyopathies; (3) fetal arrhythmias; and (4) vascular disorders.

- Structural heart disease. **Table 1** lists the multiple structural cardiac defects associated with NIHF.[1,10] Anomalies of the right heart are more common because of their direct effect on CVP. Left heart lesions may lead to increased CVP when cardiac outflow is obstructed, resulting in higher left-sided atrial and ventricular pressures and decreased flow across the foramen ovale.[5,10]Cardiac teratomas and rhabdomyosarcomas may also cause NIHF. The mechanism relates to obstruction of blood flow through the heart, either from direct mass effect, impaired cardiac function (from cardiac compression or conduction

Table 1		
Major structural cardiac defects associated with nonimmune hydrops fetalis		
Right-Sided Defects	**Left-Sided Defects**	**Other**
Double outlet right ventricle	Aortic valve abnormalities	Transposition of the great
Ebstein anomaly	Coarctation of the aorta	arteries
Hypoplastic right heart	Endocardial fibroelastosis	Truncus arteriosus
syndrome	Hypoplastic left heart	Atrioventricular canal defect
Intrauterine closure of fetal	syndrome	Endocardial cushion defect
cardiac shunts		Heterotaxy
Pulmonary stenosis or atresia		Cardiac tumors
Tetralogy of Fallot		
Tricuspid valve abnormalities		

abnormalities), or increased intrathoracic pressure (from the mass itself).[10] Obstructed cardiac blood flow leads to increased CVP and increased hydrostatic capillary pressure. Impaired venous return also causes decreased diastolic ventricular filling in the setting of already compromised cardiac function, leading to low-output cardiac failure.

- Cardiomyopathies. Primary cardiomyopathies associated with NIHF include endocardial fibroelastosis, noncompacted myocardium, Noonan syndrome, and lysosomal storage disorders.[10] Secondary cardiomyopathies include congenital infections, maternal diabetes, tachyarrhythmias, prolonged hypoxia, and high-output cardiac failure (anemia, arteriovenous malformations [AVMs], TTTS).[10,12]
- Arrhythmias. Fetal supraventricular tachycardia is the most common tachyarrhythmia associated with NIHF. Of these, accessory-pathway related atrioventricular reentrant tachycardia is seen most often (90%).[10] When the fetal heart rate is sustained at greater than 220 beats per minute (bpm), there is decreased ventricular filling, which leads to decreased cardiac output, impaired tissue oxygenation, and increased CVP. Fetal bradyarrhythmias have been associated with NIHF based on 2 proposed mechanisms: (1) increased CVP with hepatic congestion, and (2) low cardiac output with impaired tissue perfusion and oxygenation. Congenital complete AV block is most common, often with heart rates less than 65 bpm, and is associated with maternal systemic lupus erythematosus.[4,13] Other causes of congenital heart block include structural abnormalities that affect the development of the conduction pathway.
- Vascular disorders. AVMs, such as vein of Galen malformation, and hemangiomas, as in Kasabach-Merritt syndrome, are associated with NIHF as a result of high-output cardiac failure. AVMs are direct arterial-to-venous connections that act as low-resistance, high-flow circuits that "steal" blood flow from traditional circulation. To compensate, cardiac output must increase to maintain adequate perfusion to tissues. Over time, this compensation fails, leading to dilated cardiomyopathy and high-output cardiac failure with increased CVP and impaired tissue oxygenation. Hemangiomas can also have vascular shunting and/or substantial fetal hemorrhage, resulting in high-output cardiac failure. Rare vascular disorders linked to NIHF include generalized arterial calcification of infancy or arterial calcification from parathyroid disease, severe intrauterine infection, or metabolic disorders. These conditions cause refractory hypertension and cardiac failure secondary to hypertrophic cardiomyopathy and/or recurrent ischemia from calcified coronaries.[10]

Hematologic disorders Hematologic disorders causing profound anemia lead to high-output cardiac failure and tissue hypoxia. This hypoxia causes capillary tissue injury and protein leak, resulting in reduced intravascular osmotic pressure. Hypoxia also causes the redistribution of blood flow to the brain, heart, and adrenal glands, leading to both renal and liver compromise.[11] In addition, extramedullary hematopoiesis may cause increased pressure in the fetal portal and vena caval systems, leading to hepatic dysfunction and hypoproteinemia.

The cause of anemia in these cases can be divided into 2 categories: (1) excessive erythrocyte loss by hemolysis or hemorrhage, and (2) erythrocyte underproduction.[14]

- Excessive erythrocyte loss by hemolysis or hemorrhage. Hemolysis may be caused by intrinsic erythrocyte defects or, more rarely, extrinsic causes. Intrinsic erythrocyte abnormalities include the hemoglobinopathies, enzymopathies, and defects of the red cell membrane skeleton. Of the hemoglobinopathies, homozygous α^0-thalassemia is most commonly associated with NIHF. In homozygous α^0-thalassemia, there is complete lack of α-globin synthesis. Excess γ-globin chains assemble into γ_4 homotetramers or so-called hemoglobin (Hb) Bart. Hb Bart has extremely high affinity for oxygen and is associated with severe fetal tissue hypoxia.[14] The diagnosis is confirmed with hemoglobin electrophoresis. Homozygous α^0-thalassemia occurs predominantly in southeast Asia and accounts for up to 53% to 81% of cases of NIHF.[14] Fetal death usually occurs in the late second through midthird trimester of pregnancy or within a few hours after birth.-Inherited enzymopathies, including glucose 6-phosphate dehydrogenase deficiency (G6PD), pyruvate kinase deficiency, and glucose phosphate isomerase deficiencies, rarely lead to NIHF.[12] Red blood cell membrane defects, such as hereditary spherocytosis, are also not strongly associated with NIHF.Excessive erythrocyte loss by hemorrhage or hemolysis may occur in the setting of fetal hemangiomas, AVMs, fetal tumors (especially sacrococcygeal teratomas), TTTS, and fetomaternal hemorrhage. Fetomaternal hemorrhage may be caused by placental malformations and/or umbilical cord disorders. Severe, acute fetomaternal hemorrhage usually results in intrauterine death, whereas chronic fetomaternal hemorrhage may lead to anemia and the development of NIHF.[10]

- Erythrocyte underproduction. Red blood cell production is inhibited in the setting of bone marrow infiltration or bone marrow depression by infection.[14] Transient myeloproliferative disorder and congenital leukemia are both associated with trisomy 21 and can cause profound anemia because of marrow infiltration.[15] In addition, intrauterine parvovirus infection can cause bone marrow depression, leading to the destruction of erythroid progenitor cells, impairment of reticulocytosis, and severe anemia.[9,14,16] The risk of poor outcome is highest when the infection occurs at less than 20 weeks of gestation.[4]

Urinary/renal disorders Urinary conditions associated with NIHF include urethral obstruction from stenosis or atresia at the level of the ureteropelvic junction, bladder neck, or urethra; posterior urethral valves; and prune belly syndrome. Obstructive uropathy leads to urinary retention and increased pressure in the bladder, with transudation of urinary fluid and potentially bladder wall rupture. It also leads to renal dysplasia and renal failure. Other renal disorders known to be associated with NIHF include renal agenesis and dysgenesis, renal vein thrombosis, and congenital nephrosis.[1,17]

The exact mechanism of urinary/renal disorders leading to NIHF remains unclear, and it may be important from a prognostic point of view to distinguish between true NIHF versus isolated urinary ascites. It has been postulated that renal disorders lead to an imbalance of interstitial fluid production, lymphatic vessel overload, and CHF. Other suggested mechanisms include oligohydramnios with restricted fetal mobility, bladder distention with decreased cardiac output, and urine transudation (with osmotic disturbances in the abdominal cavity).[10]

Placental/umbilical cord disorders Placental tumors that have been linked to NIHF include chorioangioma and choriocarcinoma. Placental chorioangiomas are highly vascularized and can function as arteriovenous shunts, leading to high-output cardiac failure.[4,10] Choriocarcinomas are highly malignant tumors that can metastasize to fetal organs as well as to the mother. It has been proposed that choriocarcinomas impair the integrity of the maternal-fetal barrier in the placenta, leading to chronic fetomaternal hemorrhage and high-output cardiac failure.

Umbilical cord disorders, such as angiomyxoma, true knots, umbilical artery aneurysm, and umbilical vein thrombosis, are rare causes of NIHF. These abnormalities may lead to placental ischemia, edema, and impaired maternal-fetal gas exchange. The increased umbilical venous pressure impairs venous return from the placenta to the fetus, leading to low-output heart failure.

Twin-twin transfusion syndrome The monochorionic placenta in a twin pregnancy may be the site of arteriovenous communication between the 2 fetal circulations. In the setting of an arteriovenous communication, 1 twin's venous drainage enters the circulation of the second twin,[12] and this has important hemodynamic and hematologic consequences. The donor twin may develop hydrops caused by severe anemia, hypovolemia, and renal compromise. In comparison, the recipient twin has polycythemia and increased circulating blood volume, leading to volume overload, hypertension, and impaired myocardial function. All these factors contribute to cardiac failure and the development of NIHF.

Causes of increased intrathoracic pressure
Any cause of increased intrathoracic pressure may lead to obstruction of venous flow and increased CVP.[9,10] Causes of increased intrathoracic pressure include thoracic congenital anomalies and neurologic/musculoskeletal disorders.

Thoracic congenital anomalies Space-occupying lesions within the thoracic cavity may compress the lungs and heart, shifting the mediastinum and reducing venous return.[10] The location and size of the mass dictate the degree of pulmonary hypoplasia and obstruction of venous return. Examples of intrathoracic masses or congenital anomalies include congenital diaphragmatic hernia, congenital pulmonary adenomatoid malformation (CPAM), bronchopulmonary sequestration, mediastinal teratoma, and chylothorax.

Congenital high airway obstruction sequence has also been linked to the development of NIHF. It results from aplasia or intrinsic obstruction to the formation of the upper airway (larynx or trachea) during development,[18] which leads to the inability of fetal lung fluid to exit the lungs, resulting in dilatation of the airways, lung hyperinflation, and flattening of the diaphragms. Increased CVP occurs because of lung overdistention and impedance of venous return, causing low-output cardiac failure.

Neurologic/musculoskeletal disorders Neurologic disorders that lead to either hypomobility or hypotonia may lead to the development of NIHF. It is postulated that a lack of respiratory movements with limited diaphragm excursion can lead to an increase in intrathoracic pressure. Decreased fetal limb and body movements also cause impaired lymph drainage and resultant interstitial fluid accumulation. Examples include spina bifida, congenital myotonic dystrophy, fetal akinesia, and several genetic syndromes (Pena-Shokeir, multiple pterygium syndrome, arthrogryposis multiplex congenita).[1,9,10] Specific examples of skeletal dysplasias that involve the thorax include achondroplasia, camptomelic dysplasia, and short rib polydactyly syndromes.

Reduction in Intravascular Osmotic Pressure

A reduction in intravascular osmotic pressure leads to fluid extravasation, resulting in edema, ascites, and/or effusions.[10] A hypoproteinemic state can evolve under several pathophysiologic conditions, including liver injury, renal failure, and impaired capillary integrity. Liver injury can occur as a direct result of infection or anoxia or may be secondary to hepatic congestion, such as in the setting of increased CVP. Renal impairment, such as congenital nephrotic syndrome, can lead to excessive protein loss in the urine and a hypoproteinemic state. In addition, capillary membrane damage can lead to protein efflux into the interstitial space and reduced intravascular osmotic pressure.

Inborn errors of metabolism

Lysosomal storage diseases have been implicated in the development of NIHF.[19] These diseases include mucopolysaccharidoses, oligosaccharidoses, sphingolipidoses, mucolipidoses, lysosomal transport defects, and multiple sulfatase deficiency.[9] Other nonlysosomal diseases have also been associated, such as glycogenosis, fatty acid oxidation defects, cholesterol biosynthesis defects, and congenital disorders of glycosylation. Postulated mechanisms include hypoproteinemia as a result of liver failure, visceromegaly secondary to accumulation of storage material with resultant obstruction of venous return, and decreased erythropoiesis from marrow infiltration.[4,9]

Gastrointestinal disorders

A variety of gastrointestinal disorders have been implicated in NIHF, and multiple mechanisms have been identified. Reduced intravascular osmotic pressure is thought to develop when there is infarcted bowel and inflammation, leading to impaired capillary integrity. In these settings, there is protein loss into the peritoneal cavity and development of ascites. Examples of gastrointestinal obstruction include stenosis, atresia, midgut volvulus, imperforate anus, intussusception, and meconium ileus. Hepatic disorders, such as cirrhosis, hepatic necrosis, polycystic disease, hepatoblastoma, hepatic harmartomas, and biliary atresia, have also been reported in association with NIHF, most likely caused by hypoproteinemia.[4]

Obstruction of Lymphatic Flow

Impaired lymphatic drainage as a primary cause occurs when there is any structural anomaly of lymphatic development causing obstruction of proper lymphatic flow. Examples include congenital pulmonary lymphangiectasia, lymphatic dysplasia syndrome, and cervical or cystic hygromas.[9,10] Lymphatic malformations are often part of chromosomal abnormalities/syndromes.

Chromosomal abnormalities/syndromes

The most common genetic cause of NIHF is aneuploidy: monosomy X, trisomy 21, and trisomy 18.[6,9] NIHF before 24 weeks of gestation is usually related to aneuploidy.[20] Other potential causes include tetraploidy, triploidy, and chromosomal deletions and duplications.

Many mechanisms have been postulated for the development of NIHF in the setting of chromosomal abnormalities. There may be incomplete formation of the lymphatic system, such as in monosomy X. Cardiovascular or hematologic abnormalities may contribute as well as hypoalbuminemia related to liver dysfunction. There may not be 1 single pathway but multiple pathways contributing to NIHF.

Multiple syndromes have also been associated with NIHF. Noonan syndrome is frequently reported and results from a single gene defect.[6] Noonan syndrome is associated with lymphatic dysplasia as well as cardiac abnormalities, such as pulmonary valve stenosis and hypertrophic cardiomyopathy.

Damage to Peripheral Capillary Integrity

Capillary wall integrity may be compromised in the setting of hypoxia, such as in CHF, as well as in the setting of sepsis.[10] In these situations, there is damage to the glycocalyx layer, leading to increased capillary endothelial permeability.[9]

Infection

Several infections have been linked to the development of NIHF, including those caused by bacterial, viral, parasitic, and spirochetal organisms.[10] These include parvovirus, cytomegalovirus, herpes simplex virus, *Treponema pallidum*, hepatitis B virus, *Toxoplasma gondii*, adenovirus, enterovirus, varicella, rubella, respiratory syncytial virus, human immunodeficiency virus, and *Listeria monocytogenes*.[9,10,12] Ultrasonography findings, such as microcephaly, intracranial calcifications, ventriculomegaly, hepatosplenomegaly, and intrauterine growth restriction increase concern for an infectious cause.[9]

THE PRENATAL COURSE
Diagnostic Evaluation

Often, one of the causes described earlier is diagnosed and prenatal management includes repeated evaluation for hydrops. Other times, NIHF may be the initial presenting finding. Once NIHF has been identified, it is important to determine the underlying cause and assess whether there is a potential therapeutic approach. Prenatal and postnatal evaluation can determine the cause in up to 60% to 85% of cases.[5,21] **Fig. 2** provides an algorithm for diagnostic evaluation.[4]

First, a detailed maternal history to ascertain inherited diseases, consanguinity, drug exposures, and recent infections must be performed. Maternal blood type, Rh(D) antigen status, and indirect Coombs test should be collected to exclude immune hydrops as a cause. Once NIHF is suspected, referral should be made to maternal-fetal medicine if available. Detailed fetal ultrasonography should be performed to examine for structural, placental, and umbilical cord abnormalities. Middle cerebral Doppler studies should be conducted to assess for fetal anemia. Monochorionic twins should be examined for presence of TTTS. A fetal echocardiogram should be performed to monitor for cardiac arrhythmias and structural abnormalities. The cardiovascular profile score can be used to monitor cardiac status in newly diagnosed or in worsening hydrops cases, which can assist in management and timing of delivery.[22] In all cases of NIHF, amniocentesis to examine fetal karyotype and/or chromosomal microarray should be offered. Whole-exome sequencing is being used more frequently in the prenatal setting and has yielded promising results in finding pathogenic variants in cases of NIHF.[23] Viral titers (immunoglobulin [Ig] M and IgG) for cytomegalovirus, toxoplasmosis, and parvovirus should be performed if there is clinical suspicion based on ultrasonography findings or if no other cause has been ascertained. Maternal complete blood count should be collected to examine for microcytic anemia that could be caused by underlying thalassemia. A Kleihauer-Betke test can be performed to assess for fetomaternal hemorrhage.

If all testing is negative, additional testing of amniotic fluid for skeletal dysplasias, metabolic storage disorders, and erythrocyte enzymopathies may be performed.[4] A review of 678 cases of NIHF showed that nearly 30% of cases initially classified as idiopathic were caused by underlying lysosomal storage disorders on more comprehensive work-up.[20]

Maternal Complications

NIHF is associated with preterm delivery in up to 66% of cases.[4] Mirror syndrome, also known as Ballantyne syndrome, is a rare disorder in which women can develop generalized edema that mirrors the hydropic fetus. It is most closely associated with hypertension and proteinuria, which occurs in up to 60% and 40% of cases respectively. It is

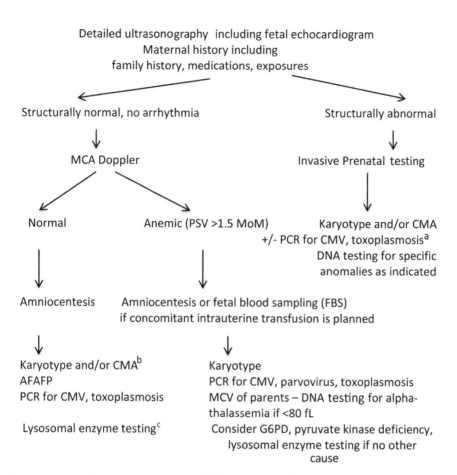

Fig. 2. Prenatal diagnostic evaluation. AFAFP, amniotic fluid alpha fetoprotein; CMA, chromosomal microarray; CMV, cytomegalovirus; MCA, middle cerebral artery; MCV, mean corpuscular volume; MoM, multiple of the median; PCR, polymerase chain reaction; PSV, peak systolic velocity. Assuming negative indirect Coombs test, thereby excluding alloimmunization. [a] CMV/toxoplasmosis testing if fetal anomalies suggest infection. [b] Either amniocentesis or fetal blood sampling. [c] Available in some laboratories. (*From* Society for Maternal-Fetal Medicine (SMFM), Norton ME, Chauhan SP, et al. *Society for maternal-fetal medicine (SMFM) clinical guideline #7: nonimmune hydrops fetalis.* Am J Obstet Gynecol. 2015 Feb;212(2):127-39. https://doi.org/10.1016/j.ajog.2014.12.018. Epub 2014 Dec 31; with permission.)

also associated with increased creatinine level, transaminitis, pulmonary edema, anemia, headaches, and visual disturbances.[4] Preeclampsia and mirror syndrome share many clinical features, and patients have been found to have similar increases in soluble fms-like tyrosine kinase (sFlt-1) and soluble endoglin (sEng), suggesting similar pathophysiology. Mirror syndrome generally resolves if hydrops resolves or following delivery. A retrospective cohort study that examined 337 cases of hydrops found that hydrops was associated with an increased risk of preeclampsia with severe features. The same study also found statistically increased rates of eclampsia, acute renal failure, pulmonary edema, postpartum hemorrhage, blood transfusion, preterm birth, and neonatal death.[24]

Antenatal Management

Management of NIHF depends on the cause, gestational age at diagnosis, and availability of antenatal or postnatal therapies. Consultation and management with maternal-fetal medicine specialists are recommended. Fetal therapies include intrauterine transfusions for fetal anemia, medication for cardiac arrhythmias, drainage of fluid collections, corticosteroids for some CPAMs, and fetoscopic laser ablation for TTTS. There are centers that, under the right conditions, also offer open fetal surgical resection of masses.[25,26] Prompt referral to centers specialized in these fetal interventions is highly recommended. Expectant management can be undertaken if the cause is unknown, but careful monitoring for mirror syndrome and preeclampsia should be performed.[4] Antepartum fetal surveillance should be considered if the suspected cause is not lethal, viability has been reached, and if the patient desires neonatal resuscitation. Antenatal corticosteroids should be given per standard obstetric guidelines if there is concern for preterm delivery and the underlying cause of NIHF is not thought to be lethal.[4]

Delivery Recommendations

Because of the wide array of potential causes for NIHF, timing of delivery is largely based on expert opinion and needs to be individualized. Delivery is generally recommended if NIHF is diagnosed at or worsening at 34 weeks' gestation. There is no evidence that delivery before 34 weeks improves outcomes because neonatal resuscitation is more difficult. Delivery should be considered by 37 weeks if there are no clinical signs of worsening fetal or maternal health. If there is concern for mirror syndrome, delivery is usually indicated.[4]

Mode of delivery depends on the underlying cause and condition of the fetus. If the cause is thought to be treatable and there is worsening fetal condition, prompt delivery by cesarean section may be required. If a palliative approach to care has been chosen, vaginal delivery is preferred. If there is large ascites or effusions, aspiration may need to be performed before delivery to minimize risk of dystocia and aid in postnatal resuscitation.[4]

Delivery for a fetus with NIHF should be performed at a center with a level III/IV neonatal intensive care unit (NICU) if resuscitation is preferred. If hydrops is not diagnosed until delivery or if delivery occurs at a center without proper NICU facilities, transfer to an appropriate center should be performed as soon as medically stable.[4]

Parental Choices and Shared Decision Making

With the diagnosis of NIHF comes the possibility of multiple options that might vary depending on the gestational age of the fetus and health of the mother. Options that should be offered include termination of pregnancy, fetal interventions if available, and expectant management with either a trial of neonatal intervention or palliative care. Antenatal consultation should be multidisciplinary and include obstetrics and gynecology; maternal-fetal medicine; neonatology; and, depending on the underlying cause, pediatric or surgical subspecialists. A coordinated, integrated team approach is needed so that the family receives consistent messaging. Any decision needs to balance maternal and fetal risks.

A plan of action should be created according to the family's wishes. This plan could include referral for termination with follow-up or the development of a formalized palliative care plan.[27] The palliative care plan could include resuscitation and a trial of therapy with or without neonatal limits depending on how the baby responds.[28,29] Counseling should include the possible redirection to comfort care if the patient is not responding to shorten futile intensive care and minimize suffering for both the baby and the parents.[30] Sharing that withdrawal of support is an option if neonatal management is not effective is an important concept to reduce suffering and promote best interests. The palliative care team may be a much-needed resource for families, providing additional psychosocial support to parents outside of the primary medical team.

If NIHF is a new diagnosis and delivery imminent, there is enough uncertainty that, although offering palliative care is a possible choice, resuscitation and evaluation will help provide more information as to the possible cause and whether it is a treatable or reversible condition. If resuscitation is planned, specific expectations regarding the delivery room and postnatal management, such as intubation and needle aspirations, should be reviewed. It is important to relay to families that their babies may not survive even with extensive resuscitation. If the baby does survive delivery, families should be aware that the NICU stay can be very long, emotionally draining, and mentally challenging.

THE NEONATAL COURSE
Delivery Room Management

A skilled neonatal resuscitation team trained in neonatal resuscitation program is critical.[12] Tasks should be assigned to all members to improve communication and streamline care. Issues with ventilation and oxygenation are expected because of pulmonary compression and possible pulmonary hypoplasia as a result of pleural effusions and/or ascites. Often, prompt intubation is necessary. If there is no or minimal improvement with intubation, it may be necessary to drain fluid. Before delivery, the team should be prepared to perform thoracenteses, an abdominal paracentesis, and even a pericardiocentesis. Surfactant administration should be considered if premature. Placement of an umbilical venous line may be necessary, especially in the setting of poor hemodynamics and need for epinephrine and fluid replacement.

Ongoing Neonatal Management

Therapeutic intervention in the immediate postdelivery phase should be targeted toward adequate physiologic support, continued diagnostic evaluation, and potential therapeutic treatment to reverse NIHF.

Respiratory support

It may be difficult to achieve adequate ventilation and oxygenation, even when intubated, until existing pleural or ascitic fluid is drained.[31] Unilateral or bilateral chest tubes or a peritoneal drain may need to be placed to improve pulmonary mechanics. Any fluid obtained should be sent for analysis. Early therapy with octreotide could be considered in the setting of a chylothorax or chylous ascites, although optimal dosing and duration are unknown.[32] Long-term management of drains depends on the cause and how the infant responds to therapy, including nutrition.

Cardiovascular support

An electrocardiogram (ECG) and echocardiogram should be obtained to evaluate for rhythm disorders, anatomy, and myocardial contractility. A pericardial effusion may be present and impair myocardial function, necessitating either a pericardiocentesis or pericardial drain placement to improve cardiac output. Poor cardiac output may be further supported by vasoactive medications, such as epinephrine, dopamine, or milrinone, or fluid administration because of potential intravascular depletion in NIHF. In the setting of intractable hypotension, stress-dose steroids should be considered for adrenocortical insufficiency.[33]

Fluid management

Fluid and electrolyte management is complex in infants with NIHF. These infants have free water excess and normal total body sodium. Fluid restriction is key, combined with frequent monitoring of serum electrolytes and total output. There is a risk for intravascular depletion, because fluid losses from pleural and peritoneal cavities may be high. Fluid replacement should then be considered with either normal saline or fresh frozen plasma. Albumin infusion is generally not recommended outside the setting of overwhelming continuous albumin loss.[34] When feeding can eventually begin, special formulas may be necessary, especially in the setting of a primary lymphatic issue.

Diagnostic evaluation

Further diagnostic work-up should be undertaken as an expansion of the prenatal work-up.

General evaluation A comprehensive physical examination should always be the first step. Examination findings, such as bruits or murmurs, may be critical in guiding additional work-up. Basic laboratory tests should be obtained and are listed in **Box 1**. Initial imaging should include a chest radiograph.

Expanded evaluation Further laboratory work depends on the suspected cause (see **Box 1**). If pleural fluid is obtained, evaluation should be done to determine whether the effusion is transudative or exudative. Diagnosis of a chylous effusion is based on findings of fluid with a total cell count greater than 1000 cells/mL with greater than 80% lymphocyte predominance and a triglyceride concentration of greater than 1.1 mmol/L (if feeding).[11,35]

Genetic testing may also be undertaken, with the first step usually being a microarray.[23] A genetics consultation is key for more expansive testing.[23] Analysis for lysosomal storage diseases may be pursued if suspicion is high and cause remains unknown. Blood should be set aside for genetic testing before any blood product administration.

Imaging can be extensive and should always be conducted in a stepwise approach based on likely cause (see **Box 1**).

Therapy

There are many known causes of NIHF but not all have potential treatments. Most medical care is supportive with a wait-and-see philosophy while additional work-up for reversible and treatable conditions is pending. For some significant anemias, a blood transfusion corrects the underlying problem and supportive care may allow for tissue recovery. For cardiac arrhythmias, a variety of antiarrhythmics, such as digoxin, propranolol, or flecainide, may be used as therapy.[13] Surgical options may be available for certain tumors, lymphatic malformations, thoracic or urinary tract abnormalities, and cardiac defects.

Mortality and Outcomes

Perinatal mortality for NIHF remains extremely high, ranging from 35% to 98%.[1,2,36] The earlier the diagnosis of NIHF, the higher the risk of mortality, with diagnosis

---

Box 1
Initial diagnostic evaluation for nonimmune hydrops fetalis

Comprehensive physical examination

General evaluation:
• Complete blood count with differential
• Blood culture
• Type and screen
• Arterial or capillary blood gas
• Complete metabolic panel (includes serum albumin)
• Conjugated and unconjugated bilirubin
• Newborn screen
• Total protein and lactate dehydrogenase (LDH) (if obtaining pleural fluid)
• Chest radiograph

Pleural fluid analysis:
• Cell count and culture
• Triglyceride level
• Total protein
• LDH

Hematologic evaluation:
• Direct Coombs
• G6PD testing (if indicated)
• Hemoglobin electrophoresis (if indicated)
• Osmotic fragility testing (if indicated)

Cardiac evaluation:
• Cardiology consultation
• ECG
• Echocardiography

Infectious evaluation:
• Parvovirus IgM antibody in blood; could send DNA polymerase chain reaction (PCR) blood (if available through laboratory)
• *T gondii* testing:
  ○ IgA and/or IgM and IgG antibody testing in blood; or
  ○ IgG and/or IgM antibody testing in cerebrospinal fluid (CSF); or
  ○ PCR of blood, CSF, pleural fluid, and/or ascitic fluid
      And:
  ○ Maternal testing, including serologies and differential agglutination (of acetone [AC]-fixed versus that of formalin [HS]-fixed tachyzoites) test (AC/HS test) and avidity testing
• Rubella testing:
  ○ IgM and IgG antibody testing in blood (could send avidity testing if available)
  ○ Maternal testing should also be undertaken
• Urine cytomegalovirus
• Herpes simplex virus DNA PCR
  ○ Surface specimens from mouth, nasopharynx, conjunctivae, and anus
  ○ Surface specimens of skin vesicles
  ○ CSF
  ○ Blood
• HIV DNA PCR
• Syphilis testing:
  ○ Rapid plasma regain/Venereal Disease Research Laboratory (VDRL) titer in blood with comparison with maternal titers
  ○ CSF VDRL if possible or proven congenital syphilis
• Further work-up pending clinical suspicion for other infectious causes

Genetic evaluation:
• Genetic consultation
• Skeletal survey (to evaluate for anomalies associated with genetic or chromosomal syndromes and skeletal dysplasias)

- Microarray
- Single-gene sequencing or genotyping/multiple gene sequencing or genotyping through panels/testing for specific deletions or duplications (as indicated)
- Whole-exome sequencing (if indicated)
- Inborn errors of metabolism testing; consider sending for lysosomal storage diseases (if indicated)

Placental evaluation:
- Pathology

Additional imaging:
- Chest computed tomography (CT) or MRI (if concerned for CPAM, bronchopulmonary sequestration)
- Cranial ultrasonography with Doppler flows, head CT, or MRI/magnetic resonance (MR) angiography (if concerned for AVM or to assess for intracranial calcifications)
- Abdominal ultrasonography (to evaluate for liver hemangiomas, presence of ascites, anomalies of kidney/ureters, and other masses)
- Conventional transnodal lymphangiography or MRI, either noncontrast heavily weighted T2 imaging or dynamic-contrast MR lymphangiography (to evaluate for lymphatic malformations)

before 24 weeks' gestation associated with a survival rate of only 4% to 6%. Other factors associated with mortality include lower gestational age at time of delivery (<34 weeks), serum albumin level less than 2 g/dL, low 5-minute APGAR (appearance, pulse, grimace, activity, and respiration) score, severe acidemia, and need for high levels of support during the first day of life (defined as high levels of inspired oxygen support and treatment with high-frequency ventilation).[31,37,38] Studies show conflicting results as to whether anatomic distribution of fluid leads to increased mortality, with some studies showing increased survival in fetuses with fluid in only 2 compartments.[2,39,40] Predictors of survival include fetal treatment (whether medically, percutaneously, or fetoscopically) and resolution of hydrops.[2]

The cause of NIHF has a significant influence on survival. When evaluating both fetal and live-born infant outcomes, a recent meta-analysis showed that infants with chromosomal abnormalities had the highest mortality (99%), followed by infants with genetic syndromes/inborn errors of metabolism. Infants with infections or placental issues had the lowest mortality.[41] For cardiovascular disorders, survival depended greatly on the individual disorder/defect, with vascular disorders having the highest mortality and arrhythmias having the lowest.

Neurodevelopmental outcomes of infants with NIHF have not been extensively studied. In general, neonatal neurodevelopmental follow-up should be recommended because these infants are often born prematurely and have complex neonatal courses, placing them at risk for developmental delays.

SUMMARY

NIHF is a final common pathway of fetuses struggling from multiple possible underlying disease states. Over the years, diagnosis has improved but a significant number of idiopathic cases remain. Some of these disorders are amenable to treatment in utero, others require neonatal systemic support and time to heal, but morbidity and mortality remain high. Multidisciplinary prenatal and postnatal counseling about all options and levels of care are critical to help families make the best decisions for their fetuses and future children.

DISCLOSURE

All authors attest that they have no commercial or financial conflicts of interest or funding resources to disclose.

Best Practices

What is the current practice?

NIHF

Best practice/guideline/care path objectives
- After NIHF identified, begin diagnostic evaluation to determine cause.
- Assess whether there is a fetal therapeutic intervention, with referral as necessary.
- Timing of delivery depends on gestational age and maternal/fetal condition; generally indicated if diagnosed/worsening at later than 34 weeks.
- Skilled neonatal resuscitation team critical for delivery

What changes in current practice are likely to improve outcomes?

- Improved prenatal diagnosis of chromosomal abnormalities and lysosomal storage disorders.
- Continued improvements in postnatal diagnosis and management.
- Improved communication between medical team and family regarding expectations and goals of care.

Major recommendations

- After initial diagnosis, evaluation should include antibody screen to rule out immune hydrops, targeted ultrasonography and echocardiography, middle cerebral artery Doppler studies, and fetal karyotype/microarray (grade 1C).
- Multidisciplinary prenatal management with obstetrics/gynecology, maternal-fetal medicine, neonatology, and other pediatric or surgical subspecialists (depending on cause) is recommended.
- Management options depend on gestational age and health of mother, which include termination, fetal intervention if applicable, and expectant management with either neonatal intervention or palliative care.
- Preterm delivery generally indicated for obstetric indications. Delivery later than 37 weeks or if diagnosis/worsening condition after 34 weeks (grade 1C).
- Delivery should occur at center with access to level III or IV NICU with transfer of care if necessary (grade 1C).
- Therapeutic intervention in immediate postdelivery phase targeted toward adequate physiologic support, continued diagnostic evaluation (see **Box 1**), and potential therapeutic treatment to reverse NIHF.

Summary statement

Multidisciplinary counseling and shared decision making is critical to supporting families through pregnancy decisions, potential fetal therapeutic interventions, neonatal management decisions, and at times accepting or transitioning to palliative care.

REFERENCES

1. Steurer M, Peyvandi S, Baer R, et al. Epidemiology of live born infants with nonimmune hydrops fetalis – insights from a population-based dataset. J Pediatr 2017; 187:182–8.
2. Derderian S, Jeanty C, Fleck S, et al. The many faces of hydrops. J Pediatr Surg 2015;50:50–4.

3. Skoll M, Sharland G, Allan L. Is the ultrasound definition of fluid collections in non-immune hydrops fetalis helpful in defining the underlying cause or predicting outcome? Ultrasound Obstet Gynecol 1991;1:309–12.

4. Society for Maternal-Fetal Medicine (SMFM), Norton ME, Chauhan SP, et al. Society for maternal fetal medicine (SMFM) clinical guideline #7: nonimmune hydrops fetalis. Am J Obstet Gynecol 2015;212:127.

5. Bellini C, Hennekam R, Bonioli E. Etiology of nonimmune hydrops fetalis: a systemic review. Am J Med Genet 2009;149A:844–51.

6. Bellini C, Donarini G, Paladini D, et al. Etiology of non-immune hydrops fetalis: an update. Am J Med Genet A 2015;167A:1082–8.

7. Bellini C, Hennekam R. Non-immune hydrops fetalis: a short review of etiology and pathophysiology. Am J Med Genet A 2012;158A(3):597–605.

8. Levick J, Michel C. Microvascular fluid exchange and the revised Starling principle. Cardiovasc Res 2010;87:198–210.

9. Yurdakok M. Non-immune hydrops fetalis. J Pediatr Neonat Individual Med 2014;3(2):e030214.

10. Randenberg A. Nonimmune hydrops fetalis part I: etiology and pathophysiology. Neonatal Netw 2010;29:281–95.

11. Bellini C, Ergaz Z, Radicioni M, et al. Congenital fetal and neonatal visceral chylous effusions: neonatal chylothorax and chylous ascites revisited. A multicenter retrospective study. Lymphology 2012;45:91–102.

12. Murphy J. Nonimmune hydrops fetalis. Neoreviews 2004;5(1):e5–14.

13. Ban J. Neonatal arrhythmias: diagnosis, treatment, and clinical outcome. Korean J Pediatr 2017;60:344–52.

14. Arcasoy M, Gallagher P. Hematologic disorders and nonimmune hydrops fetalis. Semin Perinatol 1995;19:502–15.

15. Isaacs H. Fetal hydrops associated with tumors. Am J Perinatol 2008;25:43–68.

16. Xu J, Raff T, Muallem N, et al. Hydrops fetalis secondary to parvovirus B19 infections. J Am Board Fam Pract 2003;16(1):63–8.

17. Jones D. Nonimmune fetal hydrops: diagnosis and obstetrical management. Semin Perinatol 1995;19:447–61.

18. Sanford E, Saadai P, Lee H, et al. Congenital high airway obstruction sequence (CHAOS): a new case and a review of phenotypic features. Am J Med Genet 2012;158A:3126–316.

19. Gimovsky A, Luzi P, Berghella V. Lysosomal storage disease as an etiology of nonimmune hydrops. Am J Obstet Gynecol 2015;212:281–90.

20. Lallemand A, Doco-Fenzy M, Gaillard D. Investigation of nonimmune hydrops fetalis: multidisciplinary studies are necessary for diagnosis – review of 94 cases. Pediatr Dev Pathol 1999;2(5):432–9.

21. Santo S, Mansour S, Thilaganathan B, et al. Prenatal diagnosis of non-immune hydrops fetalis: what do we tell the parents? Prenat Diagn 2011;31(2):186–95.

22. Huhta J. Guidelines for the evaluation of heart failure in the fetus with or without hydrops. Pediatr Cardiol 2004;25:274–86.

23. Mardy A, Chetty S, Norton M, et al. A system-based approach to the genetic etiologies of non-immune hydrops fetalis. Prenat Diagn 2019;39(9):732–50.

24. Burwick RM, Pilliod RA, Dukhovny SE, et al. Fetal hydrops and the risk of severe preeclampsia. J Matern Fetal Neonatal Med 2019;32(6):961–5.

25. Grethel E, Wagner A, Clifton M, et al. Fetal intervention for mass lesions and hydrops improves outcome: a 15-year experience. J Pediatr Surg 2007;42:117–23.

26. Van Mieghem T, Al-Ibrahim A, Deprest J, et al. Minimally invasive therapy for fetal sacrococcygeal teratoma: case series and systematic review of the literature. Ultrasound Obstet Gynecol 2014;43:611–9.

27. Leuthner S. Fetal palliative care. Clin Perinatol 2004;31:649–65.

28. Leuthner S, Lamberg-Jones E. The fetal concerns program: a model for perinatal palliative care. MCN Am J Matern Child Nurs 2007;32:272–8.

29. Munson D, Leuthner S. Palliative care for the family carrying a fetus with a life-limiting diagnosis. Pediatr Clin North Am 2007;54:787–98.

30. Kenner C, Press J, Ryan D. Recommendations for palliative and bereavement care in the NICU: a family-centered integrative approach. J Perinat 2015;35:519–23.

31. Takci S, Gharibzadeh M, Yurdakok M, et al. Etiology and outcome of hydrops fetalis: report of 62 cases. Pediatr Neonatol 2014;55:108–13.

32. Zaki S, Krishnamurthy M, Malhotra A. Octreotide use in neonates: a case series. Drugs R D 2018;18:191–8.

33. Peeples E. An evaluation of hydrocortisone dosing for neonatal refractory hypotension. Neonatology 2017;111:415–22.

34. Shalish W, Olivier F, Aly H, et al. Uses and misuses of albumin during resuscitation and in the neonatal intensive care unit. Semin Fetal Neonatal Med 2017;22:328–35.

35. White M, Bhat R, Greenough A. Neonatal chylothoraces: a 10-year experience in a tertiary neonatal referral centre. Case Rep Pediatr 2019;2019:3903598.

36. Wilkins I. Nonimmune hydrops. In: Resnik R, Lockwood CJ, Moore TR, et al, editors. Creasy and Resniks maternal-fetal medicine: principles and practice. 7th edition. Philadelphia: Elsevier; 2014. p. 569–77.

37. Abrams M, Meredith K, Kinnard P, et al. Hydrops fetalis: a retrospective review of cases reported to a large national database and identification of risk factors associated with death. Pediatrics 2007;120:84–9.

38. Huang H-R, Tsay P-K, Chiang M-C, et al. Prognostic factors and clinical features in liveborn neonates with hydrops fetalis. Am J Perinatol 2007;24(1):033–8.

39. Wafelman L, Pollock B, Kreutzer J, et al. Nonimmune hydrops fetalis: fetal and neonatal outcome during 1983-1992. Biol Neonate 1999;75:73–81.

40. Wy C, Sajous C, Loberiza F, et al. Outcome of infants with a diagnosis of hydrops fetalis in the 1990s. Am J Perinatol 1999;16:561–70.

41. Randenberg A. Nonimmune hydrops fetalis part II: does etiology influence mortality. Neonatal Netw 2010;29:367–80.

Mitochondrial DNA Depletion Syndromes

Donald Basel, MBBCh

KEYWORDS

- Mitochondria • External ophthalmoplegia • Pseudo-obstruction • Depletion

KEY POINTS

- Mitochondrial disorders can present at any age.
- Mitochondrial disorders can affect a single system or present as a multisystem disease.
- Mitochondrial disorders are primarily inherited as autosomal disorders.
- Hallmark features include progressive visual, hepatic, renal, neurologic, or cardiovascular symptoms.

INTRODUCTION

Mitochondria tend to get a bad reputation in today's health literate world. It seems that every blog, vlog, and social media health forum is attributing any unexplained clinical symptom to mitochondrial dysfunction. The reason for this is partly that mitochondrial dysfunction can present in many insidious ways that are not classically attributable to the typical encephalomyopathies that characterize mitochondrial disease (**Fig. 1**). Another reason relates to the challenges in making a clear diagnosis of a mitochondrial disease.[1] This article creates a category of diagnosis uncertain in order to limit the confusion created by the possibility of a mitochondrial diagnosis in the electronic medical record. Mitochondrial disorders can manifest at any age and affect any number of organ systems, from an isolated system to a complex multisystem disorder. Many are identified by unique acronyms that add to their medical mystique; NARP (neuropathy, ataxia, and retinitis pigmentosa), MELAS (mitochondrial myopathy, encephalopathy, lactic acidosis, and stroke-like episodes), LHON (leber hereditary optic neuropathy), and MNGIE (mitochondrial neurogastrointestinal encephalomyopathy) to name but a few. This article addresses some of the general aspects of mitochondrial disorders and focuses specifically on a subset of disorders relating to mitochondrial DNA depletion.

Mitochondria can be considered evolutionary remnants of a prokaryotic symbiotic relationship within a eukaryotic cell and each cell contains between 1000 and 2000 mitochondria, which creates a unique conundrum in that not all mitochondria function

Department of Pediatrics, Division of Genetics, Medical College of Wisconsin, 9000 West Wisconsin Avenue, MS #716, Milwaukee, WI 53226, USA
E-mail address: dbasel@mcw.edu

Clin Perinatol 47 (2020) 123–141
https://doi.org/10.1016/j.clp.2019.10.008
0095-5108/20/© 2019 Elsevier Inc. All rights reserved.
perinatology.theclinics.com

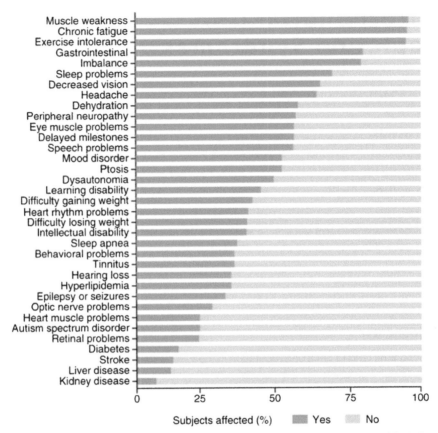

Fig. 1. Mitochondrial disease subject cohort, experienced symptoms. (*Modified from* Zolkipli-Cunningham Z, Xiao R, Stoddart A, et al. Mitochondrial disease patient motivations and barriers to participate in clinical trials. PLoS ONE 13(5):e0197513.)

equally (heteroplasmy) and that mitochondria contain their own unique plasmid genome, mitochondrial DNA (mtDNA). For normal function of mitochondria, the mtDNA encodes for 13 protein subunits of the respiratory chain, whereas nuclear genes code for the remaining subunits of the approximately 70-peptide complex.[2] This contribution is represented in **Fig. 2**, which displays the contribution to the 5 subunits of the respiratory chain complexes located in the inner mitochondrial membrane.

Mitochondrial disorders can thus be inherited in an autosomal fashion (dominant or recessive), or as maternally inherited mitochondrial genes. About 20% of all mitochondrial diseases are inherited maternally, whereas the remainder are autosomal. The incidence of mitochondrial diseases has been estimated at 1:8500.[3]

SPECTRUM OF MITOCHONDRIAL DISEASE

Mitochondrial disease represents a broad spectrum of clinically heterogeneous disorders that manifest as a result of abnormal energy production through oxidative phosphorylation in the respiratory chain (**Figs. 2** and **3**). In the perinatal period the typical presentation is that of a hypotonic neonate or infant who may additionally have metabolic dysregulation, lactic acidosis in particular. The systemic features, aside from reduced tone, could include cardiomyopathy, which may be either dilated or

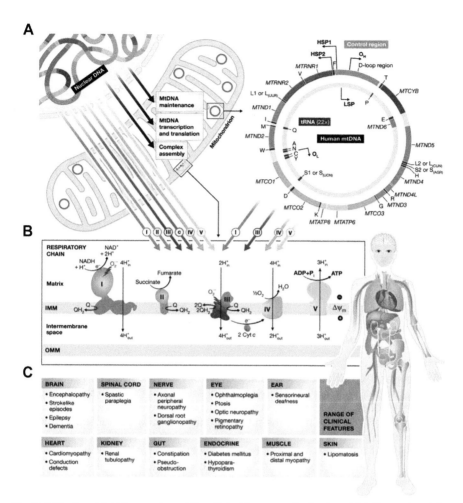

Fig. 2. Mitochondrial biogenesis and the clinical features of mitochondrial disease in adults. (*A*) Nuclear and mitochondrial genomics, (*B*) respiratory chain complexes indicating oxidative phosphorylation producing ATP, (*C*) multisystem disease spectrum. (*From* Chinnery PF. Mitochondrial disease in adults: what's old and what's new?. EMBO Mol Med. 2015 Dec;7(12):1503-12. https://doi.org/10.15252/emmm.201505079; with permission.)

hypertrophic and may be severe enough to present with cardiorespiratory failure. Poor respiratory muscle function frequently contributes to the severity of the acidosis and general poor condition. Encephalopathy and seizures are a common complication of severe perinatal mitochondrial dysfunction. Common clinical features of mitochondrial disease in older children or adults include nonspecific muscle, cardiac, endocrine, and neurologic signs. The more common clinical findings include migraine, progressive external ophthalmoplegia, optic atrophy, pigmentary retinopathy, sensorineural deafness, exercise intolerance, cardiomyopathy, seizures, encephalopathy/dementia, ataxia, and diabetes mellitus. **Fig. 2** shows the primary metabolic function within the mitochondria: producing energy-rich ATP molecules through the respiratory chain as well as the spectrum of generalized and systemic manifestations that are seen in mitochondrial dysfunction.[4,5]

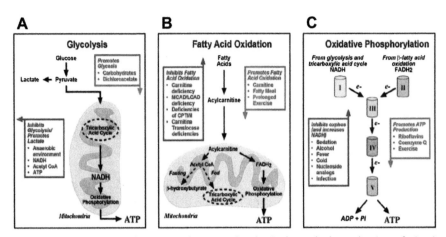

Fig. 3. The major source of energy-rich ATP molecules is through the reduction of nicotinamide adenine dinucleotide (NADH) and flavin adenine dinucleotide ($FADH_2$) molecules, which are produced in the tricarboxylic acid cycle (TCA) cycle from acetyl coenzyme A derived from glycolysis and fatty acid oxidation. The transport of electrons through the electron transport chain (ETC) results in ATP production, which is necessary for cellular function.

MITOCHONDRIAL DNA DEPLETION SYNDROMES (MTDPS)

All currently recognized mitochondrial depletion disorders are inherited in an autosomal manner. The concept of depletion comes from the lack of the ability of the mitochondrial genetic machinery to adequately replicate the mtDNA, which, in simplistic terms, means that the number of mitochondria gradually decreases until a critical mass is reached, at which point the remaining mitochondria cannot support normal cellular function and cell death ensues. The mechanism involves either deficiencies in mitochondrial nucleotide synthesis or more directly in mtDNA replication. This process should not be confused with mtDNA deletion disorders.

Mitochondrial DNA depletion syndromes represent a wide spectrum of mitochondrial disease and are categorized into 15 distinct forms based on their genetic causes.[6–34] They are subtyped into neurogastrointestinal[6,7,12,13] (**Table 1**), hepatocerebral[10–13,16–19,34] (**Table 2**), myopathic[8,9,26,27] (**Table 3**), cardiomyopathic[24,25,28–30] (**Table 4**), and encephalomyopathic[15,16,20–23,31–33] (**Table 5**) phenotypes.[4]

Most of these disorders present with failure to thrive in early infancy in addition to the broad primary organ system involvement for which they are classified. Subtypes 1 and 11 are the only forms that typically present beyond the neonatal or infant period (represented in **Tables 1** and **3**). These disorders all highlight the common theme of all mitochondrial disease: variability. There are variable ages of onset with variable clinical phenotypes within each phenotypic subset, and even though the disorders are broadly subtyped into different forms, there is phenotypic overlap across the spectrum of the disorders. Many share features of cardiac dysfunction, muscle hypotonia, and encephalopathy despite their subgrouping. The prognostic outlook for these early-onset disorders is poor, with early childhood demise being the anticipated norm.

UNDERSTANDING THE PATHOPHYSIOLOGY OF MITOCHONDRIAL DISORDERS

The underlying mechanism of disease depends on how the functions of the mitochondria are affected. In primary mitochondrial disorders, intrinsic dysfunction within the

Table 1
Mitochondrial DNA depletion syndromes: neurogastrointestinal subtypes

Title	MTDPS1[6,7]	MTDPS4B[12,13]
Inheritance	Autosomal recessive	Autosomal recessive
Age of onset	Second to fifth decade	Infancy or late childhood
Growth	Failure to thrive	Failure to thrive
Head and Neck		
Head	—	—
Face	—	—
Ears	Hearing loss, sensorineural	Hearing loss
Eyes	External ophthalmoplegia, progressive Ptosis	External ophthalmoplegia, progressive
Cardiovascular	—	—
Respiratory	—	—
Gastrointestinal	Gastrointestinal dysmotility Nausea/vomiting Malabsorption Constipation, chronic Chronic intestinal pseudo-obstruction Diverticulosis/diverticulitis Intestinal perforation	Gastrointestinal dysmotility — Malabsorption Constipation, chronic Chronic intestinal pseudo-obstruction — —
Liver	—	Hepatic dysfunction/failure
Genitourinary	—	—
Musculoskeletal	Mitochondrial myopathy Distal limb muscle weakness	Mitochondrial myopathy Diffuse muscle weakness
Skin, nails, and hair	—	—
Neurologic	—	Hypotonia
CNS	Leukoencephalopathy	Seizures Developmental delay Ataxia
CNS MRI features	Hypodensity of cerebral white matter seen on MRI	White matter abnormalities
Peripheral nervous system	Sensorimotor neuropathy Axonal demyelinating neuropathy Areflexia	Sensory neuropathy — —
Behavioral/psychiatric manifestations	—	—
Endocrine features	—	—
Hematology	—	—
Immunology	—	—
Laboratory abnormalities	Lactic acidosis Decreased activity of thymidine phosphorylase Increased serum thymidine Increased serum deoxyuridine	— — — —

(continued on next page)

Table 1 (continued)		
Title	MTDPS1[6,7]	MTDPS4B[12,13]
Muscle studies	Ragged red fibers mtDNA depletion: < 45% Decreased ETC on muscle biopsy Numerous abnormal mitochondria with loss of cristae	Ragged red fibers — Decreased ETC on muscle biopsy —
Miscellaneous	Progressive disorder —	Progressive disorder Variable severity
Gene	TYMP	POLG
OMIM number	603041	613662
Other names	MNGIE	Alpers-Huttenlocher syndrome

Abbreviations: CNS, central nervous system; ETC, electron transport chain/oxidative phosphorylation; MNGIE, myoneurogastrointestinal encephalopathy; MTDPS, mitochondrial DNA depletion syndromes; OMIM, Online Mendelian Inheritance in Man; POLG, DNA polymerase-gamma; TYMP, thymidine phosphorylase.

mitochondria is responsible for catabolic failure. This failure of the catabolic process can be broadly considered under the umbrella of energy metabolism, which includes glycolysis and beta-oxidation of fatty acids combined with the tricarboxylic acid (TCA) cycle and the oxidative phosphorylation pathway (electron transport chain [ETC]) to generate ATP (see **Fig. 3**).[35]

The major source of energy-rich ATP molecules is through the reduction of nicotinamide adenine dinucleotide (NADH) and flavin adenine dinucleotide ($FADH_2$) molecules, which are produced in the TCA cycle from acetyl coenzyme A derived from glycolysis and fatty acid oxidation. The transport of electrons through the ETC results in ATP production, which is necessary for cellular function.

BIOMARKERS FOR MITOCHONDRIAL DISEASE

The logical expectation would be that there are numerous options for using various biochemical markers for mitochondrial dysfunction. Analysis of plasma amino acids, acyl carnitines, and various other markers has proved to be less than ideal when screening for the presence of mitochondrial disease because these metabolites are often abnormal in disease states not directly linked to primary mitochondrial dysfunction. The biggest challenge with many of the putative biomarkers in mitochondrial disease is the general lack of longitudinal studies and difficulties accessing samples from affected organ systems.

Aside from metabolite analysis, additional biomarkers for mitochondrial disease include the natural history of the clinical presentation and the clinical phenotyping examination, with imaging studies of the brain using MRI, magnetic resonance spectroscopy (MRS), PET, or functional MRI.

The invasive nature of accessing affected tissue frequently limits the utility of performing ETC studies even though this is generally one of the most helpful assays in the diagnostic evaluation. Given the ease of sequencing, invasive testing is frequently reserved after sequencing has failed to yield a clear causal association or if there is a variant of unknown significance that could be interpreted as pathogenic if there are

Table 2
Mitochondrial DNA depletion syndromes: hepatocerebral subtypes

Title	MTDPS3[10,11]	MTDPS4A[12,13]	MTDPS15[34]
Inheritance	Autosomal recessive	Autosomal recessive	Autosomal recessive
Age of onset	Neonatal	Infancy	Neonatal
Growth	Failure to thrive	Failure to thrive	Failure to thrive
Head and Neck			
Head	Microcephaly	—	—
Face	—	—	—
Ears	—	—	—
Eyes	Nystagmus	Visual disturbances	—
	Disconjugate eye movements	Cortical blindness	—
	Optic dysplasia	—	—
Cardiovascular	—	—	—
Respiratory	—	—	—
Gastrointestinal	Poor feeding	—	Ascites
	Vomiting	Vomiting	—
	Portal hypertension	—	—
	Ascites	—	—
	Splenomegaly	—	—
Liver	Hepatic dysfunction/failure	Hepatic dysfunction/failure	Progressive liver failure
	Hepatomegaly	Hepatomegaly	Cirrhosis/cholestasis/steatosis
	Cirrhosis/cholestasis/steatosis	Cirrhosis/cholestasis/steatosis	—
Genitourinary	—	—	—
Musculoskeletal	—	—	Contractures of the lower limbs
Skin, nails, and hair	—	—	—
Neurologic	—	Hypotonia	—
CNS	Seizures	Seizures, refractory	—
	Encephalopathy	Developmental delay	Cognitive impairment, moderate to profound
	Cerebral atrophy	Psychomotor regression, episodic, often associated with common childhood infections	—
	Hyperreflexia	Ataxia	—
	—	Dementia	—
	—	Myoclonus	—
CNS MRI features	—	Cerebral/cerebellar atrophy	Cerebellar hypoplasia
	—	Pseudolaminar spongiform changes	—
Peripheral nervous system	Peripheral neuropathy	—	—
Behavioral/psychiatric manifestations	—	—	—

(continued on next page)

Table 2 (continued)			
Title	**MTDPS3[10,11]**	**MTDPS4A[12,13]**	**MTDPS15[34]**
Endocrine features	Hypoglycemia	—	Hypoglycemia
Hematology	Coagulopathy Thrombocytopenia	— —	Coagulopathy —
Immunology	—	—	—
Laboratory abnormalities	Lactic acidosis Hyperbilirubinemia	Lactic acidosis Increased liver function tests	Hyperbilirubinemia Abnormal liver enzymes
	Abnormal liver function tests	Increased CSF protein	Hypoalbuminemia
	Hypoalbuminemia	Methylglutaconic aciduria	Increased plasma tyrosine
	Generalized aminoaciduria	Intermittent ethylmalonic aciduria	Increased plasma methionine
	—	Intermittent dicarbonic aciduria	Abnormal urinary organic acids
Muscle studies	—	—	mtDNA depletion: <45%
	—	mtDNA depletion: < 45%	Decreased ETC on muscle biopsy
	—	Decreased ETC on muscle biopsy	Sarcoplasmic abnormalities
	—	—	Numerous abnormal mitochondria with loss of cristae
Miscellaneous	Early infant demise Hepatic failure develops in first months of life	Rapidly progressive Death usually by age 3 y	Progressive disorder Death in infancy
	—	Later onset (late childhood to young adult) has been reported	—
	—	Increased sensitivity to valproic acid toxicity	—
Gene	DGUOK	POLG	TFAMA
OMIM number	251880	203700	617156
Other names	—	—	—

Abbreviations: CSF, cerebrospinal fluid; DGUOK, deoxyguanosine kinase; MTDPS, mitochondrial DNA depletion syndromes; TFAM, mitochondrial transcription factor A.

abnormal functional studies. Two plasma biomarkers have been identified that seem to offer greater correlation with mitochondrial disease: GDF-15 (growth differentiation factor 15)[36–38] and FGF-21 (fibroblast growth factor 21).[39,40] However, increases in the levels of these peptides are not pathognomonic for a mitochondrial disorder. GDF-15 levels can be increased in pregnancy, muscle disease or intense exercise training, and pulmonary hypertension, whereas FGF-21 levels can be increased in a wide range of metabolic disorders, such as diabetes, obesity, and the metabolic syndrome. Despite this, published data seem to indicate that significant increases in their levels are highly suggestive of underlying mitochondrial dysfunction.

Table 3
Mitochondrial DNA depletion syndromes: myopathic subtypes

Title	MTDPS2[8,9]	MTDPS11[26,27]
Inheritance	Autosomal recessive	Autosomal recessive
Age of onset	Infancy or late childhood	Variable: first to fourth decade
Growth	—	Failure to thrive
Head and Neck		
Head	—	Microcephaly
Face	Facial diplegia	Facial weakness
Ears	—	—
Eyes	—	Progressive external ophthalmoplegia
	—	Ptosis
Cardiovascular	—	Dilated cardiomyopathy
	—	Arrhythmias
Respiratory	Respiratory insufficiency caused by muscle weakness	Respiratory insufficiency, severe, caused by muscle weakness
Gastrointestinal	—	Loss of appetite
	—	Abdominal fullness
	—	Nausea
	—	Diarrhea
Liver	—	—
Genitourinary	—	Renal colic
Musculoskeletal	Mitochondrial myopathy Proximal muscle weakness Gowers sign Loss of ability to walk in early childhood	Mitochondrial myopathy Fatigue/exercise intolerance Muscle atrophy, generalized Spinal deformities: scoliosis, kyphosis, rigidity
Skin, Nails, and Hair	—	—
Neurologic	Hypotonia	—
CNS	—	Developmental delay
CNS MRI features	—	Cerebellar hypoplasia
Peripheral nervous system	—	Hyporeflexia
Behavioral/ psychiatric manifestations	—	—
Endocrine features	—	Hypergonadotropic hypogonadism
Hematology	—	—
Immunology	—	—
Laboratory abnormalities	Lactic acidosis Increased serum creatine kinase Aminoaciduria	— Increased serum creatine kinase —
Muscle studies	Ragged red fibers mtDNA depletion: <45% Decreased ETC on muscle biopsy	Ragged red fibers mtDNA depletion: <45% Decreased ETC on muscle biopsy

(continued on next page)

Table 3 (continued)		
Title	**MTDPS2**[8,9]	**MTDPS11**[26,27]
Miscellaneous	Progressive disorder Later onset has been reported Variable severity	Progressive disorder — —
Gene	TK2	MGME1
OMIM number	609560	615084
Other names	—	—

Abbreviations: MGME1, mitochondrial genome maintenance exonuclease 1; MTDPS, mitochondrial DNA depletion syndromes; TK2, thymidine kinase.

Table 4 Mitochondrial DNA depletion syndromes: cardiomyopathic subtypes			
Title	**MTDPS10**[24,25]	**MTDPS12A**[28–30]	**MTDPS12B**[28–30]
Inheritance	Autosomal recessive	Autosomal dominant	Autosomal recessive
Age of onset	Infancy	Neonatal	Childhood
Growth	Failure to thrive	—	Rare: obesity
Head and Neck			
Head	—	—	—
Face	—	—	—
Ears	—	—	—
Eyes	Cataracts, infantile Myopia Glaucoma	— — —	Cataracts — —
Cardiovascular	Hypertrophic cardiomyopathy	Hypertrophic cardiomyopathy	Hypertrophic cardiomyopathy
Respiratory	Respiratory insufficiency caused by muscle weakness	Respiratory insufficiency caused by muscle weakness	—
Gastrointestinal	—	Poor feeding caused by muscle weakness	—
Liver	—	—	—
Genitourinary	—	—	—
Musculoskeletal	Mitochondrial myopathy Fatigue/exercise intolerance — —	Mitochondrial myopathy Inability to walk independently — —	Mitochondrial myopathy Inability to walk independently Muscle atrophy Feet: high-arched feet/hammer-shaped toes/ Achilles contractures
Skin, nails, and hair	—	—	—
Neurologic	Hypotonia	Hypotonia, profound	—

(continued on next page)

Table 4 (continued)			
Title	MTDPS10[24,25]	MTDPS12A[28–30]	MTDPS12B[28–30]
CNS	—	—	—
—	Normal cognition	Psychomotor delay, severe	Cognitive impairment
CNS MRI features	—	—	—
Peripheral nervous system	—	Hyporeflexia	—
Behavioral/ psychiatric manifestations	—	—	—
Endocrine features	—	—	—
Hematology	Thrombocytopenia	—	—
Immunology	—	—	—
Laboratory abnormalities	Lactic acidosis (exercise)	Lactic acidosis	Lactic acidosis
	—	Increased serum and CSF lactate	—
	3-Methylglutaconic aciduria	Organic aciduria (in some patients)	—
Muscle studies	Lipid storage myopathy	Lipid storage myopathy	Ragged red fibers
	mtDNA depletion: <45%	mtDNA depletion: <45%	mtDNA depletion: <45%
	Decreased ETC on muscle biopsy	Decreased ETC on muscle biopsy	Decreased ETC on muscle biopsy
	Numerous abnormal mitochondria with loss of cristae	Numerous abnormal mitochondria with loss of cristae	Numerous abnormal mitochondria with loss of cristae
Miscellaneous	Variable phenotype	Many patients die in infancy	Slowly progressive
	High risk of death in infancy caused by cardiac failure	Patients become ventilator dependent	—
Gene	AGK	SLC25A4	SLC25A4
OMIM number	212350	617184	615418
Other names	Sengers syndrome	—	—

Abbreviations: AGK, acylglycerol kinase; MTDPS, mitochondrial DNA depletion syndromes; SLC25A4, solute carrier family 25 (mitochondrial carrier, adenine nucleotide translocator) member 4 gene.

DIAGNOSTIC EVALUATION

Typical patients coming for an evaluation for a mitochondrial disorder are likely to follow some form of diagnostic odyssey. The reason for this is the early nonspecific clinical presentation, which overlaps with many more common disorders. Affected individuals have thus usually been seen by specialists and numerous tests have been ordered as part of a general evaluation. Key investigations that are helpful in differentiating mitochondrial disorders include biochemical screening for

Table 5

Mitochondrial DNA depletion syndromes: encephalomyopathic subtypes

Title	MTDPS5[14,15]	MTDPS8A[20,21]	MTDPS9[22,23]	MTDPS13[31,32]	MTDPS14[33]
Inheritance	Autosomal recessive	Autosomal recessive	Autosomal recessive	Autosomal recessive	Autosomal recessive
Age of onset	Infancy	Infancy	Infancy	Birth or early infancy	Birth or early infancy
Growth	Failure to thrive	Failure to Thrive	Failure to Thrive	Failure to Thrive	—
Head and Neck					
Head	—	—	—	Microcephaly	—
Face	Facial diplegia	—	—	Dysmorphic facial features: elongated narrow face, epicanthic folds	—
Ears	Hearing loss, sensorineural	—	Hearing loss	Prominent ears	Sensorineural hearing loss
Eyes	Ophthalmoplegia Ptosis	External ophthalmoplegia	—	Nystagmus Cataracts Downslanting palpebral fissures	Nystagmus Optic atrophy
Cardiovascular	—	—	—	Hypertrophic cardiomyopathy Arrhythmia	Hypertrophic cardiomyopathy
Respiratory	Respiratory insufficiency caused by muscle weakness	—	Respiratory insufficiency caused by muscle weakness	—	—
Gastrointestinal	Poor feeding	Gastrointestinal dysmotility Feeding difficulties	Feeding difficulties	Gastroesophageal reflux disease Dysphagia	—
Liver	—	—	—	—	—

Genitourinary	—	Proximal renal tubulopathy	—	Renal tubular acidosis	—
Musculoskeletal	Muscle weakness Delayed motor skills Loss of ability to walk in early childhood	—	Mitochondrial myopathy Inability to sit or hold head up	Muscle atrophy Spinal deformities: scoliosis Feet: small	—
Skin, nails, and hair	—	—	Hyperhidrosis	—	—
Neurologic	Hypotonia	Hypotonia	Hypotonia, axial, severe	Hypotonia	Spasticity
CNS	Seizures Psychomotor delay, severe Movement disorder: athetoid, dystonia, hyperkinetic Spasticity Hyporeflexia	Seizures Developmental delay Ataxia Neurologic deterioration	Psychomotor delay, severe Cerebral atrophy Widening of the ventricles	Seizures Psychomotor delay, severe Movement disorder: athetoid, dystonia, hyperkinetic Ataxia Encephalopathy	Dysmetria Encephalopathy Global developmental delay Ataxia
CNS MRI features	Imaging shows signal abnormalities in basal ganglia Cerebral atrophy	—	Basal ganglia lesions	Cerebral/cerebellar atrophy Leukodystrophy: diffuse, white matter, brainstem, basal ganglia	Cerebellar atrophy
Peripheral nervous system	Axonal demyelinating neuropathy	—	—	—	Sensorimotor axonal neuropathy
Behavioral/psychiatric manifestations	Irritability/inconsolable crying	—	—	—	—
Endocrine features	—	—	Hypoglycemia	—	—
Hematology	—	—	Neutropenia	—	—

(continued on next page)

Table 5 (*continued*)

Title	MTDPS5[14,15]	MTDPS8A[20,21]	MTDPS9[22,23]	MTDPS13[31,32]	MTDPS14[33]
Immunology	—	—	—	Recurrent infections	—
Laboratory abnormalities	Lactic acidosis; Increased serum creatine kinase; Increased serum and CSF lactate; Methylmalonic aciduria; Methylglutaconic aciduria; Increased urinary carnitine esters; Aminoaciduria, intermittent	Lactic acidosis; Aminoaciduria	Lactic acidosis; Methylmalonic aciduria; Increased lactate in spinal fluid	Lactic acidosis; Abnormal liver enzymes; Increased serum ammonia; Increased serum alanine	Lactic acidosis; —; 3-Methylglutaconic aciduria; —
Muscle studies	—; —; Decreased ETC on muscle biopsy; —	Ragged red fibers; mtDNA depletion: <45%; Decreased ETC on muscle biopsy; Numerous abnormal mitochondria with loss of cristae	Ragged red fibers; mtDNA depletion: <45%; Decreased ETC on muscle biopsy; —	—; mtDNA depletion: <45%; Decreased ETC on muscle biopsy; —	—; —; —; —
Miscellaneous	Increased frequency in the Faroe Islands (carrier 1 in 25)	Progressive disorder; Occasional later onset and more variable phenotype: MNGIE (8B)	Variable phenotype; Death usually in infancy	Variable phenotype; May result in early death	—
Gene	SUCLA2	RRM2B	SUCLG1	FBXL4	OPA1
OMIM number	612073	612075	245400	615471	616896
Other names	—	—	—	—	Behr syndrome

Abbreviations: FBXL4, F-box and leucine-rich repeat protein 4; MTDPS, mitochondrial DNA depletion syndromes; OPA1, optic atrophy 1; RRM2B, ribonucleotide reductase, M2 B; SUCLA2, succinate–coenzyme A ligase ADP-forming beta-subunit; SUCLG1, alpha subunit of succinate–coenzyme A ligase .

Table 6
Mitochondrial disease criteria

Features		
Muscular	Myopathy Abnormal EMG Motor developmental delay Exercise intolerance	Maximal score for muscle is 2
Neurologic	Developmental delay or intellectual disability Speech delay Dystonia Ataxia Spasticity Neuropathy Seizures or encephalopathy	Maximal score for neurologic is 2
Multisystem	Any gastrointestinal tract disease Growth delay or failure to thrive Endocrine Immune Eye (vision) or hearing Renal tubular acidosis Cardiomyopathy	Maximal score for multisystem is 3
Total clinical	—	Total clinical score is maximal 4
Metabolic	Lactate high, at least double: (score 2) Alanine high, at least double Krebs cycle intermediates[a] Ethyl malonic and methyl malonic acid 3-Methyl glutaconic acid CSF lactate, alanine	—
Imaging/other	Leigh disease (score 2) Strokelike episodes (score 2) Lactate peak on MRS Leukoencephalopathy with brainstem and spinal cord involvement[b] Cavitating leukoencephalopathy[b] Leukoencephalopathy with thalamus involvement[b] Deep cerebral white matter involvement and corpus callosum agenesis[b]	Total metabolic and MRI is maximal 4
Total MDC score (clinical, metabolic, imaging)	—	Total score is maximal 8

Every element scores 1 unless indicated differently. The severity of each finding is not taken into account because of the progressive nature of the disease. A total score of 1 indicates unlikely mitochondrial disorder; score 2 to 4, possible mitochondrial disorder; score 5 to 7, probable mitochondrial disorder; and score ≥ 8, definite mitochondrial disorder.

[a] Krebs cycle intermediates: alpha-ketoglutarate, succinate, fumarate.
[b] Recently numerous MRI patterns characteristic of mitochondrial disease have been described in addition to Leigh syndrome, and basal ganglia with brainstem involvement. The authors now include leukoencephalopathy with brainstem and spinal cord involvement (*DARS2*), cavitating leukoencephalopathy (*LYRM7*), leukoencephalopathy with thalamus involvement (*EARS2*), deep cerebral white matter involvement, and corpus callosum agenesis (*NUBPL*).

From Witters P, Saada A, Honzik T, et al. Revisiting mitochondrial diagnostic criteria in the new era of genomics. Genet Med. 2018 Apr;20(4):444-451. https://doi.org/10.1038/gim.2017.125. Epub 2017 Oct 26; with permission.

abnormalities of the TCA cycle, lactate (often combined with pyruvate to provide a lactate/pyruvate ratio, which, if increased >20 suggests mitochondrial dysfunction). Imaging of the brain through MRI/MRS as well as muscle investigation (electromyogram/nerve conduction velocity) or, in some cases, biopsy. Measuring metabolite levels before and after exercise can be useful to delineate mitochondrial disorders from primary myopathies.

Several clinical scoring systems have been developed to aid diagnosis of mitochondrial disease: the Newcastle Paediatric Mitochondrial Disease Scale (NPMDS)[41] and the Mitochondrial Disease Criteria (MDC)[42] are among the more commonly considered (**Table 6**). Both scales apply a numerical score to the probability of the presence of mitochondrial disease based on clinical, biochemical, and neuroimaging findings. Despite a reasonably good positive predictive value, the challenge with using such criteria exemplifies the difficulties in mitochondrial diagnosis because even 12% of study subjects with low MDC scores were identified to have a mitochondrial diagnosis on genomic analysis in the Witters and colleagues[42] study.

INTERVENTION/MANAGEMENT

Mitochondrial disorders are progressive and there are currently no curative therapies available. Management is focused on the medical management of the specific organ system dysfunction (renal, hepatic, cardiac, or neurologic) as well as optimizing nutrition and physical health. Avoidance of therapeutics known to be toxic (eg, valproic acid in POLG [DNA polymerase-gamma]-related depletion disorders) to mitochondrial function are avoided, but occasionally risk benefits play into these decisions, especially when considering inotropic medications in cardiac failure. The implementation of supplements that have some evidence to support their clinical utility are recommended; however, long-term benefits and significant disease modification remains unproved.[43] The typical mitochondrial "cocktail"[3] is recommended with the intent of optimizing oxidative phosphorylation and depleting potential oxidizing radicals that could induce autophagy. Investigational agents are being evaluated for targeting mitochondrial dysfunction. In the context of mitochondrial depletion associated with thymidine kinase, nucleosides have been shown to have some success in stabilizing the progression of the disease. Sodium pyruvate supplementation has additionally been reported to have positive health impacts for children with depletion disorders. Liver and stem cell transplants have been attempted in several centers, but the outcomes are complicated by multisystem involvement and thus this practice has been controversial unless disease is limited to the liver.[44–48]

SUMMARY

Given the broad clinical spectrum, mitochondrial disorders should be considered when the clinical presentation includes progressive multisystem involvement. Cardinal symptoms in older children or adults include migraine, seizures, optic atrophy, sensorineural deafness, neuropathy, myopathy, diabetes, pseudo-obstruction, hepatic dysfunction, cardiomyopathy, and metabolic stroke, and these in particular raise a red flag for additional evaluation for mitochondrial disease. Any neonate with muscular hypotonia and progressive cardiorespiratory failure should be evaluated more closely for possible mitochondrial dysfunction.

DISCLOSURE

D. Basel is an unpaid member of the FDNA Scientific Advisory Board.

REFERENCES

1. Parikh S, Karaa A, Goldstein A, et al. J Diagnosis of 'possible' mitochondrial disease: an existential crisis. Med Genet 2019;56(3):123–30.
2. Larsson NG, Clayton DA. Molecular genetic aspects of human mitochondrial disorders. Annu Rev Genet 1995;29:151–78.
3. Goldstein A. The elusive magic pill: finding effective therapies for mitochondrial disorders. Neurotherapeutics 2013;10(2):320–8.
4. Chinnery PF. Mitochondrial disease in adults: what's old and what's new? EMBO Mol Med 2015;7(12):1503–12.
5. El-Hattab AW, Scaglia F. Mitochondrial DNA depletion syndromes: review and updates of genetic basis, manifestations, and therapeutic options. Neurotherapeutics 2013;10:186–98.
6. Hirano M, Silvestri G, Blake DM, et al. Mitochondrial neurogastrointestinal encephalomyopathy (MNGIE): clinical, biochemical, and genetic features of an autosomal recessive mitochondrial disorder. Neurology 1994;44:721–7.
7. Nishino I, Spinazzola A, Papadimitriou A, et al. Mitochondrial neurogastrointestinal encephalomyopathy: an autosomal recessive disorder due to thymidine phosphorylase mutations. Ann Neurol 2000;47:792–800.
8. Moraes CT, Shanske S, Tritschler H-J, et al. mtDNA depletion with variable tissue expression: a novel genetic abnormality in mitochondrial diseases. Am J Hum Genet 1991;48:492–501.
9. Saada A, Shaag A, Mandel H, et al. Mutant mitochondrial thymidine kinase in mitochondrial DNA depletion myopathy. Nat Genet 2001;29:342–4.
10. Mandel H, Szargel R, Labay V, et al. The deoxyguanosine kinase gene is mutated in individuals with depleted hepatocerebral mitochondrial DNA. Nat Genet 2001; 29:337–41.
11. Mandel H, Szargel R, Labay V, et al. The deoxyguanosine kinase gene is mutated in individuals with depleted hepatocerebral mitochondrial DNA. Nat Genet 2001; 29:337–41.
12. Milone M, Massie R. Polymerase gamma 1 mutations: clinical correlations. Neurologist 2010;16:84–91.
13. Kurt B, Jaeken J, Van Hove J, et al. A novel POLG gene mutation in 4 children with Alpers-like hepatocerebral syndromes. Arch Neurol 2010;67:239–44.
14. Carrozzo R, Dionisi-Vici C, Steuerwald U, et al. SUCLA2 mutations are associated with mild methylmalonic aciduria, Leigh-like encephalomyopathy, dystonia, and deafness. Brain 2007;130:862–74.
15. Elpeleg O, Miller C, Hershkovitz E, et al. Deficiency of the ADP-forming succinyl-CoA synthase activity is associated with encephalomyopathy and mitochondrial DNA depletion. Am J Hum Genet 2005;76:1081–6.
16. Appenzeller O, Kornfeld M, Snyder R. Acromutilating, paralyzing neuropathy with corneal ulceration in Navajo children. Arch Neurol 1976;33:733–8.
17. Spinazzola A, Santer R, Akman OH, et al. Hepatocerebral form of mitochondrial DNA depletion syndrome: novel MPV17 mutations. Arch Neurol 2008;65: 1108–13.
18. Kallio A-K, Jauhiainen T. A new syndrome of ophthalmoplegia, hypoacusis, ataxia, hypotonia and athetosis (OHAHA). Adv Audiol 1985;3:84–90.
19. Sarzi E, Goffart S, Serre V, et al. Twinkle helicase (PEO1) gene mutation causes mitochondrial DNA depletion. Ann Neurol 2007;62:579–87.

20. Bourdon A, Minai L, Serre V, et al. Mutation of RRM2B, encoding p53-controlled ribonucleotide reductase (p53R2), causes severe mitochondrial DNA depletion. Nat Genet 2007;39:776–80.

21. Shaibani A, Shchelochkov OA, Zhang S, et al. Mitochondrial neurogastrointestinal encephalopathy due to mutations in RRM2B. Arch Neurol 2009;66:1028–32.

22. Rouzier C, Le Guedard-Mereuze S, Fragaki K, et al. The severity of phenotype linked to SUCLG1 mutations could be correlated with residual amount of SUCLG1 protein. J Med Genet 2010;47:670–6.

23. Ostergaard E, Christensen E, Kristensen E, et al. Deficiency of the alpha subunit of succinate-coenzyme A ligase causes fatal infantile lactic acidosis with mitochondrial DNA depletion. Am J Hum Genet 2007;81:383–7.

24. Ostergaard E, Christensen E, Kristensen E, et al. Deficiency of the alpha subunit of succinate-coenzyme A ligase causes fatal infantile lactic acidosis with mitochondrial DNA depletion. Am J Hum Genet 2007;81:383–7.

25. Calvo SE, Compton AG, Hershman SG, et al. Molecular diagnosis of infantile mitochondrial disease with targeted next-generation sequencing. Sci Transl Med 2012;4:118ra10.

26. Calvo SE, Compton AG, Hershman SG, et al. Molecular diagnosis of infantile mitochondrial disease with targeted next-generation sequencing. Sci Transl Med 2012;4:118ra10.

27. Kornblum C, Nicholls TJ, Haack TB, et al. Loss-of-function mutations in MGME1 impair mtDNA replication and cause multisystemic mitochondrial disease. Nat Genet 2013;45:214–9.

28. Thompson K, Majd H, Dallabona C, et al. Recurrent de novo dominant mutations in SLC25A4 cause severe early-onset mitochondrial disease and loss of mitochondrial DNA copy number. Am J Hum Genet 2016;99:860–76 [Erratum appears in Am J Hum Genet 2016;99:1405].

29. Echaniz-Laguna A, Chassagne M, Ceresuela J, et al. Complete loss of expression of the ANT1 gene causing cardiomyopathy and myopathy. J Med Genet 2012;49:146–50.

30. Palmieri L, Alberio S, Pisano I, et al. Complete loss-of-function of the heart/muscle-specific adenine nucleotide translocator is associated with mitochondrial myopathy and cardiomyopathy. Hum Mol Genet 2005;14:3079–88.

31. Bonnen PE, Yarham JW, Besse A, et al. Mutations in FBXL4 cause mitochondrial encephalopathy and a disorder of mitochondrial DNA maintenance. Am J Hum Genet 2013;93:471–81 [Erratum appears in Am J Hum Genet 2013;93:773].

32. Bonnen PE, Yarham JW, Besse A, et al. Mutations in FBXL4 cause mitochondrial encephalopathy and a disorder of mitochondrial DNA maintenance. Am J Hum Genet 2013;93:471–81 [Erratum appears in Am J Hum Genet 2013;93:773].

33. Spiegel R, Saada A, Flannery PJ, et al. Fatal infantile mitochondrial encephalomyopathy, hypertrophic cardiomyopathy and optic atrophy associated with a homozygous OPA1 mutation. J Med Genet 2016;53:127–31.

34. Stiles AR, Simon MT, Stover A, et al. Mutations in TFAM, encoding mitochondrial transcription factor A, cause neonatal liver failure associated with mtDNA depletion. Mol Genet. Metab. 2016;119:91–9.

35. Clay AS, Behnia M, Brown KK. Mitochondrial disease: a pulmonary and critical-care medicine perspective. Chest 2001;120:634–48.

36. Montero R, Yubero D, Villarroya J, et al. GDF-15 is elevated in children with mitochondrial diseases and is induced by mitochondrial dysfunction. PLoS One 2016; 11(2):e0148709.

37. Desmedt S, Desmedt V, De Vos L, et al. Growth differentiation factor 15: a novel biomarker with high clinical potential. Crit Rev Clin Lab Sci 2019;56:333–50.
38. Davis RL, Liang C, Sue CM. A comparison of current serum biomarkers as diagnostic indicators of mitochondrial diseases. Neurology 2016;86:2010–5.
39. Davis RL, Liang C, Edema-Hildebrand F, et al. Fibroblast growth factor 21 is a sensitive biomarker of mitochondrial disease. Neurology 2013;81(21):1819–26.
40. Suomalainen A, Elo JM, Pietiläinen KH, et al. FGF-21 as a biomarker for muscle-manifesting mitochondrial respiratory chain deficiencies: a diagnostic study. Lancet Neurol 2011;10:806–18.
41. Phoenix C, Schaefera AM, Elsona JL, et al. A scale to monitor progression and treatment of mitochondrial disease in children. Neuromuscul Disord 2006; 16(12):814–20.
42. Witters P, Saada A, Honzik T, et al. Revisiting mitochondrial diagnostic criteria in the new era of genomics. Genet Med 2018;20(4):444–51.
43. Tarnopolsky MA. The mitochondrial cocktail: rationale for combined nutraceutical therapy in mitochondrial cytopathies. Adv Drug Deliv Rev 2008;60(13–14): 1561–7.
44. Rahman J, Rahman S. Mitochondrial medicine in the omics era. Lancet 2018; 391(10139):2560–74.
45. Kamatani N, Kushiyama A, Toyo-Oka L, et al. Treatment of two mitochondrial disease patients with a combination of febuxostat and inosine that enhances cellular ATP. J Hum Genet 2019;64(4):351–3.
46. Bulst S, Holinski-Feder E, Payne B, et al. In vitro supplementation with deoxynucleoside monophosphates rescues mitochondrial DNA depletion. Mol Genet Metab 2012;107(0):95–103.
47. Abadi A, Crane JD, Ogborn D, et al. Supplementation with α-lipoic acid, CoQ10, and vitamin E augments running performance and mitochondrial function in female mice. PLoS One 2013;8(4):e60722.
48. Saito K, Kimura N, Oda N, et al. Pyruvate therapy for mitochondrial DNA depletion syndrome. Biochim Biophys Acta 2012;1820(5):632–6.

Nonimmune Anemias

Lynn Malec, MD, MSc

KEYWORDS

- Anemia • Classification • Diagnosis • Hemolysis • Differential

KEY POINTS

- Anemia in neonates must be interpreted in relation to the patient's characteristics, including gestational age, chronologic age, and sampling technique.
- Important details regarding the family history can aid in the diagnosis when evaluating for an inherited disorder and should concentrate on a history of anemia and hemolysis (jaundice, gallstones, splenomegaly, cholecystectomy/splenectomy).
- Consideration of non–immune-mediated hemolysis, including red cell membrane disorders, enzyme disorders, and hemoglobin abnormalities, is important in the neonate.
- Rare disorders of red cell production may manifest in the neonatal period and warrant further hematologic evaluation, including consideration of bone marrow biopsy.

INTRODUCTION

Anemia that is present at birth or appearing during the first weeks of life can be broadly classified into categories of anemia caused by blood loss, hemolysis, and abnormal red cell production. A systematic approach to evaluating anemia can narrow the differential diagnosis and provide guidance on which individuals warrant more detailed hematologic evaluation. This article focuses on causes of anemia in neonates and infants outside of blood loss and isoimmunization (immune-mediated hemolytic processes such as ABO or rhesus [Rh] hemolytic disease).

DEFINING ANEMIA

Anemia is quantified by a reduction in the hemoglobin concentration or red blood cell (RBC) mass with the threshold for defining anemia when values decrease to less than the 2.5th percentile of normal. Importantly, in newborns and infants, anemia must be interpreted based on the gestational age, chronologic age, weight, sex, race, and method of blood sampling. Normative values for hemoglobin and red cell indices are based on age, as outlined in **Table 1**.

- Consideration of age: term infants are born with a relative increase in their hemoglobin caused by low oxygen saturation in the fetus. After birth, because of

Versiti Blood Research Institute, Medical College of Wisconsin, 8733 Watertown Plank Road, Milwaukee, WI 53226, USA
E-mail address: LMalec@versiti.org

Clin Perinatol 47 (2020) 143–153
https://doi.org/10.1016/j.clp.2019.09.006

Table 1
Normal pediatric values of red cell mass, hemoglobin level, red cell indices, and reticulocyte count

Age	Red Blood Cells (×10⁶/UL)	Hemoglobin (g/dL)	Hematocrit (%)	MCV (fL)	MCHC (%)	Reticulocyte Count (%)
Cord blood	—	14.0–18.8	42–69	96–125	30–34	3–7
Term newborn	5.0–6.3	18.0–21.5	51–68	96–125	30–35	3–7
1–3 d	4.1–6.1	14.0–24.0	43–68	96–125	30–38	3–7
4–7 d	4.1–6.1	14.3–22.3	42–62	96–125	30–38	—
7–14 d	4.1–6.1	12.9–20.5	39–59	88–112	30–36	—
14–60 d	3.8–5.6	10.7–17.3	33–51	70–98	30–35	—
2–5 mo	3.8–5.2	10.1–14.5	30–40	70–90	32–36	—
6–12 mo	3.8–5.2	10.0–13.2	30–39	70–90	32–36	—

Abbreviations: MCHC, mean corpuscular hemoglobin concentration; MCV, mean corpuscular volume.

increased tissue oxygenation and decline in erythropoietin production, hemoglobin concentrations decrease, reaching a nadir around 9 weeks of age, known as the physiologic nadir of infancy.

- Preterm infants are born with lower hemoglobin levels, have shorter RBC survival, and a relative impairment in erythropoietin production caused by liver immaturity. The result is an exaggerated physiologic nadir that occurs earlier and is more significant than in term infants, known as anemia of prematurity.
- Consideration of sampling method: note the method of blood sampling used in hemoglobin determination. Capillary sampling results in higher concentrations of hemoglobin compared with venous or arterial sampling because of the sluggish flow through the capillaries.
- Consideration of sex: differences in causes of anemia in neonates and infants are primarily related to the possibility of X-linked disorders manifesting in boys.

EVALUATION OF ANEMIA
History

A thorough history can provide the essential clues to aid in the diagnosis of anemia, including nonimmune anemia.

- Pregnancy/birth history: details regarding bleeding during pregnancy or delivery, and inspection of the placenta for any evidence of abnormalities, including placental or umbilical cord tear or abruption, are important for determining maternal-fetal and obstetric causes of anemia.
- Family history: family history must include a detailed history of anemia in biological mother, father, and siblings as well as history of anemia within the extended family.

Inquiry regarding a prior diagnosis of anemia, prior history of jaundice, gallstones, and/or splenomegaly should be obtained. Given the increased red cell turnover in hemolytic anemias, patients are prone to gallstones, therefore asking whether any family members have had early cholecystectomy can provide a subtle clue to an inherited anemia. In addition, given that the anemia associated with some red cell disorders is ameliorated by splenectomy, a history of splenectomy in any family members should be sought.

Physical Examination

A detailed physical examination should include careful inspection of the facies, eyes, skin, chest, and abdomen with attention to any dysmorphisms that may be related to an underlying syndrome also associated with anemia and/or marrow failure. In addition, patients should be evaluated for jaundice, scleral icterus, hepatomegaly, splenomegaly, or skin findings possibly consistent with extramedullary hematopoiesis.

Symptoms

Symptoms of anemia in newborns and infants may include pallor, lethargy, tachycardia or bradycardia, apnea, jaundice, poor feeding, and poor weight gain. The chronicity and severity of anemia should be noted in addition to close attention for any clinical history or suggestion of overt or occult bleeding.[1]

DIAGNOSTIC APPROACH
Laboratory Testing

Laboratory testing, including trends over time, should include:

- Complete blood count with attention to whether anemia exists in isolation or with abnormalities of other cell lines (increased or decreased white blood cell and platelet counts)
- Red cell indices, including the mean corpuscular volume, mean corpuscular hemoglobin concentration (MCHC), and red cell distribution width
- Reticulocyte count (absolute and/or percentage)
- Bilirubin level (with fractionation)
- Direct and indirect antiglobulin tests (Coombs test/direct antiglobulin test, and antibody screen)
- Blood smear from a fresh patient sample
  - Evidence of red cell inclusions or abnormalities can give clues to the cause of anemia and are listed in **Box 1**.
- Bone marrow evaluation: a bone marrow aspirate may be necessary to determine the cause of some disorders; however, this is rarely critical in the initial evaluation of a patient outside of concern for infantile leukemia

Diagnostic Differential

A general approach to anemia in neonates involves classification of anemia related to cause, as outlined in **Table 2**.[2] The following diagnostic categories are most relevant to neonates with anemia.

HEMOLYTIC ANEMIAS

Hemolytic anemia involves the increased destruction of erythrocytes, typically with a compensatory increase in erythrocyte production leading to increased reticulocyte levels in the peripheral blood. Most infants with hemolytic anemia have accompanying hyperbilirubinemia. The cause of nonimmune hemolytic anemias can be broadly classified as follows.

Inherited Red Blood Cell Membrane Defects

Mutations in the genes encoding the RBC membrane cytoskeleton, including ankyrin, spectrin, band 3, and protein 4.2, can result in inherited hemolytic anemias, which are

Box 1
Classification of neonatal/infantile anemia based on pathophysiology

1. Decreased RBC production

Infection
   Congenital infections: cytomegalovirus, rubella, parvovirus
   Postnatal/acquired infections

Bone marrow failure syndromes
   Congenital red cell aplasia:
      Diamond-Blackfan anemia
   Anemia accompanied by other cytopenias:
      Fanconi anemia
      Dyskeratosis congenita
      Reticular dysgenesis
      Pearson syndrome

Marrow replacement/infiltration
   Congenital leukemia

2. Increased RBC destruction

Non–immune mediated
   Congenital disorders
      Red cell membrane disorders
         Hereditary spherocytosis
         Hereditary elliptocytosis
         Hereditary stomatocytosis
         Hereditary pyropoikilocytosis
      Red cell enzyme defects
         Glucose-6-phosphate dehydrogenase (G6PD) deficiency
         Pyruvate kinase deficiency
         Other rarer enzyme deficiencies
      Thalassemia syndromes
         α-Thalassemia
         γ-Thalassemia
         β-Thalassemia
      Hemoglobinopathies
         Sickle cell disease
      Unstable hemoglobinopathies
      Congenital dyserythropoietic anemia
      Infection
      Metabolic
         Galactosemia
         Osteopetrosis
   Acquired disorders
      Infection
      Disseminated intravascular coagulation

Immune mediated
   Rh, ABO, or other RBC antigen incompatibility
   Drug induced

3. Blood loss

Obstetric
   Placental bleeding
   Rupture/trauma of umbilical cord
   Malformation of the placenta and/or cord

Occult hemorrhage
   Maternofetal
   Twin-to-twin transfusion
   Internal: intracranial, extracranial, intra-abdominal
   Iatrogenic blood loss from venous/arterial sampling

Table 2
Finding of red cell inclusions on peripheral blood smear

Red Cell Inclusion	Cause of Finding	Differential Diagnosis
Heinz bodies	Denatured hemoglobin	Evidence of oxidative damage
Howell-Jolly bodies	Nuclear remnants	Splenectomy and/or ineffective erythropoiesis
Basophilic stippling	Residual RNA on polysomes	Thalassemia, lead, enzymopathies
Pappenheimer bodies	Ferritin (iron) aggregates	Sideroblastic anemia

discussed later. Careful attention to the family history of anemia, including a history of gallstones, splenomegaly, and cholecystectomy, is important.

- Hereditary spherocytosis (HS): HS is the most common inherited nonimmune hemolytic anemia and typically has an autosomal dominant (AD) inheritance (approximately 75% of cases with AD inheritance, 20%–25% are sporadic mutations, and <5% are autosomal recessive), occurring in approximately 1 in 1500 to 1 in 5000 live births. The pathophysiology is related to an intrinsic red cell defect in the membrane, leading it to be inefficiently tacked to the cytoskeleton and resulting in poor deformability as red cells pass through the spleen and red cell removal. This condition results in a hemolysis with variable degree of anemia based on mutation (with approximately 15% of patients with compensated hemolysis without anemia).[3]
  - Key features in the neonatal period include neonatal jaundice in the first 24 hours of life and exacerbation of anemia during the newborn nadir, although 40% to 50% of neonates do not develop significant neonatal jaundice with mild HS.
  - Laboratory data include anemia and reticulocytosis, with typically more subtle increases in bilirubin and lactate dehydrogenase levels. An increase in the mean corpuscle hemoglobin concentration (>36% caused by relative cellular dehydration) often solidifies the diagnosis in older children; however, an increased MCHC is less reliable in neonates and infants compared with older children.
  - Classically, the diagnosis is made using osmotic fragility testing for lysis of RBCs suspended in solutions of decreasing osmolality, with increased hemolysis noted in hypotonic saline. Because of the poor sensitivity of this testing in young infants, flow cytometry–based eosin-5-maleimide uptake has aided in the diagnosis of HS in infants.
  - Treatment includes serial monitoring of blood counts and transfusion as needed based on the trajectory of anemia.[4] The need for phototherapy, or rarely exchange transfusion, for hyperbilirubinemia occurs in the newborn period. Infants with more significant anemia (typically related to a genetic mutation conferring more significant baseline hemolysis), may need to be transfused episodically, especially in the first year of life, but often transfusion needs decline thereafter.
- Hereditary elliptocytosis: elliptocytosis occurs in approximately 1 in 4000 live births, with increased incidence in some populations, including those of African descent. Severity of disease range widely, from being asymptomatic in neonates and infants to causing intrauterine death. Elliptocytosis is further subcategorized as follows:
  - Heterozygous hereditary elliptocytosis, hereditary elliptocytosis with hemolysis, spherocytic hereditary elliptocytosis, south east Asian ovalocytosis

o Diagnosis is solidified with evaluation of characteristics elliptocytes on review of the peripheral blood smear
o Neonates and infants with elliptocytosis rarely require serial transfusion unless there is a family history of more significant phenotypic anemia
- Hereditary pyropoikilocytosis: this is a rare cause of severe hemolytic anemia in newborns/infants and has a strong association with hereditary elliptocytosis. Most patients have severe hemolysis in infancy and then typically more mild symptoms later in life.
    o Key features include significant anemia in the neonatal period with reticulocytosis
    o The diagnosis can be solidified by review of a well-prepared blood smear, which shows red cells with bizarre shapes and sizes (anisopoikilocytosis) with red cell fragmentation and microspherocytes.

Red Blood Cell Enzymopathies

Red cell enzymes are used for energy production and other essential red cell functions; anemias associated with enzyme disorders can vary widely, from those that cause a significant, chronic anemia to those that cause acute, intermittent declines in hemoglobin level.

- Glucose-6-phosphate dehydrogenase (G6PD) deficiency: the most common red cell enzyme disorder is G6PD deficiency, which affects millions of individuals worldwide. Hemolysis occurs in response to oxidative stress in the setting of infection, medications, and certain dietary and environmental exposures. Depending on the specific mutation, anemia can be low grade and chronic or more acute after exposure to an oxidant. G6PD deficiency can be detected on newborn screen and confirmed with a quantitative level.
    o Review of peripheral blood smear can reveal red cell inclusions, known as Heinz bodies, which are denatured hemoglobin, as well as blister cells.
- Pyruvate kinase deficiency: inherited in an autosomal recessive pattern, pyruvate kinase (PK) deficiency causes an error of the glycolytic pathway leading to reduction of ATP production and loss of red cell membrane permeability.[5] The severity of hemolysis in PK deficiency is highly variable, although it is similar within families. Although less common than G6PD deficiency, PK deficiency is the commonest cause of a chronic hemolytic anemia from an RBC enzyme deficiency.
    o PK deficiency is asymptomatic in the heterozygous state, but can lead to severe neonatal hemolysis and severe hyperbilirubinemia in the homozygous state.
    o In the setting of significant hemolysis, neonates may also have cholestasis as part of the presentation (which is typically self-resolving).
    o The diagnosis of PK deficiency can be made through determination of PK levels in red cells as well as DNA sequencing.
- Other RBC enzymopathies: other less common RBC enzymopathies exist that can lead to intermittent or persistent hemolysis. When unexplained hemolytic anemia exists, evaluation for these disorders through testing of enzyme levels and/or DNA sequencing in a dedicated laboratory offering testing for rare red cell disorders can aid in the diagnosis.

Hemoglobin Abnormalities

Broadly, hemoglobin abnormalities can be classified as those that involve decreased globin production resulting in thalassemia, structural hemoglobin changes resulting in qualitative abnormalities of hemoglobin (including the sickling syndromes), and changes in heme and globin binding leading to unstable hemoglobinopathies. Some hemoglobin abnormalities manifest during infancy, whereas others may be diagnosed later in life.

- Thalassemia: this is a group of hereditary disorders that cause disruption of the normal ratio of globin production necessary for normal hemoglobin production. The pathophysiology is related to decreased production of a globin chain, most typically α or β chains, which leads to a globin chain imbalance with ultimate precipitation the chain that is in relative excess. This process causes damage to the red cell membrane in addition to ineffective red cell production.[6]

Because of the changes that occur in fetuses and newborns related to globin chain synthesis (**Fig. 1**), unique findings can exist in neonates that are different than those seen in older children.

  ○ Basic thalassemia nomenclature: thalassemias are named based on the genetic defect; α-thalassemia is caused by a defect in the α -globin, β-thalassemia is caused by a defect in the β-globin, and γ-thalassemia caused by a defect in the γ-globin. In addition, thalassemias are named based on clinical severity, with minor thalassemia resulting in mild anemia/asymptomatic trait state, intermedia in moderate anemia with intermittent red cell transfusion needs, and major caused by severe anemia and transfusion dependence.
  ○ Globin production throughout development: the timing of presentation of thalassemia is related to the severity conferred by the genetic defect and the production of globin genes during the intrauterine and neonatal periods.
    ■ α-Globin production begins early in gestation and the αchain is common to all forms of hemoglobin present at birth. γ-Chain production also begins in utero and is ultimately replaced by production of β-globin chains beginning around 32 weeks' gestation.
      - The major forms of hemoglobin include:
        ○ Hemoglobin F: fetal hemoglobin is composed of 2 α chains and 2 γ chains.
        ○ Hemoglobin A: the major form of adult hemoglobin is composed of 2 α chains and 2 γ chains.
        ○ Hemoglobin A2: the minor form of adult hemoglobin is composed of 2 α chains and 2 δ chains.

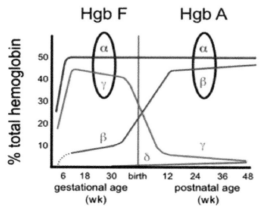

Fig. 1. Globin production based on gestational weeks and postnatal age. Hgb, hemoglobin.

○ α-Thalassemia: α-thalassemia is caused by 1 or more α chain mutations, which are most typically gene deletions. With abnormal α-globin production, γ-globin genes form a tetramer known as hemoglobin Bart. α-Thalassemia can be detected on newborn screen by the presence of Hemoglobin Barts. Individuals with α-thalassemia have persistent microcytic anemia. Work-up to determine the cause of microcytic anemia can include hemoglobin electrophoresis and genetic testing to identify common genetic mutations in α gene.

○ β-Thalassemia: β-thalassemia is cause by 1 or more typically point mutations in the β-globin genes. Although hemoglobin A usually constitutes less than 30% of the normal hemoglobin at birth, under certain circumstances, such as intrauterine blood loss, this can be greater.

■ β-Thalassemia is classified depending on the severity of symptoms; thalassemia major (also known as Cooley anemia), thalassemia intermedia, and thalassemia minor.

■ Signs and symptoms of anemia appear within the first 2 years of life, and typically within the first year, when hemoglobin A production typically predominates.

○ γ-Thalassemia: given the production of γ-globin in utero to form fetal hemoglobin, mutations in this gene can lead to γ-thalassemia, which can be apparent in fetuses or newborns. γ-Thalassemia results in transient microcytic hemolytic anemia, which may mimic hemolytic disease of the newborn.

■ Treatment includes supportive transfusion given that anemia is transient and improves after β-globin production increases, leading to increasing concentrations of hemoglobin A.

• Structural hemoglobinopathies: genetic mutations exist that confer qualitative abnormalities in hemoglobin. The most widely known include those that cause decreased solubility, including hemoglobin S and hemoglobin C. Common patterns of hemoglobin on newborn screen, their interpretation, and recommendations for follow-up are listed in **Table 3**.

Fragmentation Syndromes

Red cell fragmentation syndromes, also known as microangiopathic hemolytic anemia (MAHA), are defined by endothelial damage leading to platelet thrombosis and eventual vessel obstruction. A hallmark of the disorder is shearing of red cells as they pass through the vasculature. Evidence of MAHA is supported with clinical and laboratory evidence of hemolysis in addition to the presence of red cell fragmentation, known as schistocytes, on review of the peripheral blood smear. MAHA is not a diagnosis but a symptom of an underlying disorder. Important causes of MAHA to consider in neonates/infants include:

• Thrombotic thrombocytopenia purpura (TTP): TTP in pediatrics is rare, accounting for less than 10% of all TTP cases. In young children, TTP is almost always related to a genetic mutation rather than the formation of autoantibodies, as is the case with teenagers and adults. The pathophysiology of TTP is related to a decrease or absence of ADAMTS13 (a disintegrin and metalloproteinase with a thrombospondin type 1 motif, member 13), a key metalloprotease that is essential for the normal cleavage of von Willebrand factor (VWF). Without ADAMTS13, ultralarge multimers of VWF exist that can induce platelet thrombosis and microthrombi in the vasculature, leading to red cell shearing and destruction. Hallmarks of this disorder include anemia and thrombocytopenia, as well as renal dysfunction, fever, and possible mental status changes.

Table 3
Interpretation and recommendations based on hemoglobin findings on newborn screen

Pattern	Interpretation	Recommendation
FA	Normal	None
F only	Premature infant, β-thalassemia major	Repeat testing if persistent only F, confirmatory testing and hematology referral
AF	Likely after blood transfusion	Repeat testing
FS	Hemoglobin SS, sickle β-thalassemia, sickle HPFH	Hematology referral
FSA	Sickle β-thalassema	Hematology referral
FAS	Sickle cell trait, sickle β-thalassemia	Repeat testing at 3 mo to rule out sickle β-thalassemia
FSC	Hemoglobin SC disease	Hematology referral
FC	Hemoglobin C disease, hemoglobin C β-thalassemia	Hematology referral
FE	Hemoglobin E disease	Hematology referral
FA + variant	Hemoglobin variant trait	Education and genetic counseling
FA Barts	Silent α-thalassemia carrier, α-thalassemia trait, hemoglobin H disease, hemoglobin H Constant Spring	If Barts <10%, patient needs education and genetic counseling; if Barts >10%, patient needs further testing for evaluation of hemoglobin H (hematology referral)

Abbreviations: A, adult hemoglobin (Hb A); C, hemoglobin C; E, hemoglobin E; F, fetal hemoglobin (Hb F); HPHF, hereditary persistence of fetal hemoglobin; S, sickle hemoglobin (Hb S).

- ○ TTP should be considered in newborns/infants with hyperbilirubinemia, hemolytic anemia, and thrombocytopenia when there is evidence of spherocytes (indicating microangiopathy) on review of the peripheral blood.
- ○ Diagnosis of TTP is solidified with evidence of low or absent ADAMTS13 activity levels; confirmation of mutations in ADAMTS13 conferring a diagnosis of TTP are also typically sought.
- ○ Treatment consists of supplementation of ADAMTS13 through use of fresh frozen plasma (FFP), with frequent FFP infusions during a time of crisis and FFP infusions typically every 2 to 3 weeks as routine prophylaxis.
- • Disseminated intravascular consumption (DIC): DIC is characterized by aberrant, systemic activation of blood coagulation, which results in generation and deposition of fibrin. This fibrin deposition leads to microvascular thrombi in various organs and can contribute to organ dysfunction. Because of consumption of blood clotting proteins and platelets, DIC can result in life-threatening hemorrhage. Clinical manifestations include coagulopathy, bleeding, renal dysfunction, hepatic dysfunction, and possible thromboembolism.
  - ○ Key differentiators between DIC and TTP include normal coagulation studies (prothrombin time [PT] and partial thromboplastin time [PTT]) in TTP given there is no consumption of clotting factors with TTP. In addition, when differentiating DIC versus liver disease, factor VIII levels are normal or increased in liver disease, whereas they are decreased because of consumption in DIC.

- o Treatment of DIC includes treatment of the underlying disorder leading to DIC, which in newborns and infants is usually infection. In addition, treatment includes use of platelet transfusion in severe thrombocytopenia, FFP in bleeding, and cryoprecipitate if fibrinogen level is less than 100 mg/dL (and bleeding).
- Other disorders causing microangiopathy that are rare but should be considered as a possible cause of red cell shear include:
- o Cavernous hemangioma or hemangioendothelioma
- o Renal artery stenosis
- o Severe coarctation of the aorta

Disorders of Impaired Red Cell Production

Certain inherited bone marrow failure syndromes and other disorders of red cell production can manifest in the newborn period and are a rare but important consideration of the cause of unexplained anemia in neonates.

- Bone marrow failure syndromes: the inherited bone marrow failure syndromes are a group of rare disorders in which there is typically some degree of aplastic anemia, meaning a failure of the bone marrow to produce RBCs. Some conditions have other cytopenias at the time of diagnosis, whereas others have predominant anemia. In addition, some disorders are associated with congenital anomalies, making a thorough physical examination an important part of the evaluation. Specific disorders include:
- Diamond-Blackfan anemia (DBA): DBA is a congenital red cell aplasia that typically presents in infancy. Genetic mutations in ribosomal protein genes have been implicated with wide genetic heterogeneity among those with a similar phenotype. An estimate 25% of patients with DBA have evidence of anemia at birth. Hemoglobin values as low as 9.4 g/dL along with low reticulocyte count may be seen in the first days of life.
- o Compared with other bone marrow failure syndromes, DBA typically has anemia/red cell aplasia without other abnormalities in the blood counts.
- o Congenital abnormalities are present in approximately 40% of patients, including thumb abnormalities (bifid thumb, hypoplastic thenar eminence), craniofacial dysmorphisms (microcephaly, hypertelorism), cardiac defects, genitourinary abnormalities, craniofacial malformations, and cleft palate.
- o Key features in addition to anemia with reticulocytopenia include macrocytosis, increased fetal hemoglobin level, increased adenosine deaminase level in the blood.
- Other bone marrow failure syndromes include Fanconi anemia (FA), dyskeratosis congenital, and reticular dysgenesis. These syndromes do not classically cause anemia in the newborn period but typically manifest with cytopenias in infants and older children.
- Pearson syndrome: Pearson syndrome is a cause of impaired red cell production that may manifest in the neonatal period. The syndrome is thought to be related to mitochondrial DNA deletion, and is characterized by sideroblastic anemia and vacuolization of the bone marrow precursor cells.
- Congenital dyserythropoietic anemia (CDA): CDA is a rare inherited disorder hallmarked by ineffective erythropoiesis resulting in decreased red cell production and anemia. There are 3 major forms of CDA, with CDA type I having severe macrocytic anemia that presents in the neonatal period, often accompanied by a history by intrauterine growth restriction.

REFERENCES

1. Brugnara C, Platt OS. The neonatal erythrocyte and its disorders. In: Orkin SH, Fisher DE, Look T, et al, editors. Nathan and Oski's hematology and oncology of infancy and childhood. 7th edition. Philadelphia: WB Saunders; 2015. p. 52.
2. Brugnara C, Oski FA, Nathan DG. Diagnostic approach to the anemic patient. In: Orkin SH, Fisher DE, Look T, et al, editors. Nathan and Oski's hematology and oncology of infancy and childhood. 7th edition. Philadelphia: WB Saunders; 2015. p. 293.
3. Widness JA. Pathophysiology of anemia during the neonatal period. Neoreviews 2008;9(11):e520.
4. Ohls RK. Evaluation and treatment of anemia in the neonate. In: Christensen RD, editor. Hematologic problems of the neonate. 1. Philadelphia: WB Saunders; 2000. p. 137–70.
5. Gallagher PG. Red cell membrane disorders 2005. p. 13–8. American Society of Hematology Education Book, Hematology.
6. Tse WT, Lux SE. Red blood cell membrane disorders. Br J Haematol 1999; 104(1):2–13.

Neonatal Metabolic Crises

A Practical Approach

Katie B. Williams, MD, PhD[a], Patrice K. Held, PhD[b],
Jessica Scott Schwoerer, MD[c],*

KEYWORDS

- Metabolic disorder • Crisis • Newborn • Neonate

KEY POINTS

- Metabolic disorders often present with severe neonatal crisis that mimics more common newborn illnesses.
- Basic laboratory analysis may provide clues about an underlying metabolic disorder, but even infants with severe metabolic decompensation may have normal routine laboratory evaluations.
- Initial management of metabolic disorders, regardless of specific cause, involves removing the offending nutrient (often found in breast milk or milk-based formula) and providing a high glucose infusion with isotonic fluids to reverse catabolism.
- Advanced biochemical and molecular testing are combined to confirm a diagnosis of a metabolic disorder and guide ongoing treatment.

INTRODUCTION

Metabolic disorders arise from a disruption in the metabolism of nutrients or basic cellular functions. Individual conditions are rare, but collectively metabolic disorders are estimated to occur in 1 in 800 to 2500 births,[1,2] higher than the incidence of type 1 diabetes among non-Hispanic Caucasians in the United States.[3] Despite their collective frequency, metabolic disorders remain challenging to diagnose.

Metabolic disorders can present at any age, but the most severe presentations are typically neonates in crisis. Symptoms of a neonatal metabolic crisis are often nonspecific and mimic symptoms of far more common conditions such as central nervous system infection, epilepsy, sepsis, hypoxic ischemic encephalopathy, respiratory distress, congenital heart disease, or pyloric stenosis. Basic laboratory analysis may suggest a metabolic disorder or may be normal, even in infants

[a] Department of Pediatrics, University of Wisconsin Hospital and Clinics, 1500 Highland Avenue, Madison, WI 53705, USA; [b] Department of Pediatrics, Wisconsin State Laboratory of Hygiene, University of Wisconsin School of Medicine and Public Health, 465 Henry Mall, Madison, WI 53706, USA; [c] Department of Pediatrics, Division of Genetics and Metabolism, University of Wisconsin Hospital and Clinics, 1500 Highland Avenue, Madison, WI 53705, USA
* Corresponding author.
E-mail address: jscottschwoerer@pediatrics.wisc.edu

Clin Perinatol 47 (2020) 155–170
https://doi.org/10.1016/j.clp.2019.10.003   perinatology.theclinics.com

with severe metabolic derangements. More advanced laboratory analysis is often needed, although optimized testing strategies are often complex, may be confounded by the physiologic adaptations to critical illness, and often require several days for results. In addition, it may be difficult to obtain sufficient blood sample volumes from neonates for testing.

Newborn screening has greatly improved the timely diagnosis of metabolic disorders, although neonates may still present symptomatically before these results become available; in addition, normal results do not exclude the possibility of a metabolic disorder. Programs in the United States screen for 31 to 70 conditions, depending on the state,[4] but there are several hundred different types of metabolic disorders. Thus, it is critical to maintain a high index of suspicion for metabolic disorders in the sick neonate, especially those that are not following the expected course for more common illnesses.

This article presents a practical approach to the newborn with suspected metabolic disease, beginning with initial management strategies to stabilize the critically ill newborn and an outline of how basic laboratory tests and clinical assessments can lead to a differential diagnosis, followed by a discussion of how advanced laboratory testing can diagnose specific inborn errors of metabolism. Lastly, a summary of the most common disorders that may present in the neonatal period is provided. This review is not all-inclusive and cannot serve as a substitute for consultation with a biochemical geneticist. However, the aim is to provide health care providers in emergency medicine, primary care, and neonatology with a guide for testing to enable the more rapid identification of neonates with metabolic disorders and initial treatment strategies to stabilize the newborn.

APPROACH TO THE NEONATE WITH A SUSPECTED METABOLIC DISORDER

Newborns with metabolic disorders often appear well at birth, without signs or symptoms of illness for the first few days of life. However, they may decompensate rapidly with symptoms including poor feeding, vomiting, lethargy, and irritability. Infants with metabolic disorders do not commonly have syndromic facial features, but may have other findings to suggest an underlying metabolic disorder, such as a full fontanelle, opisthotonic posturing, hepatomegaly, or petechiae.

Initial Management

Regardless of the specific metabolic disorder, the initial management is typically standardized. First, breast milk or formula feedings may need to be held until a more definitive diagnosis is made, because breast milk or milk-based formulas often contain the offending nutrients that precipitate or exacerbate the metabolic crisis. Many metabolic disorders can be managed with partial breast milk consumption after the infant is stabilized; as such, breastfeeding mothers are encouraged to pump and store breast milk until more diagnostic information is available. Second, the neonate should be administered dextrose-containing fluids. Catabolism is often the precipitating factor in metabolic crisis, so it is important to provide a high glucose infusion rate to reverse this process. Several metabolic disorders cause cerebral edema; therefore, isotonic fluids such as normal saline are recommended and hypotonic fluids are avoided so as to minimize the risk of this potentially fatal complication. The dextrose-containing isotonic fluids should be administered until the newborn is stabilized and/or a diagnosis is achieved.

Using Basic Laboratory Analysis to Establish a Differential Diagnosis

Basic laboratory analysis should include a point-of-care glucose, complete metabolic profile with hepatic transaminases, complete blood count with differential, total and direct bilirubin, ammonia, creatine kinase, and urine ketones (**Box 1**). Newborn screening should be completed, if not already performed, and all testing should be expedited if possible.

Results from basic laboratory analysis can often yield clues about a metabolic disorder and help to establish a differential diagnosis (**Table 1**). Hypoglycemia with low urinary ketones is often the hallmark finding in symptomatic newborns with hyperinsulinemic hypoglycemia and fatty acid oxidation disorders. However, any metabolic disorder or critical illness resulting from nonmetabolic causes can lead to poor feeding and hypoglycemia, so this finding can be nonspecific. Acidosis and cytopenias may be due to organic acidemias. Hyperbilirubinemia and elevated hepatic transaminases are common in symptomatic infants with impaired carbohydrate metabolism caused by galactosemia or hereditary fructose intolerance. Hyperammonemia is the characteristic finding in urea cycle disorders but may also be caused by organic acidemias or liver dysfunction. Healthy newborns typically have elevated creatine kinase levels, even up to 10 times the normal limit; these levels should typically normalize during the first 4 days of life.[5] Severe, persistently elevated creatine kinase may be due to rhabdomyolysis, which can be seen in fatty acid oxidation disorders.

Clinical features may also provide clues about an underlying metabolic disorder. Encephalopathy and seizures may be due to fatty acid oxidation disorders, organic acidemias, amino acid disorders, or urea cycle disorders. Cardiomyopathy is associated

---

Box 1
Recommended laboratory evaluation for the neonate with a suspected metabolic disorder

Basic Laboratory Evaluation

Point-of-care glucose

Complete metabolic profile including hepatic transaminases

Blood gas or serum bicarbonate

Electrolytes

Lactate

Complete blood count with differential

Total and direct bilirubin

Ammonia

Creatine kinase

Urine ketones

Expedited newborn screen (if not already performed)

Advanced Laboratory Evaluation

Plasma acylcarnitine profile

Free and total carnitine levels

Plasma amino acids

Urine organic acids

Enzymatic testing (only for certain disorders)

Table 1
Differential diagnosis of neonatal metabolic crises based on basic laboratory findings and clinical features

Presenting Laboratory Findings	Differential Diagnosis	Specific Disorders to Consider
Hypoglycemia and absent urine ketones[a]	Fatty acid oxidation disorders Hyperinsulinemic hypoglycemia	MCAD Deficiency VLCAD Deficiency Sulfonylurea receptor mutation Potassium channel mutation
Hyperammonemia	Urea cycle disorders Organic acidemias	OTC Deficiency Citrullinemia type 1 Argininosuccinic aciduria Propionic acidemia Methylmalonic acidemia
Acidosis	Organic acidemias	Propionic acidemia Methylmalonic acidemia
Hyperbilirubinemia and elevated hepatic transaminases	Disorder of carbohydrate metabolism Aminoacidopathies	Galactosemia Tyrosinemia
Elevated creatine kinase	Fatty acid oxidation disorders	MCAD deficiency VLCAD deficiency

Presenting Clinical Features	Differential Diagnosis	Specific Disorders to Consider
Encephalopathy and/or seizures	Fatty acid oxidation disorders Amino acid disorders Organic acidemias Urea cycle disorders	MCAD deficiency VLCAD deficiency Maple syrup urine disease Propionic acidemia Methylmalonic acidemia OTC deficiency Citrullinemia type 1 Argininosuccinic aciduria
Cardiomyopathy	Organic acidemias Lysosomal storage disorders Fatty acid oxidation disorders	Propionic acidemia Methylmalonic acidemia Pompe disease MCAD deficiency VLCAD deficiency

Abbreviations: MCAD, medium-chain acyl-coenzyme A dehydrogenase; OTC, ornithine transcarbamylase; VLCAD, very-long-chain acyl-coenzyme A dehydrogenase.
[a] Any metabolic disorder or critical illness from nonmetabolic causes can lead to poor feeding and hypoglycemia; therefore, this finding may be nonspecific.

with several fatty acid oxidation disorders, certain organic acidemias, or Pompe disease, a lysosomal storage disorder. It is important to remember that basic laboratory analysis and clinical findings may be normal, even in severe metabolic crises, and should not exclude the possibility of a metabolic disorder.

Advanced Biochemical Testing to Narrow the Differential Diagnosis

The metabolism of fats, carbohydrates, and protein involves several steps, and these pathways overlap considerably (**Fig. 1**). As a result, most metabolic disorders cannot be identified from a single laboratory test, but instead require a panel of tests and

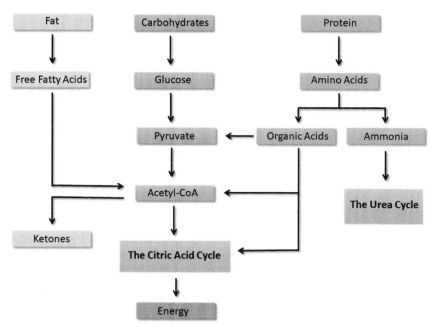

Fig. 1. Overview of metabolism. Metabolism involves several related biochemical steps to generate energy for the cell. The metabolism of fat, carbohydrate, and protein generates several intermediates that can be quantified by advanced biochemical testing. Because the metabolic pathways overlap considerably, a complete metabolic assessment often requires multiple laboratory tests and a holistic interpretation.

holistic interpretation of results. This assessment is best performed in consultation with a biochemical geneticist. Advanced laboratory testing should include a plasma acylcarnitine profile, free and total carnitine levels, plasma amino acids, and urine organic acids (see **Box 1**).

Acylcarnitines are the substrates of fatty acid oxidation. Fatty acids associate with carnitine to form acylcarnitines, which subsequently undergo fatty acid oxidation. Disorders of carnitine transport or fatty acid oxidation lead to elevations in acylcarnitines of varying carbon-chain lengths, depending on the specific enzyme deficiency, and the overall distribution of acylated species in an acylcarnitine profile, obtained under times of metabolic stress, may suggest a particular disorder or differential diagnosis. Organic acids, when in excess, can also associate with carnitine to cause elevations in specific acylcarnitine species.

Carnitine scavenges metabolic intermediates from a variety of biochemical pathways, particularly those involved in fatty acid and amino acid metabolism. Free carnitine may be depleted with a corresponding elevation in total carnitine, which is attributable to an increase in carnitine that is acyl-bound to metabolic intermediates. This characteristic pattern suggests that an underlying fatty acid oxidation defect or organic acidemia may be present.

Dietary proteins are metabolized into amino acids and are further broken down into organic acids before entering the citric acid cycle. Defects in these metabolic steps cause a characteristic pattern of amino acid or organic acid abnormalities that can be detected by analyzing plasma amino acid and urine organic acid profiles. These defects are commonly known as amino acidopathies or organic acidemias. In newborns with hyperammonemia, urine organic acids and plasma amino acids can also help to differentiate between organic acidemias and urea cycle disorders.

Some disorders, such as disorders of carbohydrate metabolism or lysosome function, will not demonstrate characteristic findings on advanced biochemical testing but can be detected by specific enzymatic or metabolite testing.

Molecular Testing to Confirm a Diagnosis

Once a particular metabolic disorder is suspected based on advanced metabolic testing and/or enzymatic testing, the diagnosis should be confirmed with a molecular assessment using single gene testing, multigene panels, or exome sequencing. If a specific disorder is not clear or the biochemical finding is associated with pathogenic variants in more than one gene, multigene panels or exome sequencing may be the most effective approach. In some infants, advanced biochemical or enzymatic testing may be challenging because of limitations in blood volume or critical illness. In such instances, multigene panels or exome sequencing may be the most appropriate initial diagnostic test. If there is a high suspicion for a particular metabolic disorder, treatment should be initiated before confirmatory molecular testing results.

DESCRIPTION OF INDIVIDUAL METABOLIC DISORDERS
Fatty Acid Oxidation Disorders

Glucose is the primary energy source for the brain, and inadequate supply can lead to seizures or neuronal cell death. The body uses 2 metabolic processes, glycogenolysis and gluconeogenesis, to prevent hypoglycemia and neurologic injury during times of poor dietary intake, illness, or increased activity. Glycogenolysis converts glycogen stores to free glucose, and gluconeogenesis converts amino acids and other substrates to free glucose. The brain uses about 50% of this combined glucose production, leaving the remaining glucose for other organs.[6] As fasting progresses, several organ systems transition to mitochondrial fatty acid oxidation to produce ketones as an energy source for the brain, sparing circulating glucose.[6]

To use the energy from fats, triglycerides must first be cleaved into free fatty acids and glycerol.[7] Circulating free fatty acids are then taken up by cells and enter the mitochondria via a carnitine transport system.[6] Once in the mitochondria, fatty acids are converted to energy via fatty acid oxidation (Fig. 2). During fasting or illness, up to 80% of the energy derived from fatty acid oxidation is used by the heart and liver. The remaining oxidation fuels hepatic ketone synthesis.[8] Newborns have limited glycogen reserves and high metabolic rate, so fatty acid oxidation plays a critical role in maintaining euglycemia.[9]

Disturbances in carnitine-mediated transport of fatty acids across mitochondrial membranes or deficiencies in the enzymes needed for fatty acid oxidation can result in fatty acid oxidation disorders. There are more than 20 different types of identified fatty acid oxidation disorders ranging from benign to severe.[10] Fatty acid oxidation disorders often present during times of fasting, illness, or stress; as such, neonatal presentation is not uncommon. The classic feature among affected individuals is hypoketotic hypoglycemia, although other signs of fatty acid oxidation disorders may include seizures, liver failure, hepatic encephalopathy, cardiomyopathy, arrhythmias, and rhabdomyolysis.[11] Regardless of biochemical etiology, fatty acid oxidation disorders are managed acutely with dextrose boluses as needed to correct hypoglycemia, followed by a continuous dextrose-containing intravenous infusion to maintain euglycemia. In newborns with proven or suspected carnitine cycle defects,

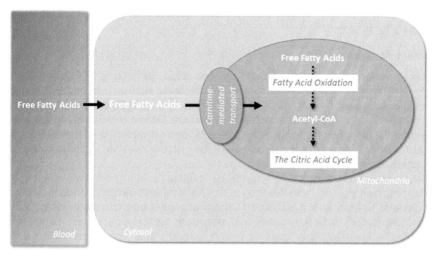

Fig. 2. Fatty acid oxidation. Circulating free fatty acids enter cells and are transported to the mitochondria via a carnitine-dependent mechanism. In the mitochondria, fatty acids are oxidized to acetyl-CoA, which fuels the citric acid cycle and generates energy for the cell. Disturbances in carnitine-mediated transport of fatty acids across mitochondrial membranes or deficiencies in the enzymes needed for fatty acid oxidation can result in fatty acid oxidation disorders.

therapeutic or empiric supplemental intravenous carnitine is also given. Once stabilized, neonatal fatty acid oxidation disorders are managed with frequent feeds to prevent catabolism and hypoglycemia, as well as long-term carnitine supplementation if carnitine deficient.

- *Medium-chain acyl-coenzyme A dehydrogenase (MCAD) deficiency.* Medium-chain acyl-coenzyme A (CoA) dehydrogenase catalyzes the first step in the oxidation of medium-length fatty acids (C6–C10). MCAD deficiency is inherited in an autosomal recessive manner and is due to pathogenic variants in the *ACADM* gene that are associated with reductions in MCAD enzyme levels to less than 10% of normal.[12] Biochemical testing typically shows elevations of medium-length acylcarnitines (C6–C10) with prominent octanoylcarnitine (C8) on acylcarnitine profile analysis.[13] Urine organic acids show a characteristic pattern of elevated medium-length dicarboxylic acids (C6>C8>C10) with inappropriately low ketones.[14] During an acute metabolic event, urine acylglycines will show elevations in hexanoylglycine, suberylglycine, and at times propionylglycine.[11] Medium-chain triglyceride oil contains medium-chain fatty acids and is contraindicated in MCAD deficiency.
- *Very-long-chain acyl-CoA dehydrogenase (VLCAD) deficiency.* Very-long-chain acyl-CoA dehydrogenase catalyzes the first step in the oxidation of long-chain fatty acids (C14–C20). VLCAD deficiency is inherited in an autosomal recessive manner owing to pathogenic variants in the *ACADVL* gene. Symptomatic newborns may present with hypoglycemia, multiorgan failure, hypertrophic or dilated cardiomyopathy, pericardial effusion, arrhythmia, hepatomegaly, or rhabdomyolysis.[15] Acylcarnitine profiles typically show elevations in C14:1, C14:2, C14, and C12:1.[16] Unlike MCAD deficiency, urine organic acid analysis is not informative for patients with VLCAD deficiency. In addition to dextrose-containing fluids,

medium-chain triglyceride oil and formula with lower fat content are often necessary for treatment.

Amino Acid Disorders

Dietary proteins are first metabolized into amino acids, the building blocks of proteins. Amino acids can then be recycled to form new proteins, such as lean body tissue, hormones, or enzymes, or used as an energy source. A vitamin B_6-dependent deamination removes the amino group from the amino acid, and the remaining carbon skeleton can enter the glycolytic pathway or the citric acid cycle to generate adenosine triphosphate. Certain amino acids can also be converted into glucose through gluconeogenesis.[7]

Several disorders are due to enzyme deficiencies that interfere with the normal metabolism of one or more amino acids. As a result, certain amino acids can accumulate to high levels and lead to medical issues that can be chronic, acute, or a combination of both. Amino acid disorders typically cause a characteristic pattern of abnormalities on plasma amino acid analysis. Long-term treatment of amino acid disorders focuses on limiting the intake of the offending amino acid(s) through specialized diets and metabolic formulas. Most amino acid disorders cause progressive symptoms over time, but certain disorders, such as maple syrup urine disease, can present acutely with metabolic crises in newborns.

- *Maple syrup urine disease (MSUD)*. MSUD is an autosomal recessive condition caused by disruption of the branched-chain α-ketoacid dehydrogenase (BCKAD) complex. BCKAD is a thiamine-dependent enzyme complex that catalyzes the second step in the degradation of the branched-chain amino acids leucine, isoleucine, and valine (**Fig. 3**). The branched-chain amino acids are essential, and typically constitute 20% to 30% of dietary amino acids.[17] Excess branched-chain amino acids are metabolized mainly in skeletal muscle, heart, adipose tissue, and kidney, with lesser contributions from the intestines and liver.[17] BCKAD complex is composed of 4 subunits, and pathogenic variants in

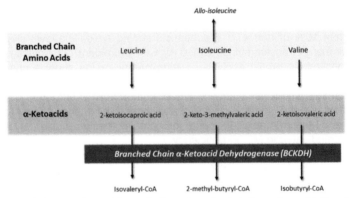

Fig. 3. Branched-chain amino acid metabolism. Branched-chain amino acids (leucine, isoleucine, and valine) are metabolized by the branched chain α-ketoacid dehydrogenase (BCKDH) complex. Maple syrup urine disease is caused by pathogenic variants in one of several genes that disrupt the function of the BCKDH complex, leading to the toxic accumulation of leucine, their respective α-ketoacids and hydroxyacid derivatives, and allo-isoleucine, the presence of which is pathognomonic for the disease.

one of several genes (*BCKDHA, BCKDHB,* or *DBT*) can lead to disruption in enzyme function,[18] leading to the toxic accumulation of leucine and associated α-ketoacids and hydroxyacid derivatives.

Newborns with classic MSUD present in the first few days of life with poor feeding, vomiting, irritability, lethargy, and rapidly progressive encephalopathy that may include seizures, opisthotonic posturing, and bicycling or posturing maneuvers. Symptomatic newborns may have a characteristic maple syrup odor in the urine and cerumen, lending to the disorder's name. Untreated newborns may have a full fontanelle on physical examination and diffuse cerebral edema or metabolic strokes on neuroimaging.[10] Despite the significant abnormalities in amino acid metabolism and severe encephalopathy, basic electrolytes are typically uninformative.[11] Amino acid analysis will show elevations in the branched-chain amino acids, particularly leucine, and the presence of allo-isoleucine, which is pathognomonic for MSUD.[19] Isoleucine and valine levels may be elevated, normal, or reduced. Treatment of affected newborns includes intensive nutritional therapy (enteral, parenteral, or both) to reverse catabolism while restricting leucine intake, and treatment of cerebral edema when present.[18]

Organic Acidemias

Organic acids are the physiologic intermediates of amino acid catabolism, fatty acid oxidation, synthesis of cholesterol and fatty acids, and the citric acid cycle.[10] Several metabolic disorders arise from impaired metabolism of one or more of these cellular processes, leading to the accumulation of one or more organic acids rather than the biochemical precursor amino acid or fatty acids. Organic acidemias can present with chronic, progressive symptoms over time, but may present with severe neonatal crises. The characteristic laboratory findings in organic acidemias include metabolic acidosis with an increased anion gap. In the acute setting, management includes dextrose-containing fluids to reverse catabolism and ongoing acidosis. Long-term management focuses on limiting intake of the offending amino acid(s) through dietary measures and supplemental vitamins and metabolic intermediates.

Propionic and methylmalonic acidemia are 2 disorders of fatty acid and amino acid metabolism that can present with severe neonatal crisis. Specifically, odd-chain fatty acids and several amino acids (valine, methionine, isoleucine, and threonine) are converted to propionyl-CoA during the course of their metabolism. Propionyl-CoA is then converted to succinyl-CoA by a 2-step enzymatic process involving propionyl-CoA carboxylase (PCC) and methylmalonyl-CoA mutase (MCM) (**Fig. 4**). Succinyl-CoA then enters the citric acid cycle to generate energy for the cell. Deficiencies in either PCC, commonly known as propionic acidemia, or MCM, commonly known as methylmalonic acidemia, can lead to severe disruption of intermediary metabolism and neonatal crises.

- *Propionic acidemia (PA).* PA is an autosomal recessive condition characterized by deficiencies in the biotin-dependent enzyme PCC and disruption in the first step of propionyl-CoA metabolism. PCC comprises 10 protein subunits, and there are more than 100 pathogenic gene variants known to cause PA.[20,21]

Newborns with PA can present with vomiting, poor feeding, seizures, and severe encephalopathy. Laboratory analysis often shows high anion gap metabolic acidosis, ketosis, lactic acidemia, and hyperammonemia. Leukopenia, thrombocytopenia, and anemia may also occur.[22] The specific deficiency of PCC leads to accumulation of free

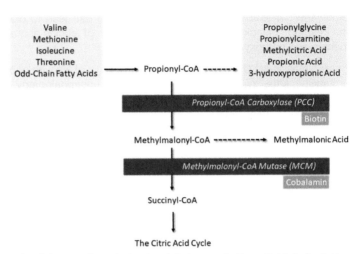

Fig. 4. Propionyl-CoA and methylmalonyl-CoA metabolism. Odd-chain fatty acids and several amino acids (valine, methionine, isoleucine, and threonine) are converted to propionyl-CoA and subsequently succinyl-CoA before entry into the citric acid cycle. Propionyl-CoA is converted to succinyl-CoA by a 2-step enzymatic process involving the biotin-dependent propionyl-CoA carboxylase (PCC) and cobalamin-dependent methylmalonyl-CoA mutase (MCM). Deficiencies in either PCC, commonly known as propionic acidemia, or MCM, commonly known as methylmalonic acidemia, can lead to severe disruption of intermediary metabolism.

propionic acid in blood and urine as well as several organic by-products, including methylcitrate, 3-hydroxypropionate, propionylglycine, and propionylcarnitine.[11] Acylcarnitine profiles show elevated propionylcarnitine (C3) and plasma amino acids show elevated glycine.[22]

During acute metabolic decompensation, affected individuals are at risk for basal ganglia stroke, which may lead to long-standing chorea and dystonia; rapid recognition and treatment of PA is crucial. Acute management of PA involves intensive nutritional management to reverse catabolism, restriction of the offending amino acids and odd-chain fatty acids, ammonia scavengers if hyperammonemia is severe, and management of coagulopathy if present.

- *Methylmalonic acidemia (MMA).* MMA is an autosomal recessive disorder caused by deficiency in the cobalamin-dependent enzyme MCM, a defect in the transport of adenosylcobalamin, or deficiency of the enzyme methylmalonyl-CoA epimerase.[23] Any of these defects disrupts the second step of propionyl-CoA metabolism and leads to the accumulation of methylmalonic acid.

Newborns with severe MMA may present similarly to those with PA (vomiting, poor feeding, lethargy, high anion gap metabolic acidosis, ketosis, lactic acidosis, and hyperammonemia). Both PA and MMA can lead to abnormal elevations in propionylcarnitine (C3), propionylglycine, 3-hydroxypropionate, and glycine. However, MMA can be distinguished from PA biochemically by elevations in serum methylmalonic acid. Elevations in homocysteine, if present, predict responsiveness to supplemental cobalamin. Acute management of MMA includes hydroxycobalamin supplementation for those patients that are cobalamin responsive, intensive nutritional therapy to reverse catabolism, restriction of the offending amino acids and odd-chain fatty acids, ammonia scavengers if hyperammonemia is severe, and management of coagulop-athy if present.[23]

Urea Cycle Disorders

Dietary amino acids in excess of a body's needs can be used as an energy source via entry into the citric acid cycle or by conversion to glucose via gluconeogenesis. In either case, the amino group must first be removed from the amino acid by a vitamin B_6-dependent deamination reaction so that the carbon skeleton can be subsequently used. The amino group then forms ammonia (NH_3), a neurotoxin.[10] The urea cycle is a hepatic multistep process that converts ammonia to urea, which can safely be excreted by the body in urine (**Fig. 5**).

Deficiencies in urea cycle enzymes can lead to severe metabolic crisis in the newborn as a result of hyperammonemia. Typically, symptomatic newborns present with poor feeding, lethargy, and progressive encephalopathy. Cerebral edema can be also be present. Ammonia levels of 150 μmol/L or, most often, higher in the setting of a normal anion gap and normal blood glucose, strongly suggest a urea cycle disor-der.[24] Although urea cycle disorders share the common feature of hyperammonemia, additional biochemical, enzymatic, and molecular testing can reveal the specific enzyme deficiency. Acute management of urea cycle disorders includes dextrose-containing fluids, reduction in enteral amino acids, supplemental arginine, ammonia scavengers, and treatment of cerebral edema if present. In some instances, liver transplant is indicated.

- *Ornithine transcarbamylase (OTC) deficiency.* OTC deficiency is the most com-mon urea cycle disorder and is an X-linked disorder caused by pathogenic variants in the *OTC* gene. OTC deficiency leads to impaired conversion of car-bamoyl phosphate to citrulline in the first step in the urea cycle. Affected

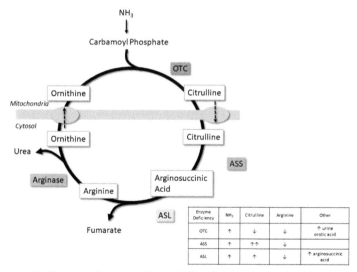

Fig. 5. Urea cycle disorders. Amino acid metabolism first involves a deamination reaction to remove the amino group from the carbon skeleton. The amino group then forms ammonia (NH_3), a neurotoxin. The urea cycle is a multistep process that converts ammonia to urea, which can be excreted by the body safely. Deficiencies in urea cycle enzymes can lead to se-vere metabolic crisis in the newborn as a result of hyperammonemia.

males typically present in severe neonatal crisis with a laboratory pattern of hyperammonemia, elevated glutamine, low citrulline, and low arginine, as detected by plasma amino acid analysis. Urine organic acid analysis typically shows elevated orotic acid.[25] Carrier females typically have a variable phenotype depending on the skewing of X-inactivation, but more commonly present outside of the neonatal period.

- *Citrullinemia type 1.* Citrulline is transported out of the mitochondria and into the cytosol and converted to argininosuccinate in the second step of the urea cycle. The process is catalyzed by the enzyme argininosuccinate synthase (ASS). Deficiencies in ASS lead to citrullinemia type 1, an autosomal recessive condition caused by pathogenic variants in the *ASS* gene. Affected newborns have hyperammonemia, markedly elevated citrulline, and low arginine detected by plasma amino acid analysis.[25]
- *Argininosuccinic aciduria.* Argininosuccinate lyase (ASL) catalyzes the third step in the urea cycle, the cleavage of argininosuccinate to arginine and fumarate. Deficiencies in ASL cause argininosuccinic aciduria, an autosomal recessive condition caused by pathogenic variants in the *ASL* gene. Affected newborns have hyperammonemia, elevated citrulline, and increased argininosuccinic acid measured by plasma amino acid analysis.[25]

Disorders of Carbohydrate Metabolism

Dietary carbohydrates are the primary fuel source for cells, particularly in nerve and red blood cells.[7] Complex carbohydrates and disaccharides are first metabolized into monosaccharides such as glucose, galactose, and fructose. Monosaccharides can then be converted to glycogen for energy storage or metabolized into pyruvate before entry into the citric acid cycle. Disorders of carbohydrate metabolism arise from perturbations in glycogen synthesis, glycogen degradation, or the metabolism of disaccharides. Although many disorders of carbohydrate metabolism present at a later age, disorders of galactose metabolism present in the newborn period with metabolic crisis.

Galactose is a monosaccharide with a structure similar to glucose, except for reversal of the -OH and -H positions on carbon 4.[10] Although isolated galactose does not typically occur naturally in many foods, it is commonly found combined with glucose to form the disaccharide lactose, which is the major carbohydrate in mammalian milk, including human breast milk and dairy products.[7] In the intestinal brush border membrane, lactose is hydrolyzed to glucose and galactose by lactase before absorption via a glucose-galactose cotransport protein.[11] Galactose can then be epimerized to glucose in a 3-step process and subsequently used to synthesize glycogen. Galactose can also be used directly by the liver to synthesize glycolipids and glycoproteins, components of cell membrane receptors and myelin in the central nervous system. Although most individuals ingest dietary galactose in the form of lactose, the body also produces small amounts of this important sugar endogenously.[10]

Typically, galactose is metabolized to glucose by a multistep process called the Leloir pathway (**Fig. 6**).[7,26] First, galactose is converted to galactose-1-phosphate by the galactokinase (GALK) enzyme. Second, galactose-1-phosphate is converted to glucose-1-phosphate by uridine diphosphate (UDP)-glucose and the enzyme galactose-1-phosphate uridylyltransferase (GALT), producing UDP-galactose in the process. Lastly, UDP-galactose is recycled back to UDP-glucose by UDP-galactose-4-epimerase (GALE). There are 3 known inborn errors of galactose metabolism, all inherited in autosomal recessive manner.

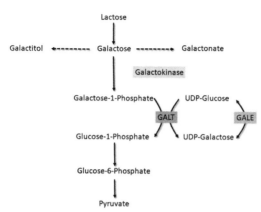

Fig. 6. Galactose metabolism. Galactose is metabolized by a multistep process called the Leloir pathway. GALE, uridine diphosphate (UDP)-galactose-4-epimerase; GALT, galactose-1-phosphate uridyltransferase.

- *Classic galactosemia.* The most severe form, classic galactosemia, is due to GALT deficiency, which leads to an accumulation of galactose-1-phosphate, galactitol, and galactonate. Untreated newborns may present with severe neonatal metabolic crisis including poor feeding, vomiting, diarrhea, jaundice, liver failure, abnormal hemostasis, hemolytic anemia, renal tubular disease, cataracts, and sepsis caused by gram-negative organisms, particularly *Escherichia coli*.[10,11] Untreated classic galactosemia is fatal in the newborn period but can be identified by newborn screening programs. Newborn screening identifies babies with classic galactosemia by metabolite testing (galactose, galactose 1-phosphate, or both) and/or GALT enzyme levels in red blood cells. Newborns with classic galactosemia may also show elevations in phenylalanine and tyrosine attributable to liver dysfunction, which may also be identified by newborn screening.[11] Newborns with galactosemia are treated with a lactose-free formula (typically a soy-based formula), which can reverse cataracts and liver and kidney disease.[10] Early recognition of classic galactosemia and prompt treatment with lactose-free formula can prevent poor outcomes in the acute setting.
- *Other forms of galactosemia.* Duarte galactosemia variants lead to 50% residual GALT enzyme function and alone are typically benign.[11,27] Individuals with one classic galactosemia variant and one Duarte variant have approximately 25% GALT enzyme activity.[27] These individuals may be identified by newborn screening but do not require therapy. GALE deficiencies are typically benign, but rarely there are newborns with intermediate-to-profound GALE deficiency who present with symptoms of classic galactosemia.[28,29] GALK deficiencies lead to accumulations in galactose, which is then converted to galactitol and galactonate, which then can cause cataracts that may be present as early as the newborn period. GALK deficiencies typically do not cause a neonatal crisis, although pseudotumor cerebri has been reported.[30]

Lysosomal Storage Disorders

Lysosomes are organelles that contain digestive enzymes and are an integral part of the intracellular recycling process of various cellular substrates including glycoproteins, mucopolysaccharides, oligosaccharides, and lipids.[10] Lysosomal storage disorders arise from deficiencies in or abnormal cellular location of one or more digestive enzymes, leading to an accumulation of the enzymatic substrate. Over time, the increasing storage of substrates impairs the function of the affected cells and organs. Numerous lysosomal storage disorders have been described with a wide range of phenotypic features. Pompe disease is a lysosomal storage disorder that can present with neonatal crisis.

- *Pompe disease.* Pompe disease is an autosomal recessive condition that arises from a deficiency in the lysosomal enzyme α-glucosidase (GAA) caused by pathogenic variants in the *GAA* gene. GAA enzyme activity is essential for glycogen degradation, so Pompe disease is also considered a disorder of glycogen storage and is alternatively termed glycogen storage type II or acid maltase deficiency.[10] Deficiency of GAA results in glycogen accumulation in multiple organs, each with its unique threshold for disease manifestations.[11]

Infantile Pompe disease can present with neonatal metabolic crises, although milder infantile, juvenile, and adult-onset forms also occur. Infants with classic Pompe disease have less than 1% GAA activity[11] and can present with poor feeding, hypotonia, cardiomyopathy, and characteristic abnormalities on electrocardiogram (shortened PR interval with a wide QRS complex).[31] Laboratory studies may show elevated creatine kinase, hepatic transaminases, and urine oligosaccharides.[10] Untreated infants with classic Pompe disease typically die of cardiopulmonary failure or aspiration

---

Best Practices

What is the current practice for neonatal metabolic crisis?

Best Practice/Guideline/Care Path Objective(s):
- Early recognition of neonatal metabolic crisis
- Appropriate initial stabilization therapies
- Basic laboratory evaluation to generate a differential diagnosis

What changes in current practice are likely to improve outcomes?

- Use of history and examination findings to differentiate neonatal metabolic crises from more common illnesses

- More rapid development of a differential diagnosis based on basic laboratory analysis

- Increased understanding of advanced biochemical and molecular testing that can identify the specific cause of the metabolic crisis

Major Recommendations

- Consider a metabolic disorder in infants presenting with poor feeding, vomiting, and lethargy

- If metabolic crisis is suspected, hold enteral feedings and initiate 10% dextrose-containing isotonic fluids to reduce catabolism

- Collect basic laboratories (glucose, complete metabolic profile, complete blood count, bilirubin, ammonia, creatine kinase, and urine ketones) to help determine what type of metabolic disorder is most likely

- Work with a biochemical geneticist to identify the advanced biochemical or molecular testing needed to confirm the diagnosis

Summary Statement: A thorough history, physical examination, and basic laboratory analysis can provide substantial insight into the underlying cause of severe metabolic crises.

pneumonia before 1 year of life.[11] Recombinant α-glucosidase enzyme therapy is now available, prompting many states to add Pompe disease to newborn screening panels. However, screening is not available in all states and it is difficult to differentiate between severe infantile forms and adult-onset forms by molecular genetics alone, so high clinical suspicion remains critically important.

SUMMARY

Metabolic disorders vary in etiology, severity, and age of onset, but several can present with neonatal crisis. Identifying these newborns can be challenging, as the presenting symptoms may be subtle and may often mimic more common neonatal medical issues. However, history and physical examination accompanied by basic laboratory evaluation can often provide clues to an underlying metabolic disorder. Once a specific class of disorders is suspected, advanced biochemical, enzymatic, and molecular testing can provide a more definitive diagnosis. Timely recognition of newborns with metabolic disease is critical for administering appropriate treatment, thereby reducing the morbidity that can be associated with these rare but potentially life-threatening disorders.

DISCLOSURE

The authors have nothing to disclose.

REFERENCES

1. Applegarth DA, Toone JR, Lowry RB. Incidence of inborn errors of metabolism in British Columbia, 1969-1996. Pediatrics 2000;105(1):e10.
2. Sanderson S, Green A, Preece MA, et al. The incidence of inherited metabolic disorders in the West Midlands, UK. Arch Dis Child 2006;91(11):896–9.
3. Bell RA, Mayer-Davis EJ, Beyer JW, et al. Diabetes in non-Hispanic white youth: prevalence, incidence, and clinical characteristics: the SEARCH for Diabetes in Youth Study. Diabetes Care 2009;32(Suppl 2):S102–11.
4. Baby's first test. 2019. Available at: www.babysfirsttest.org. Accessed July 1, 2019.
5. Gilboa N, Swanson JR. Serum creatine phosphokinase in normal newborns. Arch Dis Child 1976;51(4):283–5.
6. Foster DW. The role of the carnitine system in human metabolism. Ann N Y Acad Sci 2004;1033:1–16.
7. Byrd-Bredbenner C, Beshegetoor D, Moe G, Berning J. Wardlaw's perspectives in nutrition. 8th edition. New York: McGraw-Hill; 2009.
8. Rinaldo P, Matern D, Bennett MJ. Fatty acid oxidation disorders. Annu Rev Physiol 2002;64:477–502.
9. Vishwanath VA. Fatty acid beta-oxidation disorders: a brief review. Ann Neurosci 2016;23(1):51–5.
10. Sarafoglou K, Hoffman G, Roth K. Pediatric endocrinology and inborn errors of metabolism. New York: McGraw-Hill Companies; 2009.
11. Saudubray J, van den Berghe G, Walter J. Inborn metabolic diseases: diagnosis and treatment. 5th edition. Berlin Heidelberg: Springer-Verlag; 2012.
12. Hale DE, Stanley CA, Coates PM. Genetic defects of acyl-CoA dehydrogenases: studies using an electron transfer flavoprotein reduction assay. Prog Clin Biol Res 1990;321:333–48.

13. Smith EH, Matern D. Acylcarnitine analysis by tandem mass spectrometry. Curr Protoc Hum Genet 2010 [Chapter 17]:Unit 17.8.11–20.
14. Gregersen N, Kolvraa S, Rasmussen K, et al. General (medium-chain) acyl-CoA dehydrogenase deficiency (non-ketotic dicarboxylic aciduria): quantitative urinary excretion pattern of 23 biologically significant organic acids in three cases. Clin Chim Acta 1983;132(2):181–91.
15. Scott Schwoerer J, Cooper G, van Calcar S. Rhabdomyolysis in a neonate due to very long chain acyl CoA dehydrogenase deficiency. Mol Genet Metab Rep 2015; 3:39–41.
16. McHugh D, Cameron CA, Abdenur JE, et al. Clinical validation of cutoff target ranges in newborn screening of metabolic disorders by tandem mass spectrometry: a worldwide collaborative project. Genet Med 2011;13(3):230–54.
17. Stipanuk M. Biochemical and physiological aspects of human nutrition. Philadelphia: W. B. Saunders Company; 2000.
18. Strauss K, Puffenberger E, Morton H. Maple syrup urine disease. In: Adam MP, Ardinger HH, Pagon RA, et al, editors. GeneReviews [Internet]. University of Washington; 2013. Seattle (WA).
19. Mamer OA, Reimer ML. On the mechanisms of the formation of L-alloisoleucine and the 2-hydroxy-3-methylvaleric acid stereoisomers from L-isoleucine in maple syrup urine disease patients and in normal humans. J Biol Chem 1992;267(31): 22141–7.
20. Perez B, Desviat LR, Rodriguez-Pombo P, et al. Propionic acidemia: identification of twenty-four novel mutations in Europe and North America. Mol Genet Metab 2003;78(1):59–67.
21. Yang X, Sakamoto O, Matsubara Y, et al. Mutation spectrum of the PCCA and PCCB genes in Japanese patients with propionic acidemia. Mol Genet Metab 2004;81(4):335–42.
22. Shchelochkov O, Carrillo N, Venditti C. Propionic acidemia. In: Adam MP, Ardinger HH, Pagon RA, et al, editors. GeneReviews [Internet]. University of Washington; 2016. Seattle (WA).
23. Manoli I, Slaon J, Venditti C. Isolated methylmalonic acidemia. In: Adam MP, Ardinger HH, Pagon RA, et al, editors. GeneReviews [Internet]. University of Washington; 2016. Seattle (WA).
24. Summar M, Tuchman M. Proceedings of a consensus conference for the management of patients with urea cycle disorders. J Pediatr 2001;138(1 Suppl): S6–10.
25. Ah Mew N, Simpson K, Gropman A, et al. Urea cycle disorders overview. In: Adam MP, Ardinger HH, Pagon RA, et al, editors. GeneReviews [Internet]. University of Washington; 2017. Seattle (WA).
26. Leloir LF, Cardini CE. Carbohydrate metabolism. Annu Rev Biochem 1953;22: 179–210.
27. Elsas LJ, Dembure PP, Langley S, et al. A common mutation associated with the Duarte galactosemia allele. Am J Hum Genet 1994;54(6):1030–6.
28. Openo KK, Schulz JM, Vargas CA, et al. Epimerase-deficiency galactosemia is not a binary condition. Am J Hum Genet 2006;78(1):89–102.
29. Walter JH, Roberts RE, Besley GT, et al. Generalised uridine diphosphate galactose-4-epimerase deficiency. Arch Dis Child 1999;80(4):374–6.
30. Bosch AM, Bakker HD, van Gennip AH, et al. Clinical features of galactokinase deficiency: a review of the literature. J Inherit Metab Dis 2002;25(8):629–34.
31. Leslie N, Bailey L. Pompe disease. In: Adam MP, Ardinger HH, Pagon RA, et al, editors. GeneReviews [Internet]. Seattle (WA): University of Washington; 2017.

Neonatal Assessment of Infants with Heterotaxy

Gabrielle C. Geddes, MD[a,b,*], Sai-Suma Samudrala, BS[c], Michael G. Earing, MD[a,b,d]

KEYWORDS

- Heterotaxy • Situs inversus • Isomerism • Laterality defect • Situs ambiguus
- Ivemark syndrome

KEY POINTS

- Patients with heterotaxy require comprehensive anatomic assessment at birth to quantify the number and severity of congenital anomalies.
- All patients with heterotaxy should be treated with prophylactic antibiotics and vaccination for encapsulated organisms as if they have congenital asplenia.
- Prophylactic Ladd procedure for intestinal malrotation has been shown to increase morbidity and mortality in patients with heterotaxy.
- Routine molecular genetic testing should include copy number variant analysis and sequencing that at minimum covers causes of primary ciliary dyskinesia.

INTRODUCTION

In general terms, heterotaxy describes any disruption in laterality deviating from situs solitus[1]; however, the proper taxonomy of heterotaxy remains quite controversial.[2,3] In 2007, the International Society for Nomenclature of Paediatric and Congenital Heart Disease (ISNPCHD) published anatomic definitions specific to patients with heterotaxy,[1] focusing on 3 main terms: heterotaxy, isomerism, and situs ambiguus.[1] Under this classification system, *heterotaxy* describes patients whose anatomy does not fit into either a pure situs solitus or a situs inversus configuration, whereas the term, *isomerism*, refers to patients with heterotaxy whose atrial and/or pulmonary anatomy is in a symmetric mirror image configuration, and the term, *situs ambiguus* describes patients with heterotaxy whose laterality anomalies do not fit a classically anticipated embryologic pattern (**Fig. 1**).[1] Within the realm of cardiac care and prognosis, isomerism, with its emphasis on defining atrial appendages and pulmonary anatomy, has

[a] Department of Pediatrics, Medical College of Wisconsin, Milwaukee, WI, USA; [b] Herma Heart Institute, Children's Hospital of Wisconsin, 9000 West Wisconsin Avenue, MS#716, Milwaukee, WI 53226, USA; [c] Department of Cell Biology, Neurobiology and Anatomy, Medical College of Wisconsin, Milwaukee, WI, USA; [d] Section of Adult Cardiovascular Medicine, Department of Internal Medicine, Medical College of Wisconsin, Milwaukee, WI, USA
* Corresponding author. 975 West Walnut Street, IB Suite 130, Room 154, Indianapolis, IN 46202.
E-mail address: egeddes@iu.edu

Clin Perinatol 47 (2020) 171–182
https://doi.org/10.1016/j.clp.2019.10.011
0095-5108/20/© 2019 Elsevier Inc. All rights reserved.

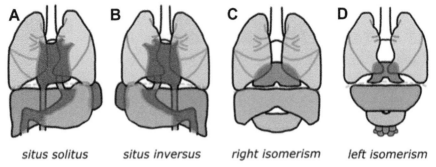

situs solitus   situs inversus   right isomerism   left isomerism

Fig. 1. Anatomic terminology. Anatomy correlating with descriptive terms frequently encountered when discussing heterotaxy. (*A*) Demonstrates normal anatomy, or situs solitus. (*B*) Demonstrates complete mirror image anatomy without malformation, or situs inversus. (*C*) Demonstrates right isomerism, which is mirror imaging of right-sided structures. (*D*) Demonstrates left isomerism, which is mirror imaging of the left-sided structures. Patients with laterality anomalies who do not fit into any of these patterns typically are characterized as having situs ambiguus. Patients with right isomerism, left isomerism, or situs ambiguus all have heterotaxy. (*Courtesy of* S. Samudrala, BS, Milwaukee WI.)

increasingly become the preferred term[1,2,4,5]; however, this label fails to appropriately capture the complexity and phenotypic diversity of laterality anomalies, often overlooking the varied systemic complications of heterotaxy, while neglecting patients with heterotaxy who have normal cardiac anatomy as well as the significant number of patients with situs ambiguus.[6–8] Despite these anatomic classifications, there is no distinction between genes causing situs inversus and genes causing heterotaxy,[9–11] suggesting that the care of patients with heterotaxy often is best customized to individual phenotypic manifestations, with a few common overarching themes.[1,2] The true incidence of heterotaxy is not known, largely due to the historical lack of consensus definitions and the unknown proportion of undiagnosed patients at the mild end of the spectrum. Heterotaxy is thought to represent up to 7% of patients with congenital heart disease and has been estimated to occur in 1 in 5000 to 10,000 live births, although the true incidence is likely higher, because many milder variants remain undiagnosed.[7,9,11–13] For the purposes of this discussion, heterotaxy is defined as a class of congenital disorders resulting from failure to establish normal left-right asymmetry during embryonic development, excluding situs inversus, as recommended by the ISNPCHD.[1] Given the phenotypic and etiologic diversity of heterotaxy, the condition does not meet criteria to be considered a syndrome, despite the frequent use of this term, and is not referred to as such.[9–11,14] Neonatal concerns for these patients, including required initial evaluation and preventative care, are discussed.[1,15] Thorough phenotyping and comprehensive care of patients with heterotaxy remain challenging, even in settings optimized for prenatal diagnosis and high-acuity neonatal management.

ANATOMIC CONSIDERATIONS

Patients with suspected heterotaxy require comprehensive anatomic assessment to confirm the diagnosis, evaluate for additional functional and anatomic abnormalities (**Table 1**), and exclude alternate diagnoses. Although the classic, prototypical features of heterotaxy follow anticipated defects of laterality, there can be phenotypic overlap between heterotaxy and a VACTERL pattern of anomalies; presuming a particular

Table 1
Anatomic assessment of neonates with heterotaxy

Organ System	Investigations	Examples of Abnormal Findings
Cardiac	Echocardiogram Electrocardiogram	Complex congenital heart disease (frequent) Arrythmias (frequent) Cardiomyopathy (rare)
Craniofacial		Cleft lip and palate (rare) Choanal atresia (rare) Laryngeal cleft (rare)
Hepatic	Abdominal ultrasound	Interrupted inferior vena cava (frequent) Congenital absence of the portal vein (rare) Biliary atresia (rare)
Intestinal	Upper gastrointestinal tract radiography[a]	Abnormal intestinal rotation (frequent) Duodenal atresia (rare)
Immunologic	Flow cytometry[a]	Low T-cell and B-cell numbers (rare)
Neurologic	Head ultrasound Brain magnetic resonance imaging[a]	Dandy-Walker malformation (rare) Neural tube defects (rare)
Pulmonary	Chest radiograph Chest computed tomography[a]	Bilateral left bronchial morphology with 2 lobes (frequent) Bilateral right bronchial morphology with 3 lobes (frequent) Tracheoesophageal fistula (rare)
Renal	Abdominal ultrasound	Horseshoe kidney (rare) Renal agenesis (rare)
Skeletal	Chest radiograph Abdominal radiograph	Vertebral anomalies (rare) Missing or extra ribs (rare)
Splenic	Abdominal ultrasound	Asplenia (frequent) Polysplenia (frequent)

Recommended diagnostic studies by system and potential abnormal findings. Rare indicates a finding is anticipated in less than 10% of patients with heterotaxy. Frequent indicates a finding is anticipated in more than 50% of patients with heterotaxy.
[a] Not routinely indicated.

combination of anomalies is consistent solely with a VACTERL association may miss laterality defects and their associated functional consequences; alternately, laterality defects with VACTERL anomalies often are associated with pathogenic variants in *ZIC3* and have an impact on care and recurrence risk, emphasizing the need for thorough phenotyping.[16–18]

Cardiac

As the first organ to express laterality, the heart frequently is involved, and abnormalities of cardiac situs typically are the first finding to suggest a diagnosis of heterotaxy.[11] More than 20% of patients with heterotaxy have cardiac anomalies beyond what would be predicted embryologically based on atrial morphology,[6] and it is likely that laterality disorders underlie a greater degree of congenital heart lesions than previously appreciated.[19] The range of structural cardiac lesions is complex and may involve atrioventricular septal lesions, conotruncal lesions, left ventricular outflow tract anomalies, right ventricular outflow tract anomalies, and anomalous pulmonary venous return.[12] Frequently, abdominal ultrasound or echocardiogram demonstrates an interrupted inferior vena cava and abnormalities of the superior vena cava.[12,20] A range of arrhythmias, including both tachyarrhythmias and bradyarrhythmias, may be seen secondary to insufficient or duplicated sinoatrial nodes resulting from mirror-imaged atrial anatomy.[8,21] The spectrum of electrophysiologic abnormalities may be broader than that which would be predicted based on atrial anatomy alone.[22] Cardiomyopathy, in particular left ventricular noncompaction, also is seen more frequently in patients with heterotaxy.[23] This variety of structural and functional anomalies makes both medical and surgical management challenging. Cardiac transplantation presents additional challenges: in addition to the inherent anatomic challenges, patients with heterotaxy may have increased risk for pulmonary hypertension, further decreasing their ability to be considered for cardiac transplantation.[24] In general, when patients with heterotaxy do undergo cardiac transplantation, they have significantly increased morbidity and mortality compared with their peers.[25]

Intestinal

More than 70% of patients have abnormal intestinal rotation.[26,27] Heterotaxy does not seem to increase the risk for acute volvulus compared with other patients with malrotation, and early data suggest that if volvulus does occur, it typically occurs in the first 6 months of life.[26,27] In patients with heterotaxy, elective Ladd procedure in asymptomatic individuals with malrotation is controversial, is independently associated with increased morbidity, and currently is not recommended.[26–29] Rarely, patients can have other intestinal anomalies, including duodenal atresia.[30]

Pulmonary

Up to 40% of patients with heterotaxy have a functional ciliopathy that may not be apparent on electron microscopy or genetic testing; however, videomicroscopy may identify ciliary motion defects or abnormal ciliary beat frequency and provide evidence of ciliary dysfunction.[31] Patients with heterotaxy, in particular those with ciliopathies, have more postoperative respiratory complications, including prolonged intubation, atelectasis, and pleural effusions; some have required tracheostomy for prolonged respiratory difficulties.[32,33] Pulmonary anomalies, with either bilateral bilobed or bilateral trilobed lungs, are common[12,20]; tracheoesophageal fistula occurs rarely and is an important consideration in an infant with recurrent pneumonia whose difficulties otherwise may erroneously be attributed to ciliary dyskinesia alone.[17]

Immunologic

The immunologic assessment of patients with heterotaxy was classically based on spleen anatomy; however, spleen anatomy is not a reliable indicator of infection risk.[34–36] The immune phenotype in heterotaxy is more complex than that seen solely with asplenia: in addition to the risk for bacteremia with encapsulated organisms, there is an increased risk for respiratory and gastrointestinal infections,[35] thought to be secondary to both anatomic asplenia and an intrinsic thymic dysfunction that is independent of acquired thymic disruption from surgical repair of congenital heart disease.[20,34,35] The authors have had 2 patients with heterotaxy who had an immunodeficiency consistent with thymic aplasia, 1 of whom was of sufficient severity to be detected on newborn screening prior to thymic disruption by sternotomy.

The immunologic management of patients with heterotaxy is highly variable.[37] The authors do not recommend attempting to discern functional or anatomic splenic status for the purposes determining the need for antibacterial prophylaxis or vaccination and instead treat all patients with heterotaxy with amoxicillin prophylaxis as well as vaccination for encapsulated organisms based on current American Academy of Pediatrics Committee on Infectious Diseases guidelines for congenital asplenia.[38] Booster vaccination may be required in the heterotaxy population more commonly than in other patients.[39] The authors have been discontinuing antibiotic prophylaxis at age 5, similar to treatment of patients with sickle cell disease, but the ideal length of prophylaxis is unknown.[40]

Hepatic

The most common hepatic finding is abnormal placement of the liver, although much more serious hepatobiliary anomalies can be present, including biliary atresia and congenital absence of the portal vein.[41–43] Liver transplantation, if indicated, requires significant planning to account for anatomic and medical complexity.[42,44–46]

Neurologic

Dandy-Walker malformation has been associated with heterotaxy but is rare.[12,18] Neural tube defects have also been described, but a true association has not been established.[12,18] The ciliary dysfunction seen in many patients with heterotaxy may be associated with neurologic dysfunction and abnormal neurodevelopmental outcomes.[20,47] Magnetic resonance imaging may demonstrate many of these findings and assist in stratifying developmental risk and prognosis, although should only be obtained for the purposes of prognostication when clinically indicated and in a stable patient.[47–49]

Renal

Renal agenesis, renal cysts, and horseshoe kidney have been noted but are not common and often are noted incidentally during abdominal ultrasound.[18,21] The authors have anecdotally observed that patients with 11 pairs of ribs are more likely to have renal dysfunction during times of critical illness, including the postoperative period from cardiac surgery.

Skeletal

Skeletal anomalies, in particular segmental anomalies of the vertebrae and ribs, are common; absent vertebrae, fused vertebrae, and hemivertebrae also are seen and sometimes may be missed on plain radiography unless such concerns are specified.[18]

Craniofacial

No specific craniofacial dysmorphisms are associated with heterotaxy. Structural anomalies that can affect the airway are rarely observed. Cleft lip and palate, micrognathia, choanal atresia, and laryngeal clefts have been seen in patients with heterotaxy but are not common manifestations.[18]

MOLECULAR TESTING AND RECURRENCE RISK
Molecular Testing

Genetic etiologies of heterotaxy are diverse.[9,50,51] Laterality also is likely uniquely sensitive to teratogenic influence.[52] The authors recommend genetic testing that assess for copy number variants as well as sequence variants in all neonates with heterotaxy, because early molecular diagnosis may significantly alter care; this is particularly true in patients who have heterotaxy due to primary ciliary dyskinesia.[53,54] At the authors' center, the most efficient, cost-effective genetic assessment to meet these goals that has been found is genomic sequencing with copy number variant analysis; alternate strategies if access to genomic sequencing is limited include a chromosomal microarray and a heterotaxy sequencing panel that includes primary ciliary dyskinesia genes. Given the frequency of variants of uncertain significance in primary ciliary dyskinesia genes in this population, pretest genetic counseling is of the utmost importance, so as to anticipate variants of uncertain significance and to reduce anxiety at time of result disclosure.

Recurrence risk

In the setting of confirmatory diagnostic genetic testing, the recurrence risk of having another child with heterotaxy can be clearly articulated. Heterotaxy has been associated with de novo, autosomal recessive, X-linked, and autosomal-dominant single-gene etiologies; as such, recurrence risks can range from less than 1% up to 50%. In families with autosomal-dominant single-gene forms of heterotaxy, there usually is variable penetrance and variable expressivity with an apparent bias toward mildly affected individuals. Variable expressivity is seen in all currently identifiable monogenic etiologies of heterotaxy, and variable penetrance also is observed. In the setting of a patient without any known family history or an identified molecular diagnosis, the authors counsel that the recurrence risk for another child with heterotaxy ranges from less than 1% to 25% and focus heavily on the potential spectrum of affected family members, including mild forms that do not result in medical concerns, up to severe forms that make survival impossible.

DIAGNOSTIC CONSIDERATIONS

When evaluating a patient for possible heterotaxy, the authors have found the most helpful clinical features to confirm a diagnosis are the presence of abnormal pulmonary venous return, abnormal intestinal rotation, and interrupted inferior vena cava. The presence of 1 or more of these features, in combination with other congenital anomalies, should be considered within the spectrum of heterotaxy and should prompt consideration of antibacterial prophylaxis and molecular testing. Although not all anatomic findings in heterotaxy result in medically actionable information, complete assessment improves anticipatory guidance and provides potential insight into underlying genetic etiologies. For example, the presence of heterotaxy and multiple midline anomalies in a VACTERL pattern in a male infant increases the suspicion of disruption of *ZIC3*, whereas a patient with renal cysts is more likely to have a ciliopathy.[16,55] Patients with VACTERL/heterotaxy overlap require different care and have a higher potential recurrence risk compared with their isolated VACTERL pattern counterparts. Although phenotypic features are helpful in suggesting potential genetic etiologies, they should not be used to narrow what genetic testing is performed on a patient.

SUMMARY

Heterotaxy is a complex multisystem disorder. There is debate regarding proper nomenclature and how to describe and classify these patients. Based on identified molecular etiologies, these classifications are mostly arbitrary. The authors advocate an individualized approach to each patient by using descriptors, such as "affected by heterotaxy characterized by," and listing each individual manifestation for completeness. Although heterotaxy classically has been associated with mortality rates as high as 50%, more recent data suggest survival has improved significantly.[7,56–60] Comprehensive anatomic and functional assessment allows for better anticipatory management of each individual's phenotypic manifestations and maximizes survival, overall health, and developmental potential. Improved understanding of best practices in infection prevention and management of patients with functional ciliopathies hold great potential in further improving mortality and morbidity, and expanded routine molecular testing will allow for novel bioinformatics approaches.

The use of prophylactic antibiotics and vaccination in patients with heterotaxy should be both more uniform and routine. Vaccination offers low potential risk and high potential benefit. Even with these precautions, the authors speculate the immunodeficiency and recurrent infection risk in these patients is more complex than currently appreciated, likely due to a combination of difficult-to-diagnose ciliary dysfunction as well as intrinsic and acquired thymic dysfunction from cyanosis and early sternotomy. Based on the authors' observation that infants who undergo sternotomy in the first 48 hours frequently have abnormal newborn screens for severe combined immunodeficiency, patients who undergo rapid surgical intervention for obstructed abnormal pulmonary venous return are a specific high-risk group. This may be unique to patients who have cyanotic cardiac lesions or a molecular predisposition to abnormal thymic development. It is possible that lower thresholds for initiating B-cell and T-cell functional assays may benefit specific populations or be required in the setting of specific clinical observations.

Given the prevalence of ciliopathies in heterotaxy, more routine utilization of mucociliary clearance therapies may help preserve pulmonary function and prevent recurrent infections. This outcome may prove especially important in patients with single ventricle physiology, because optimized pulmonary function may improve pulmonary vascular pressures and thereby improve cardiac function and decrease the risk of heart failure. Although β-agonists may promote ciliary function, further investigation will need to identify which patients may benefit most, particularly given the frequent utilization of β-blockade in patients with cardiac dysfunction.[32,61–64] Ciliopathies have additionally been implicated in hepatic fibrosis, potentially increasing the risk for post-Fontan liver disease in patients with single ventricle physiology.[65–68] Although liver transplant may be successful in these circumstances, the presence of additional anatomic anomalies, progressive multiorgan dysfunction, and complex anesthesia concerns may make surgical planning challenging.[44,45,60,69] Improved understanding and enhanced methods for the diagnosis and management of ciliopathies, as well as the relationship between ciliary function and mitochondrial function, hold considerable promise for better short-term and long-term outcomes.[31,70–73]

Molecular diagnostics will become increasingly more relevant in guiding care in this population. Early genomic testing with retention of the raw data for periodic reanalysis is critical. How to incorporate these data into a patient's chart to make them accessible and how to make the data follow a patient over time are both significant issues that need to be addressed. Novel bioinformatics approaches assessing for multigenic causes and identifying phenotypic associations need to be explored more aggressively. Leveraging techniques from other disciplines, such as those used in tumor bioinformatics, and using these to look for novel potential influences, including chromothripsis and other chromosomal rearrangements, fusion proteins, gene expression, and epigenetic regulation, will expedite enhanced understanding. At present and until these techniques are more widely available, multigenic assessments focusing on ciliopathies will result in clinically intervenable results most quickly.

Despite notable advances in both diagnosis and management, heterotaxy remains a complex and challenging entity, and significant knowledge gaps in long-term outcomes and molecular etiology persist. Complete neonatal phenotyping and molecular assessment are critical in improving both individual outcomes and global understanding of heterotaxy.

Best Practices

What is the current practice for assessment of infants with heterotaxy?

- Comprehensive anatomic assessment at birth to determine all organ systems involved
- Prophylactic antibiotics and vaccination for encapsulated organisms for all heterotaxy patients per guidelines for patients with asplenia
- Parental education and plan regarding risk for bacteremia for all heterotaxy patients
- Although assessment for intestinal malrotation can be helpful for phenotyping, prophylactic Ladd procedure can increase morbidity and mortality and should not be completed in patients with heterotaxy
- Molecular genetic testing, which at a minimum assesses for copy number variants genome-wide and sequence variants in primary ciliary dyskinesia genes, although wider genomic assessment is more appropriate

---

DISCLOSURE

The authors have nothing to disclose.

REFERENCES

1. Jacobs JP, Anderson RH, Weinberg PM, et al. The nomenclature, definition and classification of cardiac structures in the setting of heterotaxy. Cardiol Young 2007;17(Suppl 2):1–28.
2. Loomba RS, Hlavacek AM, Spicer DE, et al. Isomerism or heterotaxy: which term leads to better understanding? Cardiol Young 2015;25(6):1037–43.
3. Thiene G, Frescura C. Asplenia and polysplenia syndromes: time of successful treatment and updated terminology. Int J Cardiol 2019;274:117–9.
4. Tremblay C, Loomba RS, Frommelt PC, et al. Segregating bodily isomerism or heterotaxy: potential echocardiographic correlations of morphological findings. Cardiol Young 2017;27(8):1470–80.
5. Loomba RS, Pelech AN, Shah PH, et al. Determining bronchial morphology for the purposes of segregating so-called heterotaxy. Cardiol Young 2016;26(4):725–37.
6. Yim D, Nagata H, Lam CZ, et al. Disharmonious patterns of heterotaxy and isomerism: how often are the classic patterns breached? Circ Cardiovasc Imaging 2018;11(2):e006917.
7. Baban A, Cantarutti N, Adorisio R, et al. Long-term survival and phenotypic spectrum in heterotaxy syndrome: a 25-year follow-up experience. Int J Cardiol 2018;268:100–5.
8. Ozawa Y, Asakai H, Shiraga K, et al. Cardiac rhythm disturbances in heterotaxy syndrome. Pediatr Cardiol 2019;40(5):909–13.
9. Li AH, Hanchard NA, Azamian M, et al. Genetic architecture of laterality defects revealed by whole exome sequencing. Eur J Hum Genet 2019;27(4):563–73.
10. Catana A, Apostu AP. The determination factors of left-right asymmetry disorders-a short review. Clujul Med 2017;90(2):139–46.
11. Sutherland MJ, Ware SM. Disorders of left-right asymmetry: heterotaxy and situs inversus. Am J Med Genet C Semin Med Genet 2009;151C(4):307–17.
12. Lin AE, Krikov S, Riehle-Colarusso T, et al. Laterality defects in the national birth defects prevention study (1998-2007): birth prevalence and descriptive epidemiology. Am J Med Genet A 2014;164A(10):2581–91.

13. Fesslova V, Pluchinotta F, Brankovic J, et al. Characteristics and outcomes of fetuses with laterality defects are the current outcomes better? A single center study. J Matern Fetal Neonatal Med 2019;20:1–8.

14. Jorde L, Carey J, Bamshad M. Medical genetics. Maryland Heights (MO): Mosby Elsevier; 2010.

15. Zhu L, Belmont JW, Ware SM. Genetics of human heterotaxias. Eur J Hum Genet 2006;14(1):17–25.

16. Cowan J, Tariq M, Ware SM. Genetic and functional analyses of ZIC3 variants in congenital heart disease. Hum Mutat 2014;35(1):66–75.

17. Hashmi A, Abu-Sulaiman R, McCrindle BW, et al. Management and outcomes of right atrial isomerism: a 26-year experience. J Am Coll Cardiol 1998;31(5):1120–6.

18. Ticho BS, Goldstein AM, Van Praagh R. Extracardiac anomalies in the heterotaxy syndromes with focus on anomalies of midline-associated structures. Am J Cardiol 2000;85(6):729–34.

19. Versacci P, Pugnaloni F, Digilio MC, et al. Some isolated cardiac malformations can be related to laterality defects. J Cardiovasc Dev Dis 2018;5(2) [pii:E24].

20. Loomba RS, Ahmed MM, Spicer DE, et al. Manifestations of bodily isomerism. Cardiovasc Pathol 2016;25(3):173–80.

21. Landis BJ, Cooper DS, Hinton RB. CHD associated with syndromic diagnoses: peri-operative risk factors and early outcomes. Cardiol Young 2016;26(1):30–52.

22. Niu MC, Dickerson HA, Moore JA, et al. Heterotaxy syndrome and associated arrhythmias in pediatric patients. Heart Rhythm 2018;15(4):548–54.

23. Martinez HR, Ware SM, Schamberger MS, et al. Noncompaction cardiomyopathy and heterotaxy syndrome. Prog Pediatr Cardiol 2017;46:23–7.

24. Shibata A, Mori H, Kodo K, et al. Polysplenia syndrome as a risk factor for early progression of pulmonary hypertension. Circ J 2019;83(4):831–6.

25. Duong SQ, Godown J, Soslow JH, et al. Increased mortality, morbidities, and costs after heart transplantation in heterotaxy syndrome and other complex situs arrangements. J Thorac Cardiovasc Surg 2019;157(2):730–40.e1.

26. Ryerson LM, Pharis S, Pockett C, et al. Heterotaxy syndrome and intestinal rotation abnormalities. Pediatrics 2018;142(2) [pii:e20174267].

27. Landisch RM, Loomba RS, Salazar JH, et al. Is isomerism a risk factor for intestinal volvulus? J Pediatr Surg 2018;53(6):1118–22.

28. Abbas PI, Dickerson HA, Wesson DE. Evaluating a management strategy for malrotation in heterotaxy patients. J Pediatr Surg 2016;51(5):859–62.

29. White SC, Dean PN, McGahren ED, et al. Malrotation is not associated with adverse outcomes after cardiac surgery in patients with heterotaxy syndrome. J Pediatr Surg 2018;53(8):1494–8.

30. Dipak NK, Reddy S, Jaiswal KK, et al. Neonate with mirror image of double bubble sign. Arch Dis Child Educ Pract Ed 2019;104(2):101–2.

31. Nakhleh N, Francis R, Giese RA, et al. High prevalence of respiratory ciliary dysfunction in congenital heart disease patients with heterotaxy. Circulation 2012;125(18):2232–42.

32. Harden B, Tian X, Giese R, et al. Increased postoperative respiratory complications in heterotaxy congenital heart disease patients with respiratory ciliary dysfunction. J Thorac Cardiovasc Surg 2014;147(4):1291–8.e2.

33. Swisher M, Jonas R, Tian X, et al. Increased postoperative and respiratory complications in patients with congenital heart disease associated with heterotaxy. J Thorac Cardiovasc Surg 2011;141(3):637–44, 644.e1-3.

34. Loomba RS, Geddes GC, Basel D, et al. Bacteremia in patients with heterotaxy: a review and implications for management. Congenit Heart Dis 2016; 11(6):537–47.

35. Piano Mortari E, Baban A, Cantarutti N, et al. Heterotaxy syndrome with and without spleen: different infection risk and management. J Allergy Clin Immunol 2017;139(6):1981–4.e1.

36. Loomba RS, Pelech AN, Anderson RH. Factors influencing bacteraemia in patients with isomerism and CHD: the effects of functional splenic status and antibiotic prophylaxis. Cardiol Young 2017;27(4):639–47.

37. Loomba RS, Geddes G, Shillingford AJ, et al. Practice variability in management of infectious issues in heterotaxy: a survey of pediatric cardiologists. Congenit Heart Dis 2017;12(3):332–9.

38. Kimberlin DW, Brady MT, Jackson MA, editors. Red book. 31st edition. Itasca (IL): AAP Committee on Infectious Diseases; 2018.

39. Shao PL, Wu MH, Wang JK, et al. Pneumococcal vaccination and efficacy in patients with heterotaxy syndrome. Pediatr Res 2017;82(1):101–7.

40. Sobota A, Sabharwal V, Fonebi G, et al. How we prevent and manage infection in sickle cell disease. Br J Haematol 2015;170(6):757–67.

41. Allarakia J, Felemban T, Khayyat W, et al. Biliary atresia with an unusual abdominal orientation: a case report. Int J Surg Case Rep 2019;55:152–5.

42. Yamada Y, Hoshino K, Oyanagi T, et al. Successful management of living donor liver transplantation for biliary atresia with single ventricle physiology-from peritransplant through total cavopulmonary connection: a case report. Pediatr Transpl 2018;22(3):e13118.

43. Zhang XL, Duan XM, Wang FY, et al. An infant with abernethy malformation associated with heterotaxy and pulmonary hypertension. Chin Med J (Engl) 2017; 130(18):2257–8.

44. Youn JK, Lee JM, Yi NJ, et al. Pediatric split liver transplantation after Fontan procedure in left isomerism combined with biliary atresia: a case report. Pediatr Transpl 2014;18(8):E274–9.

45. Vallabhajosyula P, Komlo C, Wallen TJ, et al. Combined heart-liver transplant in a situs-ambiguous patient with failed Fontan physiology. J Thorac Cardiovasc Surg 2013;145(4):e39–41.

46. Haida H, Aeba R, Hoshino K, et al. Fontan completion in a patient with previous liver transplantation. Interact Cardiovasc Thorac Surg 2014;19(4):705–7.

47. Panigrahy A, Lee V, Ceschin R, et al. Brain dysplasia associated with ciliary dysfunction in infants with congenital heart disease. J Pediatr 2016;178: 141–8.e1.

48. Kelly CJ, Christiaens D, Batalle D, et al. Abnormal microstructural development of the cerebral cortex in neonates with congenital heart disease is associated with impaired cerebral oxygen delivery. J Am Heart Assoc 2019;8(5): e009893.

49. Claessens NHP, Khalili N, Isgum I, et al. Brain and CSF volumes in fetuses and neonates with antenatal diagnosis of critical congenital heart disease: a longitudinal MRI study. AJNR Am J Neuroradiol 2019;40(5):885–91.

50. Cowan JR, Tariq M, Shaw C, et al. Copy number variation as a genetic basis for heterotaxy and heterotaxy-spectrum congenital heart defects. Philos Trans R Soc Lond B Biol Sci 2016;371(1710) [pii:20150406].

51. Hagen EM, Sicko RJ, Kay DM, et al. Copy-number variant analysis of classic heterotaxy highlights the importance of body patterning pathways. Hum Genet 2016; 135(12):1355–64.
52. Sadler TW. Establishing the embryonic axes: prime time for teratogenic insults. J Cardiovasc Dev Dis 2017;4(3) [pii:E15].
53. Rubbo B, Lucas JS. Clinical care for primary ciliary dyskinesia: current challenges and future directions. Eur Respir Rev 2017;26(145) [pii:170023].
54. Lucas JS, Alanin MC, Collins S, et al. Clinical care of children with primary ciliary dyskinesia. Expert Rev Respir Med 2017;11(10):779–90.
55. Ware SM, Aygun MG, Hildebrandt F. Spectrum of clinical diseases caused by disorders of primary cilia. Proc Am Thorac Soc 2011;8(5):444–50.
56. Bhaskar J, Galati JC, Brooks P, et al. Survival into adulthood of patients with atrial isomerism undergoing cardiac surgery. J Thorac Cardiovasc Surg 2015;149(6): 1509–13.
57. Chen W, Ma L, Cui H, et al. Early- and middle-term surgical outcomes in patients with heterotaxy syndrome. Cardiology 2016;133(3):141–6.
58. Eronen MP, Aittomäki KA, Kajantie EO, et al. The outcome of patients with right atrial isomerism is poor. Pediatr Cardiol 2013;34(2):302–7.
59. Anagnostopoulos PV, Pearl JM, Octave C, et al. Improved current era outcomes in patients with heterotaxy syndromes. Eur J Cardiothorac Surg 2009;35(5):871–7 [discussion: 877–8].
60. Williams GD, Feng A. Heterotaxy syndrome: implications for anesthesia management. J Cardiothorac Vasc Anesth 2010;24(5):834–44.
61. Shiima-Kinoshita C, Min KY, Hanafusa T, et al. Beta 2-adrenergic regulation of ciliary beat frequency in rat bronchiolar epithelium: potentiation by isosmotic cell shrinkage. J Physiol 2004;554(Pt 2):403–16.
62. Bennett WD. Effect of beta-adrenergic agonists on mucociliary clearance. J Allergy Clin Immunol 2002;110(6 Suppl):S291–7.
63. Cho MJ, Lim RK, Jung Kwak M, et al. Effects of beta-blockers for congestive heart failure in pediatric and congenital heart disease patients: a meta-analysis of published studies. Minerva Cardioangiol 2015;63(6):495–505.
64. Zaragoza-Macias E, Zaidi AN, Dendukuri N, et al. Medical therapy for systemic right ventricles: a systematic review (Part 1) for the 2018 AHA/ACC guideline for the management of adults with congenital heart disease: a report of the American College of Cardiology/American Heart Association Task Force on Clinical Practice Guidelines. Circulation 2019;139(14):e801–13.
65. Rock N, McLin V. Liver involvement in children with ciliopathies. Clin Res Hepatol Gastroenterol 2014;38(4):407–14.
66. Bradley E, Hendrickson B, Daniels C. Fontan liver disease: review of an emerging epidemic and management options. Curr Treat Options Cardiovasc Med 2015; 17(11):51.
67. Hilscher MB, Kamath PS. The liver in circulatory disturbances. Clin Liver Dis 2019;23(2):209–20.
68. Gordon-Walker TT, Bove K, Veldtman G. Fontan-associated liver disease: a review. J Cardiol 2019;74(3):223–32.
69. Angelico R, Stonelake S, Perera DS, et al. Adult liver transplantation in the congenital absence of inferior vena cava. Int J Surg 2015;22:32–7.
70. Geddes GC, Stamm K, Mitchell M, et al. Ciliopathy variant burden and developmental delay in children with hypoplastic left heart syndrome. Genet Med 2016; 19(6):711–4.

71. Shapiro AJ, Leigh MW. Value of transmission electron microscopy for primary ciliary dyskinesia diagnosis in the era of molecular medicine: genetic defects with normal and non-diagnostic ciliary ultrastructure. Ultrastruct Pathol 2017; 41(6):373–85.
72. Burkhalter MD, Sridhar A, Sampaio P, et al. Imbalanced mitochondrial function provokes heterotaxy via aberrant ciliogenesis. J Clin Invest 2019;130: 2841–55.
73. Saotome M, Ikoma T, Hasan P, et al. Cardiac insulin resistance in heart failure: the role of mitochondrial dynamics. Int J Mol Sci 2019;20(14) [pii:E3552].

Neonatal and Infant Appendicitis

Christina M. Bence, MD*, John C. Densmore, MD

KEYWORDS

- Neonatal • Infant • Appendicitis • Necrotizing enterocolitis • Perforation
- Amyand hernia

KEY POINTS

- Neonatal appendicitis is a rare disease with high morbidity and mortality.
- Diagnosis is nearly always delayed because of the rarity of the disease, nonspecific symptoms that mimic other more common conditions, and unreliable imaging.
- One-third of neonatal appendicitis cases are associated with Amyand hernia, which affords similar rates of appendiceal perforation but significantly decreased mortality compared with the intra-abdominal presentation.
- Most cases of neonatal appendicitis present after the appendix has already perforated and can result in a severe intra-abdominal septic response; therefore, the mainstay of treatment is timely operative exploration with appendectomy.

INTRODUCTION
Case Presentation

A 12-month-old girl born at 37 weeks gestation presents following a 10-day history of fevers and multiple symptoms including earache, intermittent nausea and vomiting, loose stools, anorexia, and abdominal pain. She has been treated for otitis media, which her twin sister had, and subsequently urinary tract infection. Six days ago, she was started on amoxicillin and subsequently ceftriaxone for 3 days without improvement in symptoms. Rheumatology and infectious disease were consulted for 14 days of fever of unknown origin. A chest radiograph, echocardiogram, bone scan, and abdominal ultrasound (AUS) were obtained and interpreted as normal. Viral titers of enterovirus and rhinovirus were positive. Surgery was consulted on fever day 14 and a computed tomography (CT) scan of the abdomen was obtained, with the following findings: "In the right lower quadrant there are tubular fluid-filled structures with enhancing walls. I'm uncertain if this represents abnormal enhancement and wall thickening of loops of ileum or whether there could be some extraluminal fluid

Division of Pediatric Surgery, Medical College of Wisconsin, Children's Hospital of Wisconsin, 999 North 92nd Street, Suite CCC320, Milwaukee, WI 53226, USA
* Corresponding author.
E-mail address: cbence@mcw.edu

Clin Perinatol 47 (2020) 183–196
https://doi.org/10.1016/j.clp.2019.10.004
0095-5108/20/© 2019 Elsevier Inc. All rights reserved.
perinatology.theclinics.com

collection/abscesses present. The lack of intra-abdominal fat planes, and lack of oral contrast, makes determination exceedingly difficult" (**Fig. 1**). Based on peritoneal findings and the further identification of an appendicolith and abscess cavity on CT scan, the child was brought to operation and a laparoscopic appendectomy performed for perforated appendicitis. Operative findings were remarkable for a free fecalith, disseminated purulence, and early fibrinous adhesions leading to a 120-minute case and 7-day hospital stay.

CONTENT
Epidemiology

Appendicitis is the most common surgical diagnosis requiring admission for pediatric patients, yet it is exceedingly rare in neonatal and infant age groups.[1,2] The peak incidence is during the second decade with the lifetime risk of developing appendicitis falling around 8.6% for males and 6.7% for females.[2] In infants less than 1 year old the incidence is 0.38%, and in neonates less than 30 days it is even lower (around 0.04%–0.2%).[2–4] Older studies have found that infants younger than 2 years of age represent only 2% of all appendicitis cases.[5] The true incidence of appendicitis in neonates and infants is difficult to ascertain because it often mimics other more common abdominal pathologies for this age group, such as necrotizing enterocolitis (NEC), obstruction, and gastroenteritis.

Although appendicitis is generally considered an abdominal disease process, up to one-third of reported neonatal appendicitis (NA) cases present with an inflamed appendix incarcerated within an inguinal hernia, known as an Amyand hernia (AH).[6] Given the 5:1 incidence of inguinal hernias in boys versus girls, the overall 3:1 preponderance of NA in males is a product of this association with AH. Furthermore, prematurity is associated with nearly half of all appendicitis cases in neonates.[7]

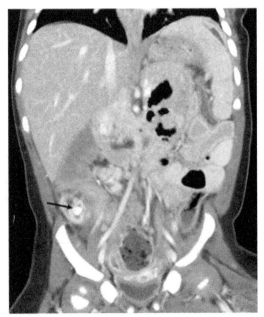

Fig. 1. CT scan demonstrating a large fecalith (*arrow*) within an abscess cavity in a 12-month-old infant found to have perforated appendicitis at operative exploration.

The perforation rate associated with neonatal and infant appendicitis is high, 70% to 85%, compared with 7% in children 5 to 12 year old.[7,8] The average time from presentation to diagnosis is greater in neonates and infants, although this does not entirely account for the high perforation rate.[7]

Clinical Presentation

One of the most challenging aspects of appendicitis in infants and neonates is the difficulty in making the correct clinical diagnosis. Most NA cases are missed until an obvious perforation requires emergent operative intervention and a perforated appendix is identified intraoperatively. The reasons for this frequent delay in diagnosis are three-fold: (1) presenting symptoms are often different from those commonly seen in older children; (2) other etiologies of abdominal pathology are more common in this age group and can present similarly; and (3) a high index of suspicion is required to perform an appropriate work-up in these small, nonverbal patients. Few case reports describe the preoperative diagnosis of NA, and the most recent literature review denotes only a 17% success rate via diagnostic imaging within the last 30 years.[7]

Appendicitis in infants and neonates can present with a variety of symptoms that should alert the provider to an abdominal source; however most are nonspecific. Abdominal distention and bilious emesis have been found over time to be the most reliable symptoms, presenting in 64% to 89% and 47% to 54% of patients diagnosed with NA, respectively (**Fig. 2**).[4,7] As the child transitions into the infant period and beyond the finding of abdominal pain is more easily recognized, documented in 35% to 81% of patients less than 3 years old.[2] Diarrhea is also found in 30% to 40% of infants with appendicitis, making gastroenteritis the most common misdiagnosis in this age group.[8]

Other nonspecific symptoms that are frequently associated with NA include refusal of feeds, fever, and general irritability. In the infant age group concurrent upper respiratory symptoms are common and often confuse the presentation.[8] There are a few clinical signs associated with neonatal and infant appendicitis that are reliable if present, but require more suspicion to identify at such a young age. These include focal right lower quadrant or iliac fossa tenderness, induration or ecchymosis over the right side, a palpable mass in the right abdomen, or an erythematous and firm right hemiscrotum.

Up to one-third of NA cases are associated with AH.[6] In these patients the presentation generally alerts more to inguinoscrotal pathology concerning for an incarcerated or strangulated inguinal hernia including a tender, nonreducible protrusion in the inguinal region with or without erythema. Because of the typical location of the

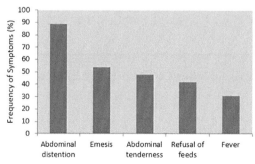

Fig. 2. Frequency of presenting symptoms in neonatal appendicitis. (*Data from* Raveenthiran V. Neonatal appendicitis (Part 1): a review of 52 cases with abdominal manifestation. J Neonatal Surg. 2015;4(1):4.)

appendix within the right lower quadrant most AH are located on the right side, although there are reports of left-sided AH associated with situs inversus, intestinal malrotation, and mobile cecum.[9] In contrast to other types of incarcerated hernia, AH does not typically present with symptoms of bowel obstruction because the true intestinal lumen is not occluded. There are reports, however, of the inflamed appendix within an inguinal hernia sac fistulizing to the scrotum and presenting as a draining inguinoscrotal wound.[10]

Imaging

Abdominal radiography is generally the first imaging study obtained in a neonate with symptoms indicative of abdominal pathology. This study is often nondiagnostic, although may demonstrate findings consistent with other intra-abdominal pathologies (eg, pneumatosis intestinalis indicative of NEC), or complications, such as obstruction or free air. In the latter scenario, no further diagnostic work-up is necessary because concern for intestinal perforation warrants emergent surgical exploration.

If an abdominal radiograph is not diagnostic, AUS should be considered as the next step in the work-up of a concerning neonatal abdomen. AUS has become the preferred initial imaging study for evaluation of appendicitis in the pediatric population because of its high specificity (>90%) and positive predictive value (98%), and its lack of exposure to ionizing radiation.[11] However, the highly variable sensitivity of AUS (40%–90%) is a result of operator-dependent abilities to visualize inflamed and normal appendices.[11,12] Ultrasound (US) of the appendix in neonates and infants is further complicated by several factors that make visualizing the appendix more difficult, and potentially limit diagnostic accuracy even when the appendix is identified (**Box 1**).

The first factor is that the shape of the appendix is different in the neonate than the older child, starting as a short, conical structure and slowly growing into a longer, narrower appendage.[13] Similarly, the outer diameter of the normal appendix increases by 0.4 mm each year up to approximately 6 to 7 years of age. Thus, the accepted cutoff of 6 mm for upper limit of normal diameter in school-aged children does not apply in infants.[13] Another factor complicating US examination of the neonatal appendix is that its intra-abdominal location is often significantly higher on the right side, sometimes even hidden underneath the liver, and is much more mobile.[14] Finally, the most common scenario of imaging postperforation with neighboring bowel edema and fluid poses a greater challenge localizing the appendix on US. In this situation it is often necessary to assess for secondary signs of appendicitis including inflammatory changes near the cecum or free fluid. For example, in one small series of laparotomy-confirmed NA, four of four preoperative US identified right-sided abdominal inflammatory masses concerning for phlegmon or abscess. These findings, in addition to stiff, fixed loops of adjacent bowel and the inability to identify an appendix,

---

Box 1
Anatomic and physiologic reasons why sonographic diagnosis of appendicitis in neonates and infants is difficult

Reason

1. Increase in normal appendiceal wall diameter until 6 to 7 years old

2. Short, conical appendiceal shape

3. Right upper quadrant/subhepatic location of appendix

4. Early perforation with free fluid or phlegmon

were reported as concerning for appendicitis and this diagnosis was later confirmed on final pathologic examination in all four cases.[14] Another NA case report describes the sonographic findings of a subhepatic, tubular structure (7 mm diameter, 25 mm length) containing heterogeneous sludge with surrounding inflammation, which was identified to be an inflamed appendix on subsequent operative exploration.[15] These radiographic findings highlight the importance of having a high index of suspicion for NA when evaluating a neonate with abdominal sepsis of unclear cause.

When findings on AUS are inconclusive in a neonate or infant with abdominal sepsis, the appropriate next step in the diagnostic work-up is difficult to determine. In older children, the combination of US followed by CT has been found to be the most effective strategy for diagnosing appendicitis, yet it is unclear how well this is extrapolated to infants.[16] Schwartz and colleagues[17] have developed a diagnostic algorithm for the work-up of NA, which involves step-wise abdominal imaging starting with abdominal radiographs, then moving onto AUS, and ultimately progressing to CT scan if a diagnosis is unclear (**Fig. 3**). The goal is to distinguish NA or another surgical emergency from NEC, the most common cause of an acute abdomen in this age group. If CT is not diagnostic for appendicitis but also does not identify signs of NEC, then the patient is taken emergently to the operating room (OR) for exploratory laparoscopy or laparotomy. Schwartz and colleagues[17] reported only one neonate that underwent a CT scan preoperatively, which was reported as normal without evidence of NEC. The patient was taken to the OR and perforated appendicitis was identified.

The feasibility and efficacy of CT for diagnosing NA is difficult to ascertain because CT imaging is rarely used in this age group and requires the patient to travel to the scanner. Transport of this type may not be feasible or safe for an acutely ill infant. Furthermore, concerns arise regarding the associated radiation exposure with CT, which may increase a patient's lifetime cancer risk.[18] In large pediatric centers, however, the addition of ALARA ("as low as reasonably achievable") principles has resulted in significantly reduced radiation doses for CT scanning that often rival abdominal radiography.[19] Yet because of the possible drawbacks to CT in the neonatal population, novel imaging strategies should also be considered. One example is the use of contrast-enhanced high-resolution US that has been introduced as a novel method of evaluating for NEC in the neonatal intensive care unit.[20] The benefits of contrast-enhanced US are that it can be performed at bedside, is noninvasive, radiation-free, and nephrotoxin-free. Furthermore, contrast-enhanced US allows for improved detection of bowel ischemia in patients being evaluated for NEC, and theoretically would be able to more easily identify the appendix and assess its viability.

Pathophysiology and Differential Diagnoses

The underlying cause of appendicitis in children and adults is generally accepted to be appendiceal luminal obstruction by stool or lymphoid tissue leading to inflammation of the appendix. Yet there are several anatomic and physiologic considerations that make this mechanism less likely in neonates and infants, which are described in **Table 1**. As the appendix elongates and narrows to its mature shape the amount of lymphoid tissue present within the submucosa increases in size and number, reaching its peak in the teenage years.[2] With the transition from neonate to infant, this relative increase in lymphoid tissue and exposure to infectious organisms manifests as a greater association with other infectious processes including gastroenteritis, upper respiratory tract infection, otitis media, pneumonia, sepsis, and urinary tract infection.[8]

In the neonatal population, the recognition of typical appendicitis is so rare that other etiologies of appendiceal inflammation and/or perforation have been theorized including ischemic, obstructive, and immunologic causes.[21] Furthermore, there is

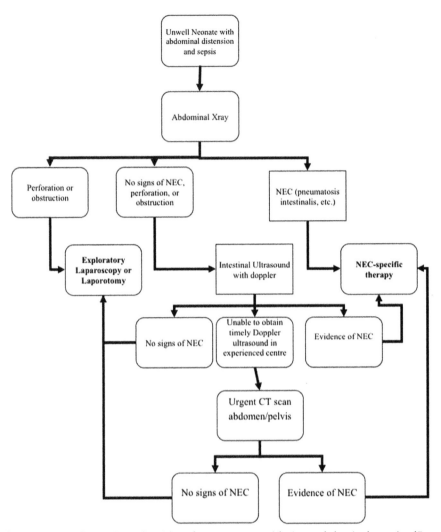

Fig. 3. Proposed imaging algorithm for neonates with intra-abdominal sepsis. (*From* Schwartz KL, Gilad E, Sigalet D, et al. Neonatal acute appendicitis: a proposed algorithm for timely diagnosis. J Pediatr Surg. 2011;46(11):2060-2064; with permission.)

Table 1	
Anatomic and physiologic reasons for the decreased incidence of appendicitis in children younger than 2 years of age	
Reason	**Explanation**
1. Broad-based (funnel-shaped) appendiceal orifice	Low risk of luminal obstruction
2. Diet of milk and soft foods	Liquid stool results in lack of fecaliths
3. Recumbent posture	Low risk of luminal obstruction
4. Infrequency of lymphatic hyperplasia	Overall lack of infectious stimuli

controversy over whether NA reflects a distinct pathologic entity or is instead a collection of secondary "appendicopathies" related to other disease states.[22] Pathologic findings of an inflamed or perforated appendix range from transmural to full-thickness appendiceal involvement, and varying degrees of necrosis and/or inflammation. Often it is impossible to distinguish primary appendicitis from secondary appendicopathies based on pathologic examination alone.[22] There are several neonatal conditions that have been associated with NA in case reports including NEC, Hirschsprung disease (HD), cystic fibrosis, meconium plug, tracheoesophageal fistula, AH, and vascular insufficiency because of perinatal asphyxia or cardiac defects.[10,23–28] Next is a discussion of the three conditions most commonly described: NEC, HD, and AH.

Necrotizing enterocolitis
There is a growing body of literature recognizing a distinct class of neonatal perforated appendicitis as a localized form of NEC.[29] The association between prematurity and NA argues that at least in a subset of cases the development of appendiceal inflammation is a result of impaired immunity, lending weight to the theory that NA is a localized NEC variant.[29] A recent review found that 44% of neonates diagnosed with appendicitis had at least one known risk factor for NEC.[7] The clinical presentation of NA is similar to that of infants with NEC, and because of the higher incidence of NEC in the neonatal population (1%–7.7% of all neonatal intensive care unit admissions) it is often the presumed diagnosis.[30] Furthermore, AUS is generally not standard in the diagnostic work-up for NEC and so the incidence of sonographic findings of appendicitis in these patients is unknown.

Based on the management algorithm for Bell stage I-IIa NEC, which involves an initial trial of expectant management with intravenous antibiotics and bowel rest, most of these patients are not brought to the OR until there is concern for perforation (eg, free air on plain radiograph or peritoneal signs on abdominal examination). Furthermore, in a subset of extremely low-birth-weight infants even perforated NEC is initially managed with intravenous antibiotics and percutaneous peritoneal drainage, further postponing laparotomy. For these reasons, the diagnosis of NA as characterized by focal appendiceal inflammation with perforation is overwhelming made intraoperatively following a delay in operative exploration.[29,31–33] In fact, a recent review found that in 44 of 52 cases of intra-abdominal NA the diagnosis was not made until laparotomy identified a perforated appendix.[7] Furthermore, pathologic examination of the surgical specimen cannot distinguish between NEC and primary NA making it difficult to distinguish between the two conditions even postoperatively.[33]

Hirschsprung disease
The association between neonatal appendiceal perforation and HD has been mentioned in the literature multiple times over the years; however, the actual number of documented cases is low. The recent review by Raveenthiran[7] reported four cases of HD coexisting with a perforated appendix out of 52 reports of NA between 1990 and 2014. Before that, Jancelewicz and colleagues[21] identified six cases of reported neonatal appendicitis in patients with a coexisting diagnosis of HD from 1967 to 1998. The proposed theory behind this association is that distal colonic obstruction results in cecal perforation, often at the appendiceal base, which represents the point of maximum tension.[23,34,35] This theory of an obstructive or mechanical cause of appendiceal perforation is further supported by the findings of periappendicitis without transmural inflammation in several of these specimens.[34,35] Although clinical correlation is necessary in determining the need for further work-up following a

diagnosis of NA, keeping HD on the differential and evaluating for colonic aganglionosis when clinically suspected is prudent. It should be noted, however, that the appendix is naturally aganglionic and so the diagnosis of HD cannot be made based on pathologic examination of the appendiceal specimen itself; rather, true colonic or rectal biopsies must be obtained.

Amyand hernia

AH is defined as an inguinal hernia containing the vermiform appendix. Although it accounts for 1% of all inguinal hernias, the likelihood of an AH presenting with acute inflammation of the incarcerated appendix is much rarer (0.1% of cases).[36] The association between AH and NA has been reported often in the literature, and is estimated to account for one-third of NA cases described.[6] AH is more common in infants than adults likely because of the higher incidence of persistent patency of the processus vaginalis and shorter, conical shape of the appendix.[37] There is still discrepancy as to whether appendicitis associated with AH is related to luminal obstruction causing inflammation and ultimately perforation, or to ischemia in the setting of a strangulated appendix.[36] The presentation of AH typically involves a tender, erythematous groin bulge on the right side with varying degrees of sepsis. The differential diagnosis includes incarcerated or strangulated inguinal hernia, hydrocele, testicular torsion, torsed appendix testis/epididymis, and epididymo-orchitis.[36–38] Because of the rarity of appendicitis associated with AH and its similarities in presentation to other common inguinoscrotal pathologies the correct preoperative diagnosis is virtually never made.[36] Furthermore, imaging, such as scrotal US to rule out testicular torsion, typically displays bowel loops within the hernia sac but often cannot distinguish the appendix from other types of intestine.[38] Regardless of an inaccurate initial diagnosis, most of the previously mentioned differential diagnoses indicate urgent surgical intervention and so a delay in appropriate management is uncommon. For the surgeon, preparation for abdominal exploration should be entertained when surgically exploring an inflamed hemiscrotum via inguinal or scrotal approach.

Operative Considerations

Abdominal appendicitis

Management of appendicitis in the neonate or infant is complex because it is often misdiagnosed initially and frequently presents with perforation. For these reasons, most reported cases of NA have been managed with open appendectomy following emergent exploratory laparotomy in the setting of obvious bowel perforation. However, it is unclear whether this strategy is appropriate in all cases, especially if the diagnosis of appendicitis is considered preoperatively. A recent meta-analysis by Fugazzola and colleagues[39] found that children with appendicitis who presented with localized appendicular abscess or phlegmon had lower rates of complications and readmission when treated initially with nonoperative management (with or without percutaneous drainage and/or delayed appendectomy) compared with initial operative management. In contrast, the patients who presented with freely perforated appendicitis had higher complication and readmission rates associated with initial nonoperative management. Neonatal and infant appendicitis presents much more commonly as free perforation with minimal walling off of a discrete abscess, which is in stark contrast to the findings in school-aged children who have a more robust omental response.[2] This frequency of free perforation, combined with the fact that NA is almost never diagnosed preoperatively in this age group, has led many surgeons to recommend prompt surgical intervention in the setting of acute abdomen when appendicitis cannot be definitively ruled out.[17,29,32]

Despite these recommendations, frequent delays in the diagnosis of NA often result in emergent exploratory laparotomy in critically ill neonates following a prolonged trial of nonoperative management. The presentation of NA often mimics that of NEC, which is generally managed nonoperatively unless there are obvious signs of bowel perforation prompting emergent operative intervention. Therefore, a high index of suspicion for NA should be kept when evaluating an infant with presumed NEC. A thorough abdominal examination looking for right-sided tenderness, erythema, or mass, and consideration of AUS or CT to evaluate the appendix, should be undertaken in neonates presenting with evidence of intra-abdominal pathology.[32] Furthermore, implementing a diagnostic algorithm to methodically differentiate between NA and NEC may aid in more timely diagnosis and surgical management.[17] Early operative intervention in patients with focal appendiceal involvement could prevent perforation and ultimately result in decreased morbidity and mortality in this patient population.[29]

Another broad consideration in the surgical management of neonatal and infant appendicitis is the role of laparoscopy. Several large pediatric studies have highlighted the benefits of laparoscopy over open appendectomy in pediatric patients including shorter length of stay, lower rates of postoperative complications including surgical site infection and ileus, and fewer readmissions. Furthermore, these benefits are maintained even for complicated appendicitis.[40] With the introduction of smaller instruments (2–3 mm), laparoscopy has been incorporated into the standard management of many neonatal conditions including pyloric stenosis, gastroesophageal reflux disease, and esophageal atresia.[41] Diagnostic laparoscopy has been used in only a handful of NA cases, but in each of these appendectomy was able to be successfully performed laparoscopically.[42–44] The limitations to laparoscopy in neonates with abdominal sepsis are that an accurate preoperative diagnosis is uncommon, and that abdominal insufflation is considered to be contraindicated in critically ill, growth-restricted neonates. However, in recent literature there have been small series that discuss the benefits of incorporating diagnostic laparoscopy into the management of the neonatal acute abdomen.[17,42,43,45] Burgmeier and Schier[43] found that of 17 neonates who underwent diagnostic laparoscopy for acute abdomen, 53% avoided an open operation either because of the definitive intervention being successfully completed laparoscopically or no further surgical intervention being required. One of these patients was found to have acute appendicitis and a laparoscopic appendectomy was performed. Success with a laparoscopic approach requires high-fidelity communication with the anesthesiologist, tolerance of lower insufflation pressures (4–6 mm Hg), and lack of resistance to conversion if the first two conditions do not provide adequate visualization.

Inguinoscrotal appendicitis

Most appendicitis cases that present as AH are managed with prompt operative intervention regardless of accurate preoperative diagnosis. Current controversy exists over the appropriate surgical management of a nonperforated, noninflamed appendix found incidentally within an inguinal hernia sac because it is unclear whether an appendectomy should be performed in all of these cases.[46] However, in the setting of obvious appendiceal inflammation or perforation, inguinal hernia repair with concurrent appendectomy is commonly described.[6,46] The question then emerges: what is the best operative approach to this condition? In general it follows the same principles as any other incarcerated inguinal hernia repair. If the diagnosis of incarcerated or strangulated hernia is made preoperatively and it is unable to be reduced, then an open inguinal approach with appendectomy through the groin and primary tissue repair of the inguinal hernia is described.[37] This approach also allows for assessment of the ipsilateral testis for viability and offers the ability to perform a concurrent orchid-opexy if an undescended testis is identified.[47,48]

If the hernia is successfully reduced preoperatively but there is concern about the viability of the bowel/appendix, then a combination of inguinal and abdominal approaches are typically used to assess the intra-abdominal contents.[6,38] Finally, laparoscopy is becoming a common approach to this condition because it allows for good visualization and assessment of the bowel and appendix while also providing the option of concurrent transabdominal laparoscopic inguinal hernia repair.

Outcomes

Although NA has been a known entity for many years, it continues to be associated with high morbidity and mortality. The driving factor behind these poor outcomes is the extremely high appendicular perforation rate in this population. The most recent literature review found a perforation rate of nearly 85% in patients diagnosed with NA at laparotomy.[7] Several reasons have been posited for this perforation risk, one of which being that appendicitis is such a difficult diagnosis to make in the neonate and often results in delayed surgical intervention. However, the data contradict this assumption because there has actually been shown to be a shorter mean delay between onset of symptoms and definitive therapy in perforated NA (3.3 days) versus uncomplicated NA (8 days).[7] This discrepancy is explained by the fact that clinical findings of perforation (eg, pneumoperitoneum) prompt earlier surgical intervention. Other reasons for the high risk of perforation in NA include a thin neonatal appendiceal wall, indistensible cecum, and long mesentery making the appendix more susceptible to ischemia.[49] Further, perforation within the neonatal abdomen often results in a more severe systemic inflammatory response because of the inadequate "walling off" of infection in the setting of minimal omentum and immature immunologic responses limiting abscess formation.[2,7]

Neonatal appendicitis is also associated with a much higher mortality rate than in the broader pediatric population. Overall the mortality rate of NA has progressively declined over the last century with a high of 78% from 1901 to 1975, 33% from 1976 to 1984, 28% from 1985 to 2000, and finally 23% from 1990 to 2014.[4,7] The major decline in mortality during the latter half of the twentieth century was likely caused by advances in antibiotic therapies and significant progress in the fields of diagnostic radiology, critical care medicine, and surgery.[7] However, the current mortality rate of 23% is much higher than that in the broader pediatric population, which cites 0.04% overall mortality for complicated appendicitis in the United States.[50]

Here again appendicitis associated with AH is distinct from that of its abdominal counterpart. Although the perforation rate of inguinoscrotal NA is still high at 50%, the mortality rate at least over the last 30 years is 0%.[38] This discrepancy in outcomes based on appendiceal location is likely caused by the fact that diagnosis of a surgical emergency is more quickly made in the setting of inguinoscrotal appendicitis, whereas acute abdominal NA is often obscured and nonoperatively managed based on a presumptive diagnosis.

SUMMARY

Neonatal appendicitis is a rare condition with a high mortality rate. Most of the time the diagnosis of NA is missed preoperatively and it is only after an exploratory operation that appendiceal involvement is identified. This is true regardless of whether the inflamed appendix is located intra-abdominally or associated with an AH. The delay in diagnosis is caused by a combination of factors including rarity of the disease; similarity in presentation to other more common neonatal conditions, such as NEC or gastroenteritis; and inadequate imaging guidelines for this age group. Because of these factors, we recommend maintaining a high index of suspicion for appendicitis in neonates and infants presenting with intra-abdominal sepsis of unclear cause. We also recommend defining an abdominal imaging algorithm similar to that published by Schwartz and colleagues[17] so that if another cause of nonoperative abdominal pathology (eg, early NEC) is not definitively identified then expedited operative exploration can be undertaken. With inclusion of the disease process in the differential diagnosis, innovation in high-resolution US and CT techniques, and improved minimally invasive approaches, the mortality rate for neonates and infants with appendicitis will further decline.

DISCLOSURE

The authors have nothing to disclose.

Best Practices

What is the current practice for neonatal and infant appendicitis?

Best practice/guideline/care path objectives
- Consider appendicitis in the differential of unexplained sepsis in neonates and infants
- Sonographic diagnosis in this population is difficult
- Appendicitis in this population is perforated at diagnosis
- One-third of neonatal cases are inguinoscrotal (Amyand hernia)
- Prompt surgical consultation and intervention may decrease the associated high morbidity and mortality

What changes in current practice are likely to improve outcomes?

- Have a low threshold to proceed to high-resolution US or CT, when feasible, and surgical consultation in unexplained neonatal and infant sepsis

- Surgeons explore neonates and infants with worsening clinical course even in setting of normal imaging

- If the diagnosis can be definitively made, nonoperative maneuvers, such as drainage and antibiotics, may be successfully used but require close clinical observation

- Inguinoscrotal appendicitis is more amenable to antibiotics and interval appendectomy

- Evaluate for Hirschsprung disease after recovery

- Recognize that many cases of neonatal appendicitis are treated as necrotizing enterocolitis

Is there a clinical algorithm? If so, please include

See **Fig. 3**

Major recommendations

- Imaging may be misleading to surgical intervention for unimproved clinical course to decrease morbidity and mortality

- Diagnostic laparoscopy may have a role in select neonates and infants

- Nonoperative approaches are more successful in contained (inguinoscrotal) appendicitis than abdominal appendicitis

- Evaluate this population for the underlying diagnosis of Hirschsprung disease via rectal biopsy

Rating for the strength of the evidence

Levels III-V

Bibliographic Sources: Refs.[7,17,35,36,42]

REFERENCES

1. HCUP National Inpatient Sample (NIS). Healthcare cost and utilization project (HCUP). Rockville (MD): Agency for Healthcare Research and Quality; 2015. Available at: www.hcup-us.ahrq.gov/faststats/landing.jsp.
2. Almaramhy HH. Acute appendicitis in young children less than 5 years: review article. Ital J Pediatr 2017;43(1):15.
3. Alwan R, Drake M, Gurria Juarez J, et al. A newborn with abdominal pain. Pediatrics 2017;140(5) [pii:e20164267].
4. Karaman A, Cavusoglu YH, Karaman I, et al. Seven cases of neonatal appendicitis with a review of the English language literature of the last century. Pediatr Surg Int 2003;19(11):707–9.
5. Cherian MP, Al Egaily KA, Joseph TP. Acute appendicitis in infants: still a diagnostic dilemma. Ann Saudi Med 2003;23(3–4):187–90.
6. Fascetti-Leon F, Sherwood W. Neonatal appendicitis and incarcerated inguinal hernia: case report and review of the literature. J Indian Assoc Pediatr Surg 2017;22(4):248–50.
7. Raveenthiran V. Neonatal appendicitis (Part 1): a review of 52 cases with abdominal manifestation. J Neonatal Surg 2015;4(1):4.
8. Marzuillo P, Germani C, Krauss BS, et al. Appendicitis in children less than five years old: a challenge for the general practitioner. World J Clin Pediatr 2015; 4(2):19–24.
9. Kaymakci A, Akillioglu I, Akkoyun I, et al. Amyand's hernia: a series of 30 cases in children. Hernia 2009;13(6):609–12.
10. Panagidis A, Sinopidis X, Zachos K, et al. Neonatal perforated Amyand's hernia presenting as an enterocutaneous scrotal fistula. Asian J Surg 2015;38(3):177–9.
11. Gongidi P, Bellah RD. Ultrasound of the pediatric appendix. Pediatr Radiol 2017; 47(9):1091–100.
12. Janitz E, Naffaa L, Rubin M, et al. Ultrasound evaluation for appendicitis focus on the pediatric population: a review of the literature. J Am Osteopath Coll Radiol 2016;5(1):5–14.
13. Trout AT, Towbin AJ, Zhang B. Journal club: the pediatric appendix: defining normal. AJR Am J Roentgenol 2014;202(5):936–45.
14. Si SY, Guo YY, Mu JF, et al. The sonographic features of neonatal appendicitis: a case report. Medicine (Baltimore) 2017;96(45):e8170.
15. Huet F, Di Maio M, Macri F, et al. Subhepatic neonatal appendicitis in premature babies: first case detected by ultrasound. Diagn Interv Imaging 2015;96(9): 969–71.
16. Wan MJ, Krahn M, Ungar WJ, et al. Acute appendicitis in young children: cost-effectiveness of US versus CT in diagnosis – a Markov decision analytic model. Radiology 2009;250(2):378–86.
17. Schwartz KL, Gilad E, Sigalet D, et al. Neonatal acute appendicitis: a proposed algorithm for timely diagnosis. J Pediatr Surg 2011;46(11):2060–4.
18. Brenner DJ, Hall EJ. Computed tomography: an increasing source of radiation exposure. N Engl J Med 2007;357(22):2277–84.
19. Shah NB, Platt SL. ALARA: is there a cause for alarm? Reducing radiation risks from computed tomography scanning in children. Curr Opin Pediatr 2008; 20(3):243–7.
20. Al-Hamad S, Hackam DJ, Goldstein SD, et al. Contrast-enhanced ultrasound and near-infrared spectroscopy of the neonatal bowel: novel, bedside, noninvasive,

and radiation-free imaging for early detection of necrotizing enterocolitis. Am J Perinatol 2018;35(14):1358–65.

21. Jancelewicz T, Kim G, Miniati D. Neonatal appendicitis: a new look at an old zebra. J Pediatr Surg 2008;43(10):e1–5.

22. Bengtsson BO, van Houten JP. Neonatal vermiform appendicopathy. Am J Perinatol 2015;32(7):683–8.

23. Stiefel D, Stallmach T, Sacher P. Acute appendicitis in neonates: complication or morbus sui generis? Pediatr Surg Int 1998;14(1–2):122–3.

24. Sahnoun L, Kitar M, Maazoun K, et al. Hirschsprung's disease presenting as neonatal appendicitis. J Neonatal Surg 2013;2(2):25.

25. Shen Z, Zheng S. Timely recognition of Amyand's hernia with appendicitis in infants. World J Pediatr 2015;11(4):392–4.

26. Ayoub BH, Al Omran Y, Hassan A, et al. The importance of timely detection and management in neonatal appendicitis. BMJ Case Rep 2014;2014 [pii: bcr2014203663].

27. Dunne B, Brown KG, Sholler G, et al. Fatal acute appendicitis in a neonate with congenital heart disease. World J Pediatr Congenit Heart Surg 2017;8(3): 411–3.

28. Pastore V, Bartoli F. A rare case of neonatal complicated appendicitis in a child with Patau's syndrome. Case Rep Pediatr 2014;2014:671706.

29. Tumen A, Chotai PN, Williams JM, et al. Neonatal perforated appendicitis attributed to localized necrotizing enterocolitis of the appendix: a review. J Neonatal Surg 2017;6(3):60.

30. Kosloske AM. Epidemiology of necrotizing enterocolitis. Acta Paediatr Suppl 1994;396:2–7.

31. Kalra VK, Natarajan G, Poulik J, et al. Isolated ruptured appendicitis presenting as pneumatosis intestinalis in a premature neonate. Pediatr Surg Int 2012; 28(4):439–41.

32. Khan RA, Menon P, Rao KLN. Beware of neonatal appendicitis. J Indian Assoc Pediatr Surg 2010;15(2):67–9.

33. Tumen A, Chotai PN, Williams JM, et al. Neonatal perforated appendicitis masquerading as necrotizing enterocolitis. J Neonatal Surg 2017;6(2):39.

34. Arliss J, Holgersen LO. Neonatal appendiceal perforation and Hirschsprung's disease. J Pediatr Surg 1990;25(6):694–5.

35. Sarioglu A, Tanyel FC, Buyukpamukcu N, et al. Appendiceal perforation: a potentially lethal initial mode of presentation of Hirschsprung's disease. J Pediatr Surg 1997;32(1):123–4.

36. Patoulias D, Kalogirou M, Patoulias I. Amyand's hernia: an up-to-date review of the literature. Acta Medica (Hradec Kralove) 2017;60(3):131–4.

37. Erginel B, Soysal FG, Celik A, et al. Neonatal perforated appendicitis in incarcerated inguinal hernia in the differential diagnosis of testis torsion. Pediatr Int 2017; 59(7):831–2.

38. Raveenthiran V. Neonatal appendicitis (part 2): a review of 24 cases with inguinoscrotal manifestation. J Neonatal Surg 2015;4(2):15.

39. Fugazzola P, Coccolini F, Tomasoni M, et al. Early appendectomy vs. conservative management in complicated acute appendicitis in children: a meta-analysis. J Pediatr Surg 2019 [pii:S0022-3468(19)30125-3].

40. Low ZX, Bonney GK, So JBY, et al. Laparoscopic versus open appendectomy in pediatric patients with complicated appendicitis: a meta-analysis. Surg Endosc 2019. https://doi.org/10.1007/s00464-019-06709-x.

41. Sinha CK, Paramalingam S, Patel S, et al. Feasibility of complex minimally invasive surgery in neonates. Pediatr Surg Int 2009;25(3):217–21.
42. Malakounides G, John M, Rex D, et al. Laparoscopic surgery for acute neonatal appendicitis. Pediatr Surg Int 2011;27(11):1245–8.
43. Burgmeier C, Schier F. The role of laparoscopy in the acute neonatal abdomen. Surg Innov 2016;23(6):635–9.
44. Dias J, Cerqueira A, Pinheiro L, et al. Acute neonatal appendicitis: the potential value of laparoscopy as a diagnostic and therapeutic tool. Case Rep Perinat Med 2013;2(1–2):83–5.
45. Smith J, Thyoka M. What role does laparoscopy play in the diagnosis and immediate treatment of infants with necrotizing enterocolitis? J Laparoendosc Adv Surg Tech A 2013;23(4):397–401.
46. Cigsar EB, Karadag CA, Dokucu AI. Amyand's hernia: 11years of experience. J Pediatr Surg 2016;51(8):1327–9.
47. Milburn JA, Youngson GG. Amyand's hernia presenting as neonatal testicular ischaemia. Pediatr Surg Int 2006;22(4):390–2.
48. Kumar R, Mahajan JK, Rao KL. Perforated appendix in hernial sac mimicking torsion of undescended testis in a neonate. J Pediatr Surg 2008;43(4):e9–10.
49. Secco IL, Costa T, Moraes ELL, et al. Neonatal appendicitis: a survival case study. Rev Bras Enferm 2017;70(6):1296–300.
50. Oyetunji TA, Nwomeh BC, Ong'uti SK, et al. Laparoscopic appendectomy in children with complicated appendicitis: ethnic disparity amid changing trend. J Surg Res 2011;170(1):e99–103.

Differentiating Congenital Myopathy from Congenital Muscular Dystrophy

Matthew Harmelink, MD

KEYWORDS

- Congenital myopathy • Congenital muscular dystrophy • Hypotonia
- Neuromuscular

KEY POINTS

- Differentiation between congenital myopathies and congenital muscular dystrophies is difficult but important to direct conversations with family.
- A structured, evidence-based approach that is timely and cost-effective can provide guidance to the clinician.
- The evaluation of neonates with congenital muscle disease requires a multidisciplinary team skilled in neonatal muscle diseases.
- There is limited class I evidence to support any diagnostic approach but enough to suggest an evaluation process.

INTRODUCTION

Differentiating between congenital myopathies (CM) and congenital muscular dystrophies (CMD) is important not only for academic purposes but also to allow better prognostication as well as evaluation of extramuscular morbidity. Although there are exceptions to this definition, traditionally, myopathies are believed to be secondary to functional defects in the muscle contractile apparatus or other intrasarcoplasmic structures, whereas dystrophies are abnormalities in muscle membrane or associated extracellular apparatus. Historically, initial differentiation was made based on histopathologic features. As the spectrum of diseases becomes both broader and also with more overlapping features, this has evolved into the use of a mixture of genotype, clinical phenotype, and muscle pathology. The clear differentiation between these 2 subsets of muscle disease is becoming blurred in neonates.

Recently, genes previously believed to be unique to each disease have been found to be present in both CM and CMD depending on the specific variant.[1] This makes phenotyping patients as well as understanding their genotype more important. This

Department of Neurology, Medical College of Wisconsin, 9000 West Wisconsin Avenue, CCC Suite 540, Milwaukee, WI 53226, USA
E-mail address: mharmelink@mcw.edu

Clin Perinatol 47 (2020) 197–209
https://doi.org/10.1016/j.clp.2019.10.005   perinatology.theclinics.com
0095-5108/20/© 2019 Elsevier Inc. All rights reserved.

article discusses how to evaluate and differentiate between the congenital muscle diseases. To avoid long lists of disease subtypes and gene lists, a few examples are included. However, this is a very rapidly expanding area and not within the scope of the article to fully discuss.

In infants, the clinical presentation for both diseases is similar. Neonates present with hypotonia and muscle weakness. Often this is associated with respiratory failure and feeding difficulties. However, depending on the disease subtype, a patient's course can vary greatly. Thus, understanding how to differentiate diseases can be useful in counseling and prognostication.

EPIDEMIOLOGY

When reviewing the incidence of pediatric neuromuscular disorders, point prevalence studies demonstrate a range from 0.68 to 2.5 per 100,000.[2–5] However, there are few specific features to be aware of regarding neonatal patients. These studies are inclusive of older onset patients who would continue to be classified as congenital. The studies are also prior to the current state of genetic testing. Because some patients do not present until a later age, this would suggest the encountered incidence is likely somewhat lower for the neonatologist. Also the fact that lowers the rate is that these studies typically included nonmyopathic disease. However, newer diagnostic techniques support a slightly higher rate. Overall, however, these numbers give a relative $\log_{10}$-type idea of incidence rate.

In addition, the population incidence varies depending on ethnic backgrounds. This phenomenon is often caused by a founder mutation. One example is, in Japan, at an incidence of 1.92 to 3.68 in 100,000 live births, Fukuyama CMD is the most common congenital muscular dystrophy; it is rare in other populations.[6] Because of the founder mutation effects, similar effects have been seen by the author in his experience on a more local level as well. As such, the individual population background of the question needs to be reviewed closely.

NOMENCLATURE

The nomenclature of the congenital muscle diseases is confusing given the evolving inclusion of genetics into pathologic diagnoses as well as variable phenotypic to genotypic correlation. Traditionally, the diseases were differentiated based on histopathologic features. However, as more related genes were identified, this differentiation has evolved. Currently, the most-straightforward classification scheme involves identification of the gene affected with the additional "-related dystrophy" or "-related myopathy". In where the form is congenital in onset, such as in this paper, use of "-related congenital muscular dystrophy" or "-related congenital myopathy" can be used.[7] However, there are many classification schemes for these diseases, especially the CMDs and CM, which Falsaperla and colleagues[8] and the author have described, respectively. For greater details, one should refer to the cited articles because it is beyond the scope of this article to discuss the various methods.[9]

For example, in infants with mutations in the RYR1 gene, both dystrophic and myopathic forms have been identified. In these cases, the disease can be labeled as RYR1-related CMD for the former and RYR1-related CM for the later.

IDENTIFYING AN INFANT WITH POSSIBLE MUSCLE DISEASE

Nearly all infants who have congenital muscle disease will be hypotonic at birth. However, the degree of hypotonia as well as the degree of weakness can vary greatly.

Differentiating between central and peripheral disease should always be done before considering a muscle disease. The incidence of infantile hypotonia is varied in the literature. In a study looking at infants older than 35 weeks gestational age but excluding those beyond 28 weeks of life or those with weakness under 2 weeks duration without nonneurologic diagnosis, 4.2% of infants admitted to a neonatal intensive care unit were noted to be hypotonic.[10] In infants who are hypotonic due to neurologic causes, approximately 60% to 80% were from a central cause and 12% to 34% were from a peripheral cause.[10–12] Of these remaining patients, 82% of cases will be related to a muscle disease.[11] There is little in the literature to indicate relative incidences between CM and CMD. Likely this is due to the overlapping features making a clear separation difficult.

Methods of differentiating central and peripheral causes are poor, with data looking at the clinical ability being unreliable. The positive predictive value of the initial physical examination for an infant localized to central hypotonia is approximately 86%. Yet, the positive predictive value in identifying peripheral hypotonia from initial examination was 52%.[10] Likely this is related to the fact that central hypotonia features are identified as "positive" features or findings that are not typically present in healthy individuals. In contrast, most peripheral hypotonia examination features are "negative" or has a lack of features. Identifying an absent feature is more difficult for our cognitive algorithms than identifying a positive feature making the peripheral disorders more difficult to diagnose. As such, suspicion of muscle disease should rely on present features that suggest muscle problems rather than a lack of features to suggest against it. This makes the examination an important resource to exclude CMD and/or CM from the differential diagnosis.

DIAGNOSTIC ALGORITHM

There are no class I evidence-based algorithms for evaluating neonates with possible muscle disease. There are a few currently published algorithms that differ somewhat based on their audience and range of ages they suggest. For the purpose of this article, we have used neonatal specific evidence to create a specific algorithm for neonates. However, be aware that the limited evidence becomes less effective in preterm infants given the paucity.

In an ideal situation, the evaluation of the neonatal muscle disease involves a multidisciplinary approach in which the pediatric neuromuscular physician/electromyographer works closely with the neonatologist, pediatric geneticist, and pathology teams to arrive at a diagnosis. The purpose of the algorithm (**Figs. 1–3**), however, is to use the currently available literature to optimize efficacy, invasiveness, and cost-effectiveness. This will let families and providers make informed decisions about interventions and goals of care. In addition, other neuromuscular causes and nonmuscle mimics can be excluded. Specifically, diseases that have current available treatments, such as spinal muscular atrophy, infantile onset Pompe disease, or myotubular myopathy, should be excluded or included early given interventions are available.

The evaluation of a neonate with suspected muscle disease can be broken down into 3 separate phases: early phase, specialist phase, and late phase. The theory behind this separation is to maximize a timely diagnosis while minimizing cost and invasive procedures. In addition, in cases where the specialist is not available, skipping the specialist step is feasible.

In the early phase of testing, these tests are inexpensive, minimally invasive with rapid turnarounds in hours to days. Specialist evaluation includes nonneonatologist involvement for testing. Late evaluations include testing that may take days to weeks

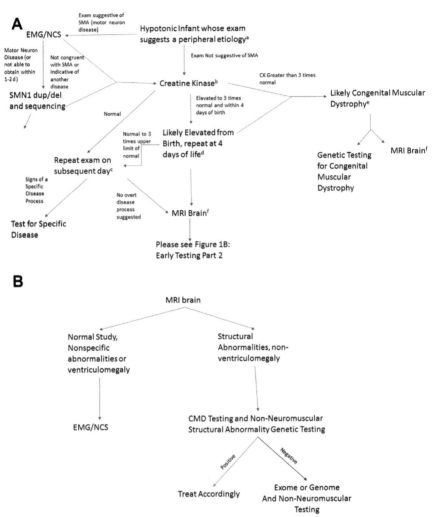

Fig. 1. (*A*) Early testing part 1. Blue lines lead to another diagnostic test, red lines are the result of nondiagnostic terminal testing, and green lines are positive diagnostic testing results. Throughout the algorithm, diagnostics is being considered, not treatment. Thus, for seizures, neurosurgical intervention, respiratory support, or other issues, the care needed to be provided should not be outweighed by diagnostic considerations. Of note, all pathways result in a brain MRI, they are separated to demonstrate the different thought processes. [a] In a hypotonic infant in whom a peripheral cause is expected, early testing should start with a creatine kinase and GAA blood spot if not part of the newborn screening process. Based on the level seen will result in the next steps of diagnosis. [b] Given the neonatal neurologic examination evolves quickly, a repeat examination on the subsequent day can help confirm the concerns before more testing is being considered. [c] The purpose of the repeat CK is to ascertain a level closer to the infants' baseline. Waiting weeks until the true baseline is not feasible, but this does allow the diagnostician to have a level closer to normal without forgoing too much time. [d] Given the low likelihood of another disease with such an elevated CK, directed genetic testing is likely the fastest way to arrive at a diagnosis. However, given the known common structural brain abnormalities, an MRI of the brain can help give more information but can be done concurrently. A normal MRI of the brain would not rule out a CMD. [e] Neuroimaging at this stage helps to differentiate

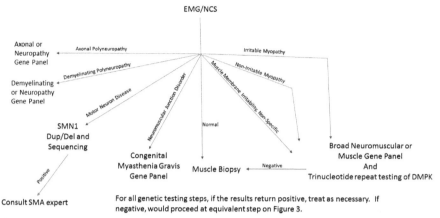

Fig. 2. Specialist and late testing (EMG/NCS available). The diagnostic algorithms at this stage are separated depending on the timely availability of a neonatal skilled electromyographer. In cases where this is available, directed testing can help avoid a muscle biopsy in many cases. Given the overlapping phenotypes and genotypes, differentiation of muscle features into myopathic or dystrophic cannot be made. As such broader panel testing is often recommended. Ideally, if there is the possibility to reflex to exome for negative results, this can help expedite care as well.

for results to return. As such, mimics and other intervenable diseases should be ruled out before awaiting this testing.

EARLY TESTING

Early testing focuses on rapid testing to exclude other causes or direct-focused genetic testing (see **Fig. 1**A, B).

Creatine Kinase

Creatine kinase (CK) is an enzyme found mostly in muscle but also seen in the heart and brain. This has been described initially in the evaluation of cardiac disease but is now also strongly associated with muscle diseases.[13] The enzyme level is not directly tested but a measurement of the by-product of the reaction it catalyzes. As such, the ranges reported do vary slightly by laboratory. In addition, CK peaks about 24 hours after any type of muscle injury and remains elevated for longer periods of time, with a half-life of 24 to 48 hours, making early "baseline" level determination in some circumstances difficult. CK can be elevated in infants after birth with reports

---

further as well as raise the suspicion of another disease in which the infant's examination was misleading to suggest a peripheral cause. [f] The MRI of the brain will help direct further care. In children in whom structural abnormalities are seen, directed nonmuscle testing along with testing for CMD, in the case of normal CK CMD, can be evaluated. For those infants without a clear cause, further studies are needed. As genetic testing is being considered, involvement of a geneticist, neuromuscular physician skilled in genetics, or similar such consultant is likely advisable to be involved to assist with interpretation and genetic counseling. (B) Early testing part 2. Blue lines lead to another diagnostic test, red lines are the result of nondiagnostic terminal testing, and green lines are positive diagnostic testing results. GAA, acid alpha-glucosidase.

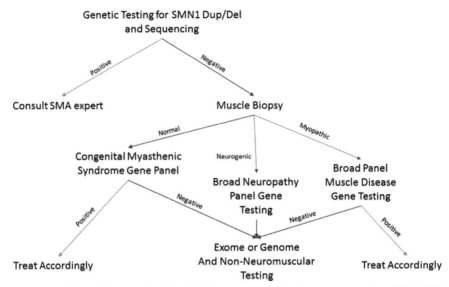

Fig. 3. Specialist and late testing (EMG/NCS not available). In circumstances where EMG/NCS is not available, exclusion of SMA should be undertaken given the currently available treatments. The earlier treatment is thought to provide better outcome. Infantile Pompe disease, which also has a therapy, should have already been excluded by either newborn screening or the GAA noted in the early testing. At this stage, the biopsy will have some proxy for the EMG/NCS in differentiating myopathic from neuropathic diseases while also providing more data about myopathic features. Again, broader panel testing is often warranted to avoid abnormal correlations. If these tests are negative, often nonneuromuscular disease with atypical neuromuscular features and broader exome-wide or genome-wide testing is needed. A specialist trained in genetics is highly recommended to be involved before ordering these tests for interpretation.

of up to 10 times the normal level of CK-MM. The level declined, in healthy neonates, to near normal by about 4 days after birth and normal activity by 6 to 10 weeks after birth.[14] There is evidence to suggest a vaginal delivery has statistically higher levels relative to cesarean sections in infants.[15]

However, persistent elevated CK is not diagnostic of primary muscle disease but rather demonstrates muscle membrane instability. Thus, neurogenic lesions can cause elevations in denervation. For example, elevation of CK in patients with type 1 spinal muscular atrophy (SMA) has been reported with 41% greater than 2 standard deviations above the logarithm used in one study; in this population, 2 patients had CK values between 300 and 1000.[16]

This test does not have a high sensitivity as many of the myopathies, and even some dystrophies may have normal CK values in neonates. Finally, the enzyme is a concentration reflective of that leaked from muscle into the serum. As such, neonates with significantly low muscle bulk can have correspondingly low CKs. Elevated levels of CK (>2–4 times normal) suggest a neuromuscular disease if drawn at an appropriate time. Levels greater than 5 to 10 times the upper limit of normal strongly suggest a CMD in a neonate in most circumstances.

Neurologic Examination

The examination of neonates with congenital muscle disease will often demonstrate noticeable hypotonia. Stretch reflexes can be variable based on the degree of weakness and are typically normal to absent in muscle disease. The exception is overt hyperreflexia, which, in the context of a patient with other signs of a peripheral disease as well, indicates a disease with mixed central and peripheral disease. This is more commonly seen in CMD. However, given the end-organ of the reflex arch is muscle, in severely weak patients, the upper motor neuron dysfunction may not be apparent on an examination. In **Table 1**, a guide to localization based on physical examination findings is shown.

The examination should be used as a localizing and exclusionary feature, as it is not predictive enough to fully exclude other diseases. The best example of this is that in one study of infants with gestational ages 27 to 37 weeks, triceps reflexes were diminished in both healthy and ill infants significantly compared with other reflexes tested.[12] Also to note is that 88% of patients with peripheral hypotonia had decreased or absent reflexes as compared with 36% of the infants with a central cause.[13]

Respiratory Features

Respiratory involvement may separate a CMD from a CM although some subtypes may have a differential in respiratory muscle weakness as compared with axial muscle weakness.

Extra Muscle Features

Extramuscular features indicate a dystrophic process but cannot exclude a myopathic process. However, certain features suggest nonmuscle diseases such as dysmorphic features.

Neuroimaging

Imaging of the muscle has little evidence to support its diagnostic use in neonates. Although there is evidence that suggests patterns of involvement in older children and adults, this has not been validated to differentiate disease in neonates.

Rather, the use of neuroimaging is supported in evaluating for extra muscle involvement. Because of the underlying hypotonia and weakness, neonates with peripheral disease can have higher risk for perinatal injuries. As such, cerebral MRI features suggest a hypoxic-ischemic injury with a sentinel event that indicates an underlying CM or CMD just as this indicates a nonneuromuscular disorder or primary acquired during delivery.[17]

However, CMD has been associated with structural brain abnormalities. Although ventriculomegaly is possible, other suggestive features include cerebellar cysts as well as nodular heterotopia, frontal pachygyria, pontine hypoplasia, microcephaly, Dandy-Walker malformation, and absence of the cerebellar vermis.[18,19] These features are most often seen in the dystroglycanopathies, whereas white matter hyperintensities on T2 MRI sequences are found in LAMA2-related CMD (also known as merosin-related CMD).[20]

That is, not to imply that the congenital myopathies do not have MRI findings but rather, outside of acquired issues such as HIE, these findings are less common. However, features of leukoencephalopathy can be seen in CM although structural abnormalities are less likely present.[21] In rare cases, however, such as reported in ACTA1-related CM, frontal lobe hypoplasia and lateral ventricular dilatation can be seen.[22]

SPECIALIST TESTING

This tier of testing involves specialists skilled at doing or analyzing testing that provides rapid results and is often needed in neonates with suspected muscle disease, often in conjugation with electromyography and nerve conduction studies (see **Fig. 2**).

Table 1
Localization of hypotonia in an infant

Sign Cause	Strength	Tone	Muscle Mass	Deep Tendon Reflexes	Infantile Reflexes	Muscle Fasiculations	Sensation
Central injury	Normal to mild weakness (or focal weakness/paralysis)	Hypotonia—axial > appendicular	Normal (initially) to decreased (develops)	Present to increased (may be hyporeflexic acutely)	Variable	Absent	Variable possible decrease
Central developmental/genetic	Normal to mild weakness	Hypotonia—axial > appendicular	Normal to decreased	Absent to increased	Variable	Absent	Normal
Anterior horn cell	Moderate to severe weakness	Hypotonia—diffuse or appendicular > axial	Normal or atrophic	Decreased to absent	Absent	Present	Normal
Peripheral nerve cell	Moderate to severe weakness	Hypotonia—diffuse or appendicular > axial	Normal or distal predominant atrophy	Decreased to absent	Absent	Absent	Variable possible normal to decrease
Neuromuscular junction	Moderate to severe weakness	Hypotonia—diffuse or appendicular > axial	Normal to decreased	Present to decreased	Absent	Absent	Normal
Muscle	Moderate to severe weakness	Hypotonia—diffuse or appendicular > axial	Normal to decreased	Decreased to absent	Absent[a]	Absent	Normal

[a] In patients with muscle disease the spectrum of reflexes is very broad. Although they may be absent, this is not the same in all cases and is related strongly to the degree of weakness. Thus in an infant who can move their limbs antigravity muscles, the reflexes would be expected to be at least 1 + by standard grading methodology.

Electrodiagnostic Testing

Electrodiagnostic testing typically involves nerve conduction studies and electromyography. In a neonate with presumed muscle disease, these tests should be done simultaneously. The nerve conduction portion allows evaluation and differentiation of motor and sensory demyelinating and axonal neuropathies as well as evaluation of neuromuscular junction defects. In regard to disorders of the neuromuscular junction, due to the immature end plate of the muscle, the sensitivity and specificity have been reported at 84% and 70%, respectively.[23] As such, they are better used to exclude neuromuscular junction disease. In most cases of genetic neuromuscular disease, these studies will be normal, as will be antibody testing, and genetic testing is the first line of testing.

The electromyography involves needle electrode placement into muscles to evaluate the spontaneous activity of muscle fibers as well as the pattern of recruitment, size, and shape of the motor units. These patterns, in combination with the nerve conduction studies, can help localize a peripheral lesion. In children, the yield has been reported to be between 80% and 91% sensitive.[24,25] However, the specificity was 67% in myopathic disorders. The metabolic myopathies were most commonly missed by electromyography (EMG).[25] This yield is not neonate specific, with the closest being a subgroup of children younger than 4 months having an EMG predicting a diagnosis 82% of the time.[26]

Electrodiagnostic testing in a neonate with possible muscle disease serves 2 purposes. First, it is used to exclude neuropathic mimics, which would suggest other disease processes. The sensitivity and specificity of EMG/nerve conduction study for neuropathic disease is high, as 95.5% is correct in diagnosing the disease.[25]

LATE TESTING

After the second line of testing is completed, more directed testing can be considered. When a clinician has reached the third tier of testing, a peripheral disease should be suggested. In addition, neuropathies and neuromuscular junctions have been ruled out, and the CMDs with high CK level have been separated from the less common CMDs with normal to mildly elevated CK as well as the CMs (see **Fig. 3**).

MUSCLE BIOPSY

A muscle biopsy is meant to give histopathologic features. This test is most definitive for distinguishing between a dystrophy and myopathy although it is not always specific enough to suggest a genotype and thus a specific disease. CM will often have intracellular structural differences such as changes in nuclear or mitochondrial structure as well as possibly clear central cores. Other common features of CM on biopsy include small muscle fiber size with possible fiber-size variations. CMD, in converse, may have some of these features but will often show signs of a more degenerative process with features of increased fibrosis.

The yield of muscle biopsy is not 100%, however. Because of the pathologic process that results in histopathologic features accumulating over time, a normal muscle biopsy cannot rule out definitively a muscle disease although other possibilities on the differential diagnosis should be strongly considered. In the cases of a normal biopsy, a repeat biopsy a year later is often warranted if the concern for a muscle disease persists. The yield of muscle biopsy in the literature is around 40%, but these are often retrospective studies that do not delineate how localization was completed. In addition, this was regarding the yield of muscle biopsy in infants, not the yield in infants with a muscle disease.[27]

However, a skilled pediatric myopathologist is needed to interpret the biopsy, as the normal values used in older children and adults may not hold true. In neonates, type 1 fibers are smaller than type 2 fibers, not following the typical pattern of adults, making differentiation of some diseases difficult but also misdiagnosis possible.[28] There are phases of evaluation that can be done from a muscle biopsy—typically, the initial stains showing ultrastructure can be completed in a few days. However, membrane staining and more specialized testing can take further time.

GENETIC TESTING

Currently, the cost and time to results for genetic testing has become much lower in the last few years. As such, genetic testing can be an appropriate testing method. However, the exact variant, unless previously described or, in cases of compound heterozygous, not well described for recessive diseases, does not always provide evidence to predict the phenotype. The classic example of this is the diagnosis of Pompe myopathy, where there is a significant rate of late-onset disease.[29] However, without knowing the predicted phenotype, patients can be inappropriately diagnosed with infantile Pompe disease when in fact they are more likely to have a late-onset disease and another current ongoing process.

TIMING THE TEST

The decision when to include genetic testing into the algorithm is somewhat variable. The time for result reporting of panel testing typically takes days to weeks. However, exomes and genomes often take longer. Yet for some tests, such as SMN1 testing in spinal muscular atrophy, test results can return in under a week.

As such, for patients who are doing well and the genetic diagnosis will not change outcomes (such as differentiating a congenital myopathy, which may improve over time, from a congenital muscular dystrophy, which will not), early testing needs to be weighed against waiting for all testing, especially the muscle biopsy to return. However, incases of infants in which prognostication will affect the families' desire for supportive care (nutritional, respiratory), genetic testing can be completed sooner.

In addition, the utility of counseling for future pregnancies should not be ignored. Families who have had children with or who died from CM or CMD may not always have had a specific diagnosis. Without a known diagnosis, they were unable to make an informed decision about their options for future pregnancies. This extends beyond the immediate family. In X-linked diseases, such as X-linked myotubular myopathy from MTM1 gene variants, the mother's sisters may also be carriers placing her son at risk of having the disease.

Finally, in some diseases such as X-linked MTM1-related CM, gene therapies are in development, which may drastically alter the course of the disease.[30]

For these reasons, given the relatively inexpensive cost of testing, the use of panel testing including both sequencing as well as duplication/deletion is advised in all cases. Because some panels are not all-inclusive of neuromuscular diseases, and phenotyping is needed, at the time when the examiner is working to differentiate CM from CMD, the testing can be sent. However, one of the more common causes of peripheral neonatal hypotonia, myotonic dystrophy, will not be typically detected on these tests due to the pathogenic nature of a trinucleotide repeat in the DMPK gene; a specific nucleotide repeat test is required.

A FUTURE NOTE ABOUT NEWBORN SCREENING

Currently in neuromuscular medicine, newborn screening has become a discussed topic given the recent advances in treatment. Interventions for SMA as well as current research in X-linked myotubular myopathy have resulted in a movement forward. There is a nationwide movement to have newborn screening for SMA in every state. However, the method of testing as well as the sensitivity and specificity vary significantly based on the exact procedure. In a similar note, as treatments become available for the congenital muscle diseases, there is discussion about how to add them to these state-wide panels. Close consultation with a knowledgeable geneticist or pediatric neuromuscular physician should be had in interpreting these testing.

DISCLOSURE

The author has the following financial disclosure: The author have served on the advisory board for Biogen, Avexis, Sarepta, and PTC. In addition, the author has provided consulting for Biogen, Blueprint Partnerships, Connected Research, ETS Consulting, Magnolia Innovation, Market Plus, and Sanderson Market Plus. The author currently on the advisory board for Emerging Therapy Solutions. The author also on the advisory board for Hopeful Together, Inc a nonprofit organization working toward a treatment of POMGnT1-related CMD. The author has grant support from Cure SMA, PPMD, and MDA. The author has an unrestricted education grant from Sarepta.

Best Practices

What is the current practice for differentiating congenital myopathy and congenital muscular dystrophy?

- Differentiation between congenital myopathies and congenital muscular dystrophies is difficult but important to direct conversations with family.
- A structured, evidence-based approach that is timely and cost-effective can provide guidance to the clinician.
- The evaluation of neonates with congenital muscle disease requires a multidisciplinary team skilled in neonatal muscle diseases.

What changes in current practice are likely to improve outcomes?

- Mixed use of laboratory, electrodiagnostic, and genetic information with a rapid movement to broad testing in patients without a clear diagnosis will improve accuracy and efficiency.
- Genetic diagnosis needs pathologic correlation given the genotype/phenotype overlays to give prognostication by an experienced clinician in neuromuscular disease.
- Dividing testing into phases allows for a systematic approach with attention to timing of results that will change management and diagnostic plans.

Major Recommendations

- Early testing should focus on excluding other causes and direct-focused testing for treatable diseases.
- The second step, specialist testing, involves more focal testing for neuromuscular disorders and differentiating between subtypes.
- Late testing focuses on the testing that is broader and takes more time to return; this is done after other diseases that are not able to be diagnosed in this manner have been excluded.

REFERENCES

1. Helbling D, Mendoza D, McCarrier J, et al. Severe neonatal RYR1 myopathy with pathologic features of congenital muscular dystrophy. J Neuropathol Exp Neurol 2019;78(3):283–7.
2. Mostacciuolo ML, Miorin M, Martinello F, et al. Genetic epidemiology of congenital muscular dystrophy in a sample from north–east Italy. Hum Genet 1996;97:277–9.
3. Hughes MI, Hicks EM, Nevin NC, et al. The prevalence of inherited neuromuscular disease in Northern Ireland. Neuromuscul Disord 1996;6:69–73.
4. Darin N, Tulinius M. Neuromuscular disorders in childhood: a descriptive epidemiological study from western Sweden. Neuromuscul Disord 2000;10:1–9.
5. Norwood FL, Harling C, Chinnery PF, et al. Prevalence of genetic muscle disease in Northern England: in-depth analysis of a muscle clinic population. Brain 2009;132:3175–86.
6. Osawa M, Sumida S, Suzuki N, et al. Fukuyama type congenital muscular dystrophy. In: Fukuyama Y, Osawa M, Saito K, editors. Congenital muscular dystrophies. Amsterdam: Elsevier Science; 1997. p. 31–68.
7. Bönnemann CG, Wang CH, Quijano-Roy S, et al. Members of International standard of care Committee for congenital muscular dystrophies. Diagnostic approach to the congenital muscular dystrophies. Neuromuscul Disord 2014;24(4):289–311.
8. Falsaperla R, Praticò AD, Ruggieri M, et al. Congenital muscular dystrophy: from muscle to brain. Ital J Pediatr 2016;42(1):78.
9. Harmelink M. Congenital myopathies In: Emedicine. 2019. Available at: https://emedicine.medscape.com/article/1175852-overview. Accessed May 30, 2019.
10. Laugel V, Cossee M, Matis J, et al. Diagnostic approach to neonatal hypotonia: retrospective study of 144 neonates. Eur J Pediatr 2008;167:517–23.
11. Birdi K, Prasad AN, Prasad C, et al. The floppy infant: retrospective analysis of clinical experience. (1990–2000) in a tertiary care facility. J Child Neurol 2005;20:803–8.
12. Richer LP, Shevell MI, Miller SP. Diagnostic profile of neonatal hypotonia: an 11-year study. Pediatr Neurol 2001;25:32–7.
13. Pauly G. Comparative study of glutamic oxalacetic transaminase and creatine phosphokinase values in the differential diagnosis of myocardial infarction. Wis Med J 1969;68(9):273–6.
14. Gilboa N, Swanson J. Serum Creatine phosophokinase in normal newborns. Arch Dis Child 1976;51(4):283–5.
15. Malamitsi-Puchner A, Minaretzis D, Martzeli L, et al. Serum levels of creatine kinase and its isoenzymes during the 1st postpartum day in healthy newborns delivered vaginally or by cesarean section. Gynecol Obstet Invest 1993;36:25–8.
16. Rudnik-Schöneborn S, Lützenrath S, Borkowska J, et al. Analysis of creatine kinase activity in 504 patients with proximal spinal muscular atrophy types I–III from the point of view of progression and severity. Eur Neurol 1998;39:154–62.
17. Kawase K, Nishino I, Sugimoto M, et al. Hypoxic ischemic encephalopathy in a case of intranuclear rod myopathy without any prenatal sentinel event. Brain Development 2015;37(2):265–9.
18. Millichap JG. Brain MRI findings in congenital muscular dystrophy. Pediatr Neurol Briefs 2006;20(3):22.

19. Brun B, Mockler S, Laubscher K, et al. Comparison of brain MRI findings with language and motor function in the dystroglycanopathies. Neurology 2017;88(7): 623–9.

20. Caro P, Scavina M, Hoffman E, et al. MR imaging findings in children with merosin-deficient congenital muscular dystrophy pilar A. AJNR Am J Neuroradiol 1999;20(2):324–6.

21. Biancalana V, Romero NB, Thuestad IJ, et al. Some DNM2 mutations cause extremely severe congenital myopathy and phenocopy myotubular myopathy. Acta Neuropathol Commun 2018;6(1):93.

22. Saito Y, Komaki H, Hattori A, et al. Extramuscular manifestations in children with severe congenital myopathy due to ACTA1 gene mutations. Neuromuscul Disord 2011;21:489–93.

23. Pitt M. Neurophysiological assessment of abnormalities of the neuromuscular junction in children. Int J Mol Sci 2018;19:624.

24. Ghosh PS, Sorenson EJ. Diagnostic yield of electromyography in children with myopathic disorders. Pediatr Neurol 2014;51(2):215–9.

25. Hellmann M, von Kleist-Retzow JC, Haupt WF, et al. Diagnostic value of electromyography in children and adolescents. J Clin Neurophysiol 2005;22(1):43–8.

26. Packer RJ, Brown MJ, Berman PH. The diagnostic value of electromyography in infantile hypotonia. Am J Dis Child 1982;136(12):1057–9.

27. Serdaroglu E, et al. G.P. 334 - Etiological yield of muscle biopsy in the newborn period. Neuromuscul Disord 2015;25(Supplement 2):S286.

28. Vogler C, Bove KE. Morphology of skeletal muscle in children. An assessment of normal growth and differentiation. Arch Pathol Lab Med 1985;109(3):238–42.

29. Ausems MG, Verbiest J, Hermans MP, et al. Frequency of glycogen storage disease type II in The Netherlands: implications for diagnosis and genetic counselling. Eur J Hum Genet 1999 Sep;7(6):713–6.

30. Elverman M, Goddard M, Mack D, et al. Long-term effects of systemic gene therapy in a canine model of myotubular myopathy. Muscle Nerve 2017;56:943–53.

Printed and bound by CPI Group (UK) Ltd, Croydon, CR0 4YY

03/10/2024

01040402-0004